Thoracic Anesthesia

Editor

PETER SLINGER

ANESTHESIOLOGY CLINICS

www.anesthesiology.theclinics.com

Consulting Editor
LEE A. FLEISHER

December 2012 • Volume 30 • Number 4

ELSEVIER

1600 John F. Kennedy Boulevard, Suite 1800 • Philadelphia, PA 19103-2899

http://www.theclinics.com

ANESTHESIOLOGY CLINICS Volume 30, Number 4
December 2012 ISSN 1932-2275, ISBN-13: 978-1-4557-5061-0

Editor: Pamela Hetherington

Anesthesiology Clinics (ISSN 1932-2275) is published quarterly by Elsevier Inc., 360 Park Avenue South, New York, NY 10010-1710. Months of issue are March, June, September, and December. Periodicals postage paid at New York, NY and at additional mailing offices. Subscription prices are $154.00 per year (US student/resident), $313.00 per year (US individuals), $383.00 per year (Canadian individuals), $496.00 per year (US institutions), $615.00 per year (Canadian institutions), $216.00 per year (Canadian and foreign student/resident), $434.00 per year (foreign individuals), and $615.00 per year (foreign institutions). To receive student and resident rate, orders must be accompanied by name of affiliated institution, date of term, and the *signature* of program/residency coordinator on institutions letterhead. Orders will be billed at individual rate until proof of status is received. Foreign air speed delivery is included in all *Clinics'* subscription prices. All prices are subject to change without notice. POSTMASTER: Send address changes to *Anesthesiology Clinics,* Elsevier Health Sciences Division, Subscription Customer Service, 3251 Riverport Lane, Maryland Heights, MO 63043. Customer Service (orders, claims, online, change of address): Elsevier Health Sciences Division, Subscription Customer Service, 3251 Riverport Lane, Maryland Heights, MO 63043. Tel: 1-800-654-2452 (U.S. and Canada); 314-447-8871 (outside U.S. and Canada). Fax: 314-447-8029. E-mail: journalscustomerservice-usa@elsevier.com (for print support); journalsonlinesupport-usa@elsevier.com (for online support).

Reprints. For copies of 100 or more of articles in this publication, please contact the Commercial Reprints Department, Elsevier Inc., 360 Park Avenue South, New York, NY 10010-1710. Tel.: 212-633-3812; Fax: 212-462-1935; E-mail: reprints@elsevier.com.

Anesthesiology Clinics, is also published in Spanish by McGraw-Hill Inter-americana Editores S. A., P.O. Box 5-237, 06500 Mexico D. F., Mexico.

Anesthesiology Clinics, is covered in *MEDLINE/PubMed (Index Medicus), Current Contents/Clinical Medicine, Excerpta Medica, ISI/BIOMED*, and *Chemical Abstracts*.

Printed and bound by CPI Group (UK) Ltd, Croydon, CR0 4YY

Transferred to digital print 2012

Contributors

CONSULTING EDITOR

LEE A. FLEISHER, MD
Robert D. Dripps Professor and Chair of Anesthesiology and Critical Care, Professor of Medicine, Perelman School of Medicine, University of Pennsylvania School of Medicine, Philadelphia, Pennsylvania

GUEST EDITOR

PETER SLINGER, MD, FRCPC
Professor of Anesthesia, Department of Anesthesia, Toronto General Hospital, University of Toronto, Toronto, Ontario, Canada

AUTHORS

KAYODE ADENIJI, BMedSci, MBBS, MRCP, DICM
Clinical Fellow, Interdepartmental Division of Critical Care, Faculty of Medicine, Toronto General Hospital, University of Toronto, Toronto, Ontario, Canada

PAUL H. ALFILLE, MD
Department of Anesthesia, Critical Care and Pain Medicine, Massachusetts General Hospital; Harvard Medical School, Boston, Massachusetts

RANDAL S. BLANK, MD, PhD
Associate Professor, Chief, Thoracic Anesthesia, Department of Anesthesiology, University of Virginia Health System, Charlottesville, Virginia

SANJEEV V. CHHANGANI, MD, MBA, FCCM
Department of Anesthesia, Critical Care and Pain Medicine, Massachusetts General Hospital; Harvard Medical School, Boston, Massachusetts

STEPHEN R. COLLINS, MD
Assistant Professor, Department of Anesthesiology, University of Virginia Health System, Charlottesville, Virginia

ANA FERNANDEZ-BUSTAMANTE, MD, PhD
Assistant Professor, Anesthesiology, University of Colorado School of Medicine, Aurora, Colorado

ION A. HOBAI, MD, PhD
Department of Anesthesia, Critical Care and Pain Medicine, Massachusetts General Hospital; Harvard Medical School, Boston, Massachusetts

J. MICHAEL JAEGER, MD, PhD
Co-Medical Director, TCV Surgical ICU, Division of Critical Care Medicine, Associate Professor, Departments of Anesthesiology and Surgery, University of Virginia Health System, Charlottesville, Virginia

DAVID W. KACZKA, MD, PhD
Assistant Professor, Harvard Medical School; Department of Anesthesia, Critical Care, and Pain Medicine, Beth Israel Deaconess Medical Center, Boston, Massachusetts

GEORGE W. KANELLAKOS, MD, FRCPC
Chief, Thoracic Anesthesia, Assistant Professor, Dalhousie Department of Anesthesia, Pain Management and Perioperative Medicine, Queen Elizabeth II Health Sciences Center, Halifax, Nova Scotia, Canada

BRUCE KILPATRICK, MBBCh, FCA(SA)
Anaesthesiologist, Department of Anaesthesia, Royal Inland Hospital, Kamloops, British Columbia, Canada

JENS LOHSER, MD, MSc, FRCPC
Associate Professor, Department of Anesthesiology, Pharmacology and Therapeutics, Vancouver General Hospital, University of British Columbia, Vancouver, British Columbia, Canada

ANDREW B. LUMB, MBBS, FRCA
Consultant Anaesthetist, Department of Anaesthesia, St James's University Hospital; Lecturer in Anaesthesia, University of Leeds, Leeds, United Kingdom

RALPH LYERLY III
Assistant Professor of Anesthesiology, Department of Anesthesiology, University of Alabama School of Medicine, Birmingham, Alabama

GUIDO MUSCH, MD
Associate Professor, Harvard Medical School; Department of Anesthesia, Critical Care and Pain Medicine, Massachusetts General Hospital, Boston, Massachusetts

ALESSIA PEDOTO, MD
Assistant Clinical Attending, Department of Anesthesiology and Critical Care Medicine, Memorial Sloan-Kettering Cancer Center, New York, New York

ALBERT PERRINO, MD
Jr Professor of Anesthesiology, Yale University School of Medicine, New Haven

FERENC PUSKAS, MD, PhD
Associate Professor, Anesthesiology, University of Colorado School of Medicine, Aurora, Colorado

CAIT P. SEARL, BSc, MA, MBChB, MRCP, FRCA
Consultant Cardiothoracic Anaesthetist and Intensivist, Freeman Hospital, Newcastle upon Tyne Hospitals NHS Foundation Trust, United Kingdom

PETER SLINGER, MD, FRCPC
Professor of Anesthesia, Department of Anesthesia, Toronto General Hospital, University of Toronto, Toronto, Ontario, Canada

ANDREW C. STEEL, BSc, MBBS, MRCP, FRCA, FRCPC, EDICM
Assistant Professor, Interdepartmental Division of Critical Care, Faculty of Medicine, Toronto General Hospital, University of Toronto, Toronto, Ontario, Canada

BRAD STEENWYK, MD
Associate Professor of Anesthesiology, Department of Anesthesiology, University of Alabama School of Medicine, Birmingham, Alabama

BREANDAN SULLIVAN, MD
Assistant Professor, Anesthesiology and Critical Care Medicine, University of Colorado School of Medicine, Aurora, Colorado

MARCOS F. VIDAL MELO, MD, PhD
Associate Professor, Harvard Medical School; Department of Anesthesia, Critical Care and Pain Medicine, Massachusetts General Hospital, Boston, Massachusetts

VERA VON DOSSOW-HANFSTINGL, MD
Department of Anesthesiology, Ludwig Maximilian University, Munich, Germany

LAURA J. WALTON, MBChB, FRCA
Specialist Trainee in Anaesthesia, Department of Anaesthesia, St James's University Hospital, Leeds, United Kingdom

Contents

lungs are hyperinflated. Low tidal volume and inspiratory pressure are surrogates for the stress and strain concept; but lung compliance, transpulmonary pressure, and chest wall elastance might differ in individual patients. In previous published studies, an increasing number of patients were treated successfully with extracorporeal support. Extracorporeal membrane oxygenation and interventional lung assist allow ultraprotective ventilation strategies. However, these assists have different technical aspects and different indications.

remains an issue in roughly 10% of cases. Algorithms for the management of OLV hypoxemia have to be adapted to the thoracoscopic approach, in particular the need for optimal surgical exposure. With appropriate planning and caution, most of the treatment modalities for OLV hypoxemia can be applied to the thoracoscopy setting, with some modifications.

Advancements in robotic-assisted thoracic surgery present potential advantages for patients as well as new challenges for the anesthesia and surgery teams. This article describes the major aspects of the surgical approach for the most commonly performed robotic-assisted thoracic surgical procedures as well as the pertinent preoperative, intraoperative, and postoperative anesthetic concerns.

Tracheal resection and reconstruction (TRR) is the treatment of choice for most patients with tracheal stenosis or tracheal tumors. Anesthesia for TRR offers distinct challenges, especially for the less experienced practitioner. This article explores the preoperative assessment, strategies for induction and emergence from anesthesia, the essential coordination between the surgical and anesthesia teams during airway excision and anastomosis, and postoperative care. The most common complications are reviewed. Targeted readership is practitioners with less extensive experience in managing airway surgery cases. As such, the article focuses first on the most common proximal tracheal resection. Final sections discuss specific considerations for more complicated cases.

Surgical resection remains a standard treatment option for localized esophageal cancer. Surgical approaches to esophagectomy include transhiatal and transthoracic techniques as well as minimally invasive techniques that have been developed to reduce the morbidities associated with laparotomy and thoracotomy incisions. The perioperative mortality for esophagectomy remains high with cardiopulmonary and anastomotic complications as the most frequent and serious morbidities. This article reviews the management of patients presenting for esophagectomy, with a focus on evidence-based anesthetic and perioperative approaches for improving outcomes.

This article describes the perioperative risks of pregnant patients with anterior mediastinal masses, and demonstrates the importance of a multidisciplinary approach for the management of high-risk patients. Mediastinal mass syndrome is defined as immediate right heart failure secondary to vascular compression when positive pressure ventilation is initiated. Greater emphasis on the potential for cardiovascular collapse (versus respiratory collapse) challenges the conventional teaching of risks associated with mediastinal masses in the adult population.

ANESTHESIOLOGY CLINICS

FORTHCOMING ISSUES

March 2013
Trauma
Yoram Weiss, MD and
Micha Shamir, MD, *Guest Editors*

June 2013
Cardiac Anesthesia
Colleen Koch, MD, *Guest Editor*

RECENT ISSUES

September 2012
Postanesthesia Care Unit
Scott A. Falk, MD, *Guest Editor*

June 2012
Neurosurgical Anesthesia
Ansgar M. Brambrink, MD, PhD, and
Jeffrey R. Kirsch, MD, *Guest Editors*

March 2012
**Surgical Palliative Care and Pain
Management**
Geoffrey P. Dunn, MD,
Sugantha Ganapathy, MBBS, and
Vincent Chan, MD, *Guest Editors*

RELATED INTEREST

Chest Surgery Clinics, February 2012 (Volume 22, Issue 1)
Current Management Guidelines in Thoracic Surgery
M. Blair Marshall, *Guest Editor*

DOWNLOAD
Free App!

Review Articles
THE CLINICS

NOW AVAILABLE FOR YOUR iPhone and iPad

Foreword

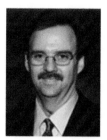

Lee A. Fleisher, MD
Consulting Editor

It has been over 4 years since an issue of *Anesthesiology Clinics* has been devoted to thoracic anesthesia. During that interval, thoracic surgery has continued to evolve, which requires evolution in the anesthetic management of patients undergoing thoracic surgery. There are changes in airway and esophageal surgery. Technology has also had a major impact on the field, including the development of robotic surgery. With a focus on increasing our value in health care, it is also important to both implement strategies to reduce perioperative risk and treat complications effectively once they occur. In this issue of *Anesthesiology Clinics*, a remarkable group of international experts in the field have written outstanding reviews to help all of us provide state-of-the-art care.

In choosing an editor for a thoracic anesthesia issue, it was easy to once again ask Peter Slinger, MD, who was the editor of the 2008 issue. Dr Slinger is currently Professor of Anesthesia at the University of Toronto and coeditor of 4 of the major texts in the field. He is currently an associate editor for the Thoracic Anesthesia section of the *Journal of Cardiothoracic and Vascular Anesthesia* and a member of the editorial board of *Anesthesia and Analgesia*. He has written and lectured extensively on the issues of 1-lung ventilation and thoracic anesthesia, and is, therefore, able to define the key issues for our readers.

Lee A. Fleisher, MD
Perelman School of Medicine
University of Pennsylvania School of Medicine
3400 Spruce Street, Dulles 680
Philadelphia, PA 19104, USA

E-mail address:
lee.fleisher@uphs.upenn.edu

Anesthesiology Clin 30 (2012) xiii
http://dx.doi.org/10.1016/j.anclin.2012.08.013   **anesthesiology.theclinics.com**

Preface

Thoracic Anesthesia

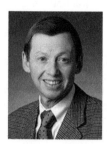

Peter Slinger, MD, FRCPC
Guest Editor

I would like to thank Dr Lee Fleisher for the invitation to compile and edit this volume of *Anesthesiology Clinics* on Thoracic Anesthesia. The volume and complexity of thoracic surgical procedures continue to increase and coincidentally the knowledge-base for anesthesiologists providing care for these patients needs to grow. This issue of *Anesthesiology Clinics* is aimed at helping clinicians keep abreast in some of the areas of progress in Thoracic Anesthesia.

In the last century the major cause of morbidity and mortality after pulmonary resection surgery was atelectasis and pneumonia. Improvements in postoperative therapy including better analgesia techniques with thoracic epidural and paravertebral analgesia have decreased the incidence of these complications to the extent that now the major cause of mortality after lung cancer surgery is acute lung injury. Thus, the initial section of this *Anesthesiology Clinics* volume examines the problem of lung injury in the context of thoracic surgery.

Article 1, by Dr Andrew Steel of the Departments of Anesthesia and Critical Care of the University of Toronto, presents recent information on the underlying pathophysiology of lung injury. The second article, by Drs Lumb and Walton, examines the role of oxygen toxicity in lung injury. Dr Lumb from the University of Leeds in England is the editor of *Nunn's Applied Respiratory Physiology*, one of the foundations of our knowledge of the interaction of anesthesia and the respiratory system. The third article by Bruce Kilpatrick and me examines the evidence that lung-protective ventilation strategies can reduce the incidence of lung injury following cardiothoracic surgery. The fourth article in this section on lung injury by Dr Vera Von Dossow-Hanfstingl presents recent advances in therapy for patients with established acute lung injury. Dr Von Dossow-Hanfstingl, who previously worked in Berlin and now in Munich, has a career interest in basic research and clinical practice relating to lung injury. We may have practically come to the end of the line of research with clever new strategies for mechanical ventilation in established cases of lung injury. It is possible that the important new advances in therapy may be some form of extracorporeal lung support.

Anesthesiology Clin 30 (2012) xv–xvi
http://dx.doi.org/10.1016/j.anclin.2012.08.002
1932-2275/12/$ – see front matter

Extracorporeal membrane oxygenation (ECMO) had a surge of interest as therapy for adult respiratory distress syndrome 30 years ago but was largely laid aside due to complications. However, ECMO and other types of lung-assist devices are experiencing a major resurgence.

The fifth article in this volume discusses the related and ever-contentious issue of fluid management in thoracic surgery. Anesthesiologists continuously walk a fine line between giving a pulmonary resection patient too much intravenous fluid intraoperatively, thus contributing to lung injury, and giving too little fluid, leading to renal dysfunction. Dr Perrino from Yale and Dr Searle from Newcastle, England, look at the role that goal-directed fluid strategies play in helping with this recurring clinical problem.

Article 6 by Dr Ferenc Puskas and coworkers from the University of Colorado, Denver, present the increasing applications of transesophageal echocardiography in noncardiac thoracic surgery. Article 7 by Dr Alessia Pedoto, from the Thoracic Anesthesia Division of Memorial-Sloane Kettering Cancer Center in New York City, is an update on the continuing controversies about double-lumen tubes in thoracic surgery.

Article 8 by Dr Jens Lohser, the Director of Thoracic Anesthesia at the Vancouver General Hospital, discusses the difficult clinical problem of hypoxemia during 1-lung ventilation for minimally invasive thoracic surgery, where the traditional therapy of continuous positive airway pressure to the nonventilated lung is usually not an option. The problems of anesthetic management for minimally invasive thoracic surgery are magnified with the recent advent of robotic thoracic surgery. In article 9 Dr Brad Steenwyck presents management suggestions based on the large clinical experience that he and his colleagues in the Anesthesia Department at the University of Alabama, Birmingham, have developed with this procedure.

Airway surgery is always a challenge for the anesthesiologist. In article 10 Dr Paul Alfille, the Director of Thoracic Anesthesia from the Massachusetts General Hospital, discusses his approach to this difficult clinical problem. In article 11 Dr Jaeger and coauthors from the University of Virginia, Charlottesville, describe the current controversies in management of anesthesia for esophageal resection. During major esophageal surgery all of the issues presented about lung injury and fluid management, in the initial articles of this volume of *Anesthesiology Clinics*, collide with the potential concern that the use of inotropes or vasopressors may contribute to ischemia of the gut anastomosis. Dr Jaeger leads us through this minefield.

In article 12 Dr George Kanellakos, the Director of Thoracic Anesthesia at Dalhousie University in Halifax, outlines a management strategy for the very difficult clinical problem of a pregnant patient who presents with an anterior mediastinal mass. In the final article Dr Vidal-Melo and coworkers from Harvard present a case-based overview of pulmonary pathophysiology in cardiothoracic anesthesia.

I hope this volume of *Anesthesiology Clinics* offers the reader a wide-based update on advances in Thoracic Anesthesia. I have been fortunate in the enthusiasm that the contributing authors have shown for this project and in their willingness to share their knowledge and time in producing this issue.

Peter Slinger, MD, FRCPC
University of Toronto
Toronto General Hospital
Toronto, Ontario, Canada

E-mail address:
peter.slinger@uhn.on.ca

The Pathophysiology of Perioperative Lung Injury

Kayode Adeniji, BMedSci, MBBS, MRCP, DICM,
Andrew C. Steel, BSc, MBBS, MRCP, FRCA, FRCPC, EDICM*

KEYWORDS

- Pathophysiology • Perioperative • ARDS • Alveolar epithelium • Stem cell
- Gene therapy

KEY POINTS

- It is important to use predicted body weight rather than actual body weight in determining tidal volume and consider using lung protective strategies even in the absence of any definite lung injury (ie, normal lungs).
- A multifaceted approach may be required to affect not only the development of acute lung injury (ALI)/acute respiratory distress syndrome (ARDS) but also to encourage its resolution. Supporting apoptosis rather than necrosis as the primary neutrophil-driven pathologic process may accelerate the re-epithelization of the alveolar/capillary barrier and thus enhance its function. Stem cell and gene therapy may play a future role in this.

INTRODUCTION

The degree of perioperative lung injury that patients sustain results from a complex interaction between their current physiologic state, comorbidities, lifestyle choices (eg, alcohol or smoking), underlying surgical diagnosis, operative approach (minimally invasive vs open technique), and ultimately their cardiopulmonary interaction with a mechanical ventilator.

The lungs of one man may bear, without injury, as great a force as those of another man can exert; which by the bellows cannot always be determined.[1] This quotation, from Fothergill's[1] description of the successful mouth-to-mouth resuscitation of an asphyxiated coal miner, indicates that an inkling of the pulmonary injury that mechanical ventilation can induce was contemplated as early as the eighteenth century. Direct lung injuries (**Table 1**) resulting from the mechanical delivery of inhalational anesthesia can be correlated with types of ventilator-induced lung injury (VILI) that ultimately result in ARDS. Ashbaugh and colleagues'[2] and Petty and Ashbaugh's[3] initial description in the late 1960 established the modern description of ARDS and, more importantly, the

Interdepartmental Division of Critical Care, Faculty of Medicine, University of Toronto, Toronto General Hospital, 585 University Avenue, Toronto, Ontario, M5G 2N2, Canada
* Corresponding author.
E-mail address: andrew.steel@uhn.ca

Anesthesiology Clin 30 (2012) 573–590
http://dx.doi.org/10.1016/j.anclin.2012.08.011
1932-2275/12/$ – see front matter © 2012 Elsevier Inc. All rights reserved.

Table 1
The close relationship between ventilator-induced lung injury and perioperative lung complications

Perioperative Lung Injuries	Types of VILI
Pneumothorax	Barotrauma
Bronchopleural fistula	
Atelectasis	Atelectrauma
ALI	Volutrauma
ARDS	Biotrauma
Pneumonia	Intubation

recognition that defining and investigating this clinical entity could pay dividends in the care of patients both in the operating room and subsequently in ICUs.[4,5]

The incidence of pulmonary complications after noncardiac surgery is comparable with that of cardiac complications (2.7% vs 2.5%, respectively).[6] Pulmonary complications, specifically respiratory failure requiring ventilation, are associated with high morbidity and mortality, increased costs, and length of hospital stay.[7] In a prospective, nested, case-control study of 4420 consecutive patients, Fernández-Pérez and colleagues[8] investigated the etiologic factors in the 238 (5.4%) postoperative pulmonary complications identified in recipients of high-risk elective surgery. ALI was the most common cause (83 [35%]) of postoperative respiratory failure and was associated with a markedly lower postoperative survival (60-day and 1-year survival, 99% vs 73% and 92% vs 56%; $P<.001$).

This review addresses primarily the pathophysiology of perioperative lung injury with reference to VILI and ARDS/ALI (terms, ARDS and ALI, used interchangeably). Readers are directed to recent publications that have comprehensively addressed the management aspects that can be used to ameliorate the development of this problem.[7,9]

DIAGNOSTIC CRITERIA

The Berlin revision of the 1994 American-European Consensus Conference definition of ARDS was conducted for reasons related to its reliability and validity[10] (**Table 2**). Particular concerns were the lack of a clear definition of the term, *acute*, that oxygenation criteria were easily manipulated by ventilator settings (eg, positive end-expiratory pressure [PEEP]), and that radiographs of patients taken in ICU are notoriously difficult to interpret. There was also the belief that the use of the term, *ALI*, originally encompassing ARDS, had led to an incorrect presumption that ALI was somehow less serious than an ARDS classification.[11]

ANATOMY OF ARDS: ENDOTHELIAL AND EPITHELIAL INJURY

The distal airway is composed of terminal respiratory and bronchiolar units lined with ciliated cuboidal and nonciliated Clara epithelial cells; the latter have a significant secretory function and the capacity to assist in ion transport.[12] The alveolar–capillary surface consists of 2 basement membrane supported barriers: the external alveolar epithelium and the internal microvascular endothelium, separated by the pulmonary interstitial space (**Fig. 1**). In health, large type I flattened epithelial cells cover 95% of the lung's surface; cuboidal type II cells make up the remainder of the area.

Tight intercellular junctions form the links between adjacent cells, ensuring a barrier, which, under normal conditions, is less permeable than the vascular endothelial barrier

Table 2
Summary of the Berlin task force definition of the acute respiratory distress syndrome

	Acute Respiratory Distress Syndrome		
	Mild	**Moderate**	**Severe**
Timing	Acute onset within 1 wk of a known clinical insult or new, worsening respiratory condition.		
Oxygenation	Pao$_2$:Fio$_2$ ratio 201–300 (with PEEP $\geq$5 cm H$_2$O)	Pao$_2$:Fio$_2$ ratio $\leq$200 (with PEEP $\geq$5 cm H$_2$O)	Pao$_2$:Fio$_2$ ratio $\leq$100 (with PEEP $\geq$10 cm H$_2$O)
Origin of edema	Respiratory failure not fully explained by cardiac failure or fluid overload		
Chest radiograph	Bilateral opacities	Bilateral opacities	Opacities involving at least 3 quadrants
Additional physiologic derangements	N/A	N/A	V$_{ECorr}$ >10 L/min or C$_{RS}$ $\leq$40 mL/cm H$_2$O
Expected mortality	10%	32%	62%

Abbreviations: C$_{RS}$, compliance of the respiratory system; Fio$_2$, inspired oxygen concentration; Pao$_2$, partial pressure of arterial oxygen; V$_{ECorr}$, corrected expired volume per minute.
    Data from The ARDS Definition Task Force, Ranieri VM, Rubenfeld GD, et al. Acute Respiratory Distress Syndrome. The Berlin Definition. JAMA 2012;307(23):2526–33.

to the movement of fluid and protein between the interstitial/vascular and alveolar spaces.[12,13] Type II cells are complex, highly metabolically active, and responsible for the synthesis and secretion of pulmonary surfactant, proliferation, and differentiation into type I cells after injury and sodium and chloride ion transport.[13,14]

There is convincing evidence that this transepithelial active salt transport in type II and, to a lesser extent, type I cells drives osmotic water movement principally through aquaporin channels (in the latter) (**Fig. 2**). It is, therefore, the primary determinant of alveolar fluid reabsorption and clearance rather than differences in hydrostatic and

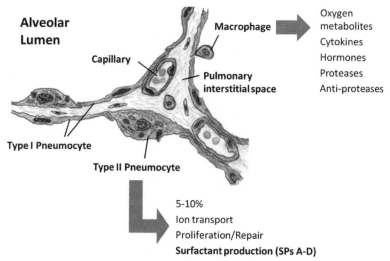

Fig. 1. The alveolar-endothelial barrier and its cellular functions. SPs-surfactant proteins.

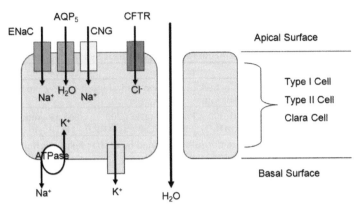

Fig. 2. Schematic of the potential transepithelial support mechanisms present on type II, Clara, and type I pulmonary epithelial cells that lead to the resorption of alveolar edema fluid. Sodium is taken up by the various epithelial sodium channels through the apical membrane of type II cells and transported basolaterally by the sodium pump (Na^+,K^+-ATPase). The relevant pathways for chloride transport are unclear but may involve CFTR. Water moving through water channels (aquaporins) located primarily on type I cells. Some water may also cross by paracellular routes. AQP_5, aquaporin 5; CNG, cyclic nucleoside-gated channel. (*Data from* Matthay MA, Robriquet L, Fang X. Alveolar epithelium: role in lung fluid balance and acute lung injury. Proc Am Thorac Soc 2005;2(3):206–13.)

protein osmotic pressures (Starling forces). The evidence for this paradigm stems from work showing.

1. Epithelial sodium channel (ENaC) are present in isolated type II and type I alveolar cells.[15,16]
2. The rate of alveolar fluid clearance is temperature-dependent, as demonstrated in ex vivo hypothermia human lung studies.
3. The inhibition of the apical transporters (by Amiloride) and distal Na^+,K^+-ATPase (by ouabian) reduced fluid clearance in human lungs and an in situ sheep preparation for measuring fluid clearance.[14,17,18]
4. That chloride uptake and cystic fibrosis transmembrane regulator (CFTR)-like transport seems to be required for β-adrenergic cyclic adenosine monophosphate–stimulated fluid clearance from the distal airspaces of the lung and can be inhibited.[19,20]
5. A series of elegant animal studies provided evidence that active ion transport must be responsible for the fluid clearance.[21,22] Anesthetized, ventilated sheep had an isomolar protein solution instilled into their airways. In the face of subsequent rising alveolar protein concentrations, it was found that protein concentrations in serum, the lung interstitium, and lymphatic drainage all decreased. The alveolar oncotic pressure was 40 cm H_2O greater than the oncotic pressure in the vascular/interstitial spaces.

It is the disruption of this endoepithelial interface by the interaction between patient, disease, and machine that is largely responsible for lung injury.

MECHANICAL VENTILATION AND ALI

In 2000, a National Heart, Lung and Blood Institute–sponsored clinical trial of 861 patients reported that a lower tidal volume ventilation strategy with a plateau pressure limit reduced mortality of ALI patients by 22% compared with (higher) conventional tidal volumes.[23] Now a significant body of evidence from experimental animal and observational and interventional human studies demonstrates the deleterious effects of inappropriate ventilatory strategies, even in functionally normal lungs. Gajic and colleagues[24,25] demonstrated that the use of high tidal volumes (>700 mL) and high peak inspiratory pressures (>30 cm H_2O) in the first 48 hours after surgical ICU admission was associated with the development of ARDS. Furthermore, they reported that 24% of 332 patients with normal lungs ventilated in ICU developed ALI within 5 days of admission. The principal risk factors for ALI were large tidal volumes, blood product transfusion, and restrictive lung physiology—all potentially intraoperative issues.[24,25] de Oliveira and colleagues[26] sampled bronchoalveolar lavage (BAL) fluid after 12 hours' ventilation and found that inflammatory markers in the fluid were significantly higher in those critically ill patients, without lung injury, who received conventional tidal volume (10–12 mL/kg) versus a protective ventilator strategy (6–8 mL/kg predicted body weight). Similar injurious ventilation strategies in major abdominal surgical patients ventilated for greater than 5 hours demonstrated increased plasma leakage into the alveoli and activation of the clotting cascade in sampled BAL.[27] High intraoperative ventilation pressures represent the strongest risk factor for ALI development (approximately 3-fold increased risk of peak inspiratory pressure ≥25 vs 15 cm H_2O) predisposing to the early (postoperative days 0–3) incidence of ALI seen in the bimodal distribution of pulmonary dysfunction postpneumonectomy.[28] Additional risks identified were excessive fluid administration, pneumonectomy, and preoperative alcohol misuse.

A retrospective study of 806 pneumonectomies found the incidence of postpneumonectomy pulmonary edema was 2.5%, with 100% mortality in those affected. There was no difference in perioperative fluid balance between postpneumonectomy ALI cases (24-h fluid balance 10 mL/kg) compared with matched pneumonectomy controls without ALI (13 mL/kg).[29] Therefore, although fluid administration may play a role in postsurgical lung injury, this study, using rigorous fluid restriction compared with other reports, suggests that limiting intraoperative fluids might only reduce but not eliminate ALI altogether.[30,31] The importance of finding low/normal pulmonary artery wedge pressures, high-protein edema fluid, and activated inflammatory cascade in these patients supports the role of endothelial damage in the postoperative lung capillary permeability that also affects the nonoperated lung.

A study by Mead and colleagues[32] in 1970 examined the intrapulmonary pressure distribution in a heterogeneous lung model that included both normal and collapsed alveoli. Tidal volume inflation resulted in the hyperinflation of those alveoli continuously accessible to ventilation (stress failure—disruption of the alveolar-capillary barrier) and cyclic recruitment/derecruitment of the collapsed units (shear stress on epithelial cells).[33,34] In the region between hyperinflated and the normal alveoli and between the continuously recruited/derecruited alveoli and the normally expanded regions, the tidal inflation opening pressure generated was amplified 4.5-fold within the pulmonary interstitum. Absolute airway pressure itself does not directly lead to injury but rather transpulmonary (alveolar minus pleural) pressures and the degree of regional lung distension.[35] The close proximity of the vascular endothelium to the pulmonary epithelial surface thus renders it susceptible to these forces generated by mechanical ventilation. The regional stress induced by positive pressure ventilation increases microvascular transmural pressures, thus disrupting capillaries and thereby altering perfusion and increasing lung injury.[36]

This phenomenon of VILI is well recognized. It encompasses a complex interaction of overdistension (volutrauma), increased transpulmonary pressure (barotrauma), the cyclic opening and closing of alveoli (atelectrauma), and the resulting detrimental inflammatory state (biotrauma) (persisting postoperative atelectasis itself is a pathologic inflammatory state[37]). Nonphysiologic ventilation (larger tidal volumes) can establish VILI in normal lungs, exacerbate existing lung injury, and sensitize the lung to further injury. This is the so-called 2-hit model,[38] which is significant with large transfusions, cardiopulmonary bypass, and associated ischemia-reperfusion injury).[39]

IMAGING FINDINGS
Chest Radiograph

Chest x-ray (CXR) features of ARDS vary widely depending on the stage of the disease. Early findings on the chest radiograph often include bilateral diffuse, predominantly peripheral, alveolar opacities with air bronchograms (consolidation) that obscure pulmonary vascular markings and are indistinguishable from pulmonary edema. These opacities progress to more extensive consolidation that can become asymmetric. Septal lines and pleural effusions by definition are initially uncommon in the absence of coexistent ventricular dysfunction.

X-ray features tend to stabilize, and radiographic worsening after 5 to 7 days usually indicates an additional concurrent disease process. In the fibrotic phase, chest radiographs may have an interstitial appearance. This is not necessarily due to fibrosis because this may completely resolve in many patients who survive.[40,41]

CT

The introduction of CT scanning has had an enormous impact on the understanding of ALI/ARDS pathophysiology and the effects of different treatment strategies.[42–44]

The CT features are[45,46]

- Predominantly dependent bilateral basal abnormalities (86%)
- Areas of consolidation with air bronchograms (89%)
- Patchy atelectasis (42%)
- Mixed ground-glass appearance and consolidation (27%)

ARDS that is due to pulmonary disease tends to be asymmetric, with a mix of consolidation and ground-glass opacification, whereas ARDS due to extrapulmonary causes has predominantly symmetric ground-glass opacification. CT scanning can be used to detect the pathologic features and complications of ARDS that are occult on chest radiographs largely because diffuse consolidation obscures other findings. It is more reliable than the chest radiograph in the detection of suspected fibrosis.

Constantin and colleagues[47] performed CT scans at zero PEEP before, during, and after recruitment maneuvers in 19 patients with early ALI/ARDS. In patients with grossly focal loss of lung aeration, hyperinflation occurred rather than recruitment. The opposite was true, however, in patients with more homogeneous lung morphology. In addition, alveolar recruitment only persisted beyond the interval of the recruitment maneuver in patients with nonfocal morphology.[44]

Ultrasound

Bouhemad and colleagues[48] studied the use of lung ultrasound (US) to evaluate recruitment. They measured the amount of recruited (or derecruited) lung when PEEP was changed from 0 cm H_2O to 15 cm H_2O (or vice versa) in 40 patients with ALI/ARDS. They developed a US-based score classifying 4 patterns of aeration, and the transition of any given region of interest from one pattern to another received a score. There was significant correlation with the amount of recruitment measured both by the pressure-volume curve and any PEEP-induced oxygenation improvement.[48] Xirouchaki and colleagues[49] went on to compare the diagnostic accuracy of US to that of CXR in 42 mechanically ventilated patients. Using comparison with CT scan, US showed a higher sensitivity and specificity (ranging between 75% and 100%) than the CXR (range, 38%–99%).

Positron Emission Tomography

Positron emission tomography has the unique ability to image functional processes in vivo. It has revealed that ALI/ARDS lungs demonstrate increased metabolic activity compared with those of controls and it is believed to reflect the presence and activity of inflammatory cells.[50,51] Diffuse increased metabolic activity is also present in regions showing normal aeration on CT scan.[52] BAL studies also show that radiographically spared, nondependent areas have substantial inflammation,[53] supporting evidence that during ALI/ARDS, despite radiographic appearances, no lung region is spared by the inflammatory process.

DIFFERENTIAL DIAGNOSIS OF ALI

The causes of ALI and ARDS are well described and summarized in **Table 3**. Differential diagnostic considerations include pneumonia (eg, due to aspiration), diffuse alveolar hemorrhage, and pulmonary edema of any cause.

PATHOPHYSIOLOGY

Classically, the physiologic elements that manifest in ARDS are rapid-onset hypoxemia, an increase in dead space ventilation, and reduced lung compliance. Together these features increase work of breathing and metabolic demand, leading to severe respiratory failure. The importance of endothelial injury and increased vascular permeability to the formation of pulmonary edema are well established, and the degree of alveolar epithelial injury is a valuable predictor of outcome.[14,53,54]

PHASES OF ALI/ARDS
Exudative Phase (Days 1–7)

Lung biopsies from ALI patients display an alveolar cellular infiltrate rich with neutrophils, macrophages, and erythrocytes. The alveolar epithelium is disrupted, and denuded basement membranes are lined by fibrin-rich hyaline exudates.[55] The

Table 3
Clinical risk factors and conditions associated with ALI and ARDS

Direct (Pulmonary) Injury	Indirect (Extrapulmonary) Injury
Pneumonia	Sepsis
Aspiration	Severe trauma
Pulmonary contusion	Cardiopulmonary bypass
Fat embolism	Drug overdose
Near drowning	Acute pancreatitis
Inhalational injury	Blood transfusion (Transfusion Related Acute Lung Injury [TRALI])
Reperfusion syndrome	Disseminated intravascular coagulopathy

morphologic hallmark of diffuse alveolar damage (DAD) is used to describe the histo-logic features of cell death, epithelial hyperplasia, inflammation, disordered coagula-tion, and fibrinolysis. In this acute phase (**Fig. 3**) the mechanisms for injury to the epithelial barrier depend on

1. Neutrophil-dependent release of injurious proteases and reactive oxygen species, and
2. Bacterial exoproducts

The acute phase of ARDS is characterized by interstitial and pulmonary edema and surfactant dysfunction and followed by inflammation.

Edema

The combined effects of increased filtration and increased permeability contribute to the development of acute edema. The transcapillary hydrostatic pressure, which is the pressure responsible for driving fluid out of the extra-alveolar pulmonary vessels, is increased in 2 ways:

1. A reduction in the interstitial pressure around the extra-alveolar vessels, resulting from increased surface tension (due to surfactant dysfunction) and the stretching of the interstitial space (by hyperinflation).
2. Elevation in extra-alveolar hydrostatic pressure in response to the decreased caliber of intra-alveolar vessels caused by the raised alveolar pressure.[56]

Epithelial injury also contributes to alveolar flooding.

1. Disruption of the epithelial barrier can lead to septic shock in patients with bacterial pneumonia.[57]
2. Loss of epithelial integrity and injury to type II cells disrupts normal fluid transport, impairing the removal of edema fluid from the alveolar space.[58]
3. Cuboidal type II alveolar cell injury impairs surfactant production and turnover.[59]

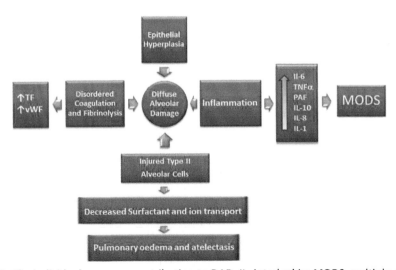

Fig. 3. The individual processes contributing to DAD. IL, interleukin; MODS, multiple organ dysfunction syndrome; TF, tissue factor; vWF, von Willebrand factor.

Surfactant

Surfactant dysfunction contributes to nonhomogeneous airspace collapse. There are several possible mechanisms:

1. Rather than simply injury-related reduction in surfactant production by type II cells,[60] surfactant release is actually initially enhanced by high-volume ventilation. Increased surface area of the alveoli, however, increases the rate at which surfactant is released into the conducting airways and this eventually exceeds the rate of production.[61]
2. High tidal volume ventilation increases the conversion of the large aggregate surfactant on epithelial cells. Eventually, the basement membrane gives way, leading to alveolar hemorrhage.[59]
3. The alveolar pulmonary edema fluid contains serum proteins and proteases that disable surfactant.[62]

Cytokines

A complex network of cytokines and other proinflammatory compounds initiate and amplify the inflammatory response in ALI/ARDS. The shear stress and stretch injury (discussed previously) induce proinflammatory cytokines (specifically, up-regulation of nuclear factor κB] from endothelial, epithelial, and macrophage cells). Damage to the cell membranes causes an increase in the intracellular calcium concentrations. This rise in calcium results in membrane deformation, which triggers the activation of genes involved in paracrine signaling, and the production of factors, such as transforming growth factor 1 and basic fibroblast growth factor. Genes responsible for the synthesis of fibronectin, collagen, and matrix metalloproteinase are also activated and up-regulated.[7,63,64] It is unclear whether these responses are directly accountable for the activation of proinflammatory genes or whether their initiation arises secondary to cell necrosis and cell membrane exposure.[64]

The mechanism of injury-induced cell death determines the pulmonary response to a noxious insult. Apoptosis (programmed cell death) occurs without the release of cell contents whereas necrosis, resulting in cell membrane disruption, causes inflammation. The inflammatory reaction is chemotactic, priming and activating polymorphonuclear leukocytes—neutrophils migrate to the lung parenchyma and macrophages migrate to the alveolar air spaces. Hyperoxia intensifies the process and modifies the balance between apoptosis and necrosis toward the former (toxic oxygen metabolites).[65]

Apoptosis plays a role in protecting the lung against mechanical stress and is vital in maintaining alveolar-epithelial integrity. It is suppressed by the key mitogen-activated protein kinase cell membrane–nucleus transduction pathway. Low mechanical stress causes primarily pulmonary apoptosis. High stress changes the balance between apoptosis and necrosis, leading to more necrosis.[7] Overexpression of mitogen-activated protein kinases, as seen in high-stretch ventilation strategies, therefore results in the inhibition of less-damaging proapoptotic mechanisms.[66]

Pulmonary versus Extrapulmonary ARDS

Although there are some conflicting data among studies, there are suggestions of different circulating cytokine profiles between types of ARDS,[67–70] suggesting different patterns of cellular injury that derive from a greater or lesser injury severity. Therefore, it is the differential activation of alveolar epithelium or versus vascular endothelial cells in pulmonary (pneumonia) versus extrapulmonary (trauma/sepsis)

ARDS, respectively. This explanation seems more biologically plausible rather than simply due to the differing pathophysiology of the inciting disease process.

It is not only the production of proinflammatory cytokines that is important but also the balance between proinflammatory and anti-inflammatory mediators (eg, interleukin [IL]-1–receptor antagonist, soluble tumor necrosis factor receptor, and autontibodies against IL-8, IL-10, and IL-11) (**Fig. 4**). It seems clear that studies of the biologic activity

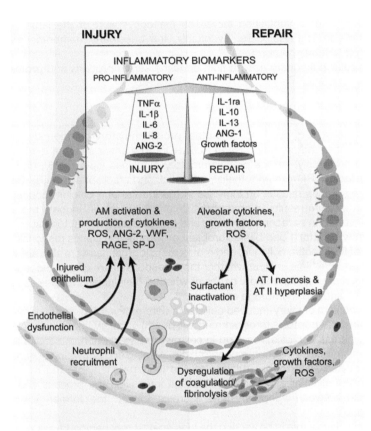

Fig. 4. Schematic demonstrating the cytokine imbalance that drives the development of ALI/ ARDS. The injured alveolus in the acute phase (*left*) and the repair phase in ALI. In the acute exudative phase, there is activation of resident alveolar macrophages, which results in production of several proinflammatory molecules. These stimulate chemotaxis and activation of neutrophils, which release a variety of mediators that further increase the proinflammatory environment of the injured alveolus and are associated with both alveolar endothelial and epithelial injury. The mechanisms that play a role repair in ALI are illustrated (*right*). Alveolar type II cells undergo hyperplasia and there is also recruitment of fibroblasts (not shown). There is release of growth factors and anti-inflammatory cytokines involved in repair. These mediators as well as cell-specific activation/injury can be measured as biomarkers. AM, alveolar macrophage; ANG, angiopoietin; AT, alveolar epithelial cell type; IL-1ra, IL-1 receptor antagonist; RAGE, receptor for advanced glycation end products; ROS, reactive oxygen species; SP-D, surfactant D. (*From* Cross LJ, Matthay MA. Biomarkers in acute lung injury: insights into the pathogenesis of acute lung injury. Crit Care Clin 2011;27(2):355–77.)

of cytokines rather than static levels of biomarkers that may not reflect tissue pathophysiology may be the key to effective immunomodulatory therapy.[53,69] Although this may suggest different disease states (**Fig. 5**), the utility of these markers in defining and changing practice in distinct patterns of ALI remains unclear other than perhaps in deciding ventilator strategy.

Gattinoni and coworkers[71] have demonstrated that the effect of PEEP on lung recruitment is associated with the percentage of potentially recruitable lung. This, in turn, varies according to inciting insult. Higher PEEP levels (>15 cm H_2O) seemed more beneficial in patients with a higher percentage of potentially recruitable lung, including mostly individuals with pneumonia-induced ARDS. Conversely, lower PEEP levels (<10 cm H_2O) seemed more advantageous in those with a lower percentage of potentially recruitable lung, as seems to occur in sepsis-induced ALI. Therefore, speculatively, lower levels of PEEP may be adequate in indirect ARDS compared with direct ARDS.[71]

Coagulopathy

The cytokine profile in ALI activates thrombotic and antifibrinolytic pathways that favor fibrin deposition with microthombosis. Lung biopsy specimens of ALI patients contain microthrombi within pulmonary capillaries in addition to capillary endothelial injury. BAL specimens from ARDS patients contain increased tissue factor and factor VIIIa (potent stimulators of the extrinsic coagulation cascade). Tissue factor activity (a procoagulant) and plasminogen activator inhibitor-1 (inhibitor of urokinase plasminogen activator [ie, fibrinolytic defect]) and thus increased alveolar fibrin deposition are revealed in serial BAL specimens in ALI.[72] Decreasing circulating protein C and increased circulating thrombomodulin are markers of this altered prothrombotic, antifibrinolytic state.[73] The role played by endothelial cell injury activation within the pulmonary microvasculature is reflected in elevated plasma levels of von Willebrand factor and plasma endothelin-1 observed in ALI patients. These markers are all associated with increased mortality and fewer ventilation-free days.[74]

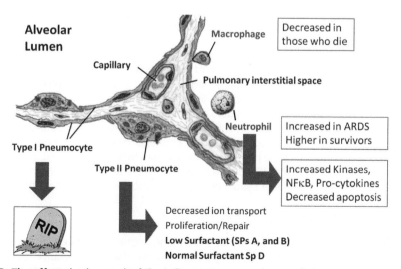

Fig. 5. The effects (*red arrows*) of the inflammatory cascade on cellular components of the alveolar capillary barrier that affect prognosis. SPs-surfactant proteins.

Physiology

Flooding of the alveolar airspaces impairs adequate ventilation resulting in hypoxemia from ventilation-perfusion mismatch and intrapulmonary shunt. Additional right-to-left shunt from reabsorption atelectasis secondary to alveolar denitrogenation may also contribute when high levels of oxygen are administered.[75] There is a reduction in thoracic compliance due to the presence of protein-rich pulmonary edema fluid, cellular infiltrate, and a reduction in functionally active surfactant. Direct injury of micro-thrombi lead to compromised blood flow of the alveoli and the subsequent damage to the pulmonary microvascular bed results in an increased physiologic pulmonary dead space fraction.[76] Patients develop hypoxia, hypercapnia, and an increased work of breathing; mechanical ventilation support is the sine qua non that follows.

Fibroproliferative Phase (Day 5—Recovery)

After the acute phase of ARDS, some patients may follow an uncomplicated course and rapid resolution of their disease. In other patients, the alveolar space becomes filled with mesenchymal cells, their products, and neovascularization (interstitial gran-ulation tissue). These patients progress to fibrotic lung injury, which can be observed histologically as early as 5 days after the initiation of ventilation.[77] This process of fibrosing alveolitis may begin even earlier in the course of the disorder promoted by early profibroinflammatory mediators, such as IL-1 and procollagen III peptide.[69,78] This biologic process correlates with worse clinical outcome and an increased risk of death.[79]

RESOLUTION

A functional, intact distal lung epithelium is associated with a better prognosis in patients with ALI/ARDS.[77] The type II cells repopulate the denuded basement membrane by proliferating and differentiating into type I cells under the control of epithelial growth factors. This restores the normal alveolar architecture and increases the fluid-transport capacity of the alveolar epithelium, allowing rapid removal of alve-olar edema. In a study of 79 ALI patients, serial measurements of pulmonary edema fluid protein in the first 4 hours after intubation demonstrated that maximal alveolar fluid clearance was associated with a better prognosis, lower mortality, and a shorter duration of mechanical ventilation.[80] Lower tidal volume and reduced airway pressure preserve near-normal alveolar fluid transport in the presence of acid-induced lung injury in rats. This suggests that protection of the alveolar epithelium may be an impor-tant mechanism to explain the mortality benefit of lung protective ventilatory strate-gies.[81] The process of fluid resorption is discussed previously.

A considerable quantity of both soluble and insoluble protein must also be removed from the air spaces. Soluble protein is likely cleared via paracellular diffusion and, to a lesser extent, via endocytosis by alveolar epithelial cells. Macrophages remove insoluble protein and apoptotic neutrophils by phagocytosis. The removal of insoluble protein is particularly important, because hyaline membranes provide a framework for the growth in the fibrous tissue associated with the poor prognosis phenotype.[82]

TRANSLATION INTO THE OPERATING ROOM

In a bid to determine the frequency at which lung protective strategies are imple-mented in response to low Pao_2/Fio_2 ratios during the intraoperative ventilator management of hypoxia, Blum and colleagues[83] performed a retrospective cohort study of 11,000 patients receiving general anesthetic over a 5-year period at a large tertiary medical center. The results suggested that anesthetists respond to hypoxemia by increasing Fio_2 and peak inspiratory pressure rather than initiating lung protective strategies. The data demonstrated, however, at least a progressive trend toward lower tidal volumes (decrease by 2 mL/kg predicted body weight), lower peak inspiratory pressure (decreased by 5 cm H_2O), and higher PEEP (increased by 2 cm H_2O). This perhaps indicates that lung protective strategies from critical care medicine are beginning to influence anesthetic management.[83]

SUMMARY: FUTURE DIRECTIONS?

Over the past 25 years, there have been several biologically plausible, ineffective pharmacologic strategies for ARDS. They have been aimed at specific therapeutic targets and used with the aim of ameliorating the perpetuating cycle demonstrated in ARDS. Some therapies, such as the direct, inhaled pulmonary vasodilators (eg, nitric oxide) transiently improve oxygenation. Others, however, such as low-dose corticosteroids in the late phases of the disease, continue to cause highly contentious debate and repeated study.[84]

Strategies that hasten the resolution of the illness may ultimately be as important as those that attenuate early inflammatory injury. Unfortunately, the trend of benefit from accelerated clearance of alveolar fluid seen in experimental models and in a single-centered trial[85] of intravenous β-agonists were not confirmed in a multicenter randomized controlled trail. The Beta Agonist Lung Injury Trial 2 study randomized patients with early ARDS to receive either salbutamol (15 μg/kg) or placebo.[86] Recruitment was stopped early after the second interim analysis because of safety concerns—salbutamol increased 28-day mortality by 34% versus 23% in the control group, respectively (risk ratio 1.47; 95% CI, 1.03–2.08).

Increasing adrenergic load in patients already under a great degree of physiologic stress and instituting a treatment to stimulate a type II alveolar cell driven process early, while the alveolar epithelium is still denuded, may have been responsible for the poor outcomes. Accelerating re-epithelialization by encouraging the proliferation of type II cells by epithelium-specific growth factor (eg, epidermal growth factor, transforming growth factor α, keratinocyte growth factor, and hepatocyte growth factor, which are all present in the edema fluid of patients with ALI/ARDS) has been shown to increase alveolar epithelium repair in rat models.[87] Multifaceted strategies directed at restoring the alveolar capillary barrier and accelerating its functional capacity merit continued clinical evaluation.[88]

It has been proposed and demonstrated in animal models that the use of pluripotential mesenchymal stem cells and embryonic stem cells can mitigate and provide a significant survival advantage[89] in bleomycin-induced and endotoxin-induced ALI. After migration, differentiation, and engraftment at the sites of acute inflammation, the proposed mechanisms of action relate to

1. Increased production of growth factors that also mobilize endogenous stem cells
2. Alterations in the local cytokine profile supporting repair and modifying the balance from proinflammatory to anti-inflammatory state (ie, enhanced production of IL-10 and blocking TNF-α and IL-1)
3. Potential to differentiate into different cell lines (lung, liver, and kidney), enhancing repair of ALI and multiple organ dysfunction syndrome[90]

Other strategies with potential include gene therapy focused on up-regulating the expression of anti-inflammatory mediators. There is, however, a potential for harm related to the lineage into which the engrafting cells could differentiate, influenced by the underlying extracellular matrix (teratoma potential) and the possibility of oncogenesis when using viral vectors for nucleotide transfer.[90,91]

REFERENCES

1. Fothergill J. Observations on a case published in the last volume of the medical essays, c. of recovering a man dead in appearance, by distending the lungs with air1. Philos Trans R Soc Lond 1744;43:275–81.
2. Ashbaugh DG, Bigelow DB, Petty TL, et al. Acute respiratory distress in adults. Lancet 1967;2(7511):319–23.
3. Petty TL, Ashbaugh DG. The adult respiratory distress syndrome. Clinical features, factors influencing prognosis and principles of management. Chest 1971;60(3):233–9.
4. Bernard GR, Artigas A, Brigham KL, et al. The American-European Consensus Conference on ARDS. Definitions, mechanisms, relevant outcomes, and clinical trial coordination. Am J Respir Crit Care Med 1994;149(3 Pt 1):818–24.
5. Matthay MA, Zimmerman GA, Esmon C, et al. Future Research Directions in Acute Lung Injury Summary of a National Heart, Lung, and Blood Institute Working Group. Am J Respir Crit Care Med 2003;167(7):1027–35.
6. Smetana GW. Postoperative pulmonary complications: an update on risk assessment and reduction. Cleve Clin J Med 2009;76(Suppl 4):S60–5.
7. Kilpatrick B, Slinger P. Lung protective strategies in anaesthesia. Br J Anaesth 2010;105(Suppl 1):i108–16.
8. Fernández-Pérez ER, Sprung J, Afessa B, et al. Intraoperative ventilator settings and acute lung injury after elective surgery: a nested case control study. Thorax 2009;64(2):121–7.
9. Beck-Schimmer B, Schimmer RC. Perioperative tidal volume and intra-operative open lung strategy in healthy lungs: where are we going? Best Pract Res Clin Anaesthesiol 2010;24(2):199–210.
10. The ARDS Definition Task Force*. Acute respiratory distress syndrome. The Berlin definition. JAMA 2012;307(23):2526–33.
11. Angus DC. The acute respiratory distress syndrome: what's in a name? JAMA 2012;307(23):2542–4.
12. Reynolds SD, Malkinson AM. Clara cell: progenitor for the bronchiolar epithelium. Int J Biochem Cell Biol 2010;42(1):1–4.
13. Matthay MA, Robriquet L, Fang X. Alveolar epithelium: role in lung fluid balance and acute lung injury. Proc Am Thorac Soc 2005;2(3):206–13.
14. Matthay MA, Folkesson HG, Clerici C. Lung epithelial fluid transport and the resolution of pulmonary edema. Physiol Rev 2002;82(3):569–600.
15. Canessa CM, Schild L, Buell G, et al. Amiloride-sensitive epithelial Na+ channel is made of three homologous subunits. Nature 1994;367(6462):463–7.
16. Johnson MD, Widdicombe JH, Allen L, et al. Alveolar epithelial type I cells contain transport proteins and transport sodium, supporting an active role for type I cells in regulation of lung liquid homeostasis. Proc Natl Acad Sci U S A 2002;99(4):1966–71.
17. Sakuma T, Okaniwa G, Nakada T, et al. Alveolar fluid clearance in the resected human lung. Am J Respir Crit Care Med 1994;150(2):305–10.
18. Sakuma T, Pittet JF, Jayr C, et al. Alveolar liquid and protein clearance in the absence of blood flow or ventilation in sheep. J Appl Physiol 1993;74(1):176–85.
19. Jiang X, Ingbar DH, O'Grady SM. Adrenergic regulation of ion transport across adult alveolar epithelial cells: effects on Cl- channel activation and transport function in cultures with an apical air interface. J Membr Biol 2001;181(3):195–204.

20. Fang X, Fukuda N, Barbry P, et al. Novel role for CFTR in fluid absorption from the distal airspaces of the lung. J Gen Physiol 2002;119(2):199–207.
21. Matthay MA, Berthiaume Y, Staub NC. Long-term clearance of liquid and protein from the lungs of unanesthetized sheep. J Appl Physiol 1985;59(3):928–34.
22. Matthay MA, Landolt CC, Staub NC. Differential liquid and protein clearance from the alveoli of anesthetized sheep. J Appl Physiol 1982;53(1):96–104.
23. Ventilation with lower tidal volumes as compared with traditional tidal volumes for acute lung injury and the acute respiratory distress syndrome. The Acute Respiratory Distress Syndrome Network. N Engl J Med 2000; 342(18):1301–8.
24. Gajic O, Dara SI, Mendez JL, et al. Ventilator-associated lung injury in patients without acute lung injury at the onset of mechanical ventilation. Crit Care Med 2004;32(9):1817–24.
25. Gajic O, Frutos-Vivar F, Esteban A, et al. Ventilator settings as a risk factor for acute respiratory distress syndrome in mechanically ventilated patients. Intensive Care Med 2005;31(7):922–6.
26. Pinheiro de Oliveira R, Hetzel MP, dos Anjos Silva M, et al. Mechanical ventilation with high tidal volume induces inflammation in patients without lung disease. Crit Care 2010;14(2):R39.
27. Choi G, Wolthuis EK, Bresser P, et al. Mechanical ventilation with lower tidal volumes and positive end-expiratory pressure prevents alveolar coagulation in patients without lung injury. Anesthesiology 2006;105(4):689–95.
28. Licker M, de Perrot M, Spiliopoulos A, et al. Risk factors for acute lung injury after thoracic surgery for lung cancer. Anesth Analg 2003;97(6):1558–65.
29. Turnage WS, Lunn JJ. Postpneumonectomy pulmonary edema. A retrospective analysis of associated variables. Chest 1993;103(6):1646–50.
30. Waller DA, Keavey P, Woodfine L, et al. Pulmonary endothelial permeability changes after major lung resection. Ann Thorac Surg 1996;61(5):1435–40.
31. Williams EA, Quinlan GJ, Goldstraw P, et al. Postoperative lung injury and oxidative damage in patients undergoing pulmonary resection. Eur Respir J 1998; 11(5):1028–34.
32. Mead J, Takishima T, Leith D. Stress distribution in lungs: a model of pulmonary elasticity. J Appl Physiol 1970;28(5):596–608.
33. Gefen A, Elad D, Shiner RJ. Analysis of stress distribution in the alveolar septa of normal and simulated emphysematic lungs. J Biomech 1999;32(9):891–7.
34. Bonetto C, Terragni P, Ranieri VM. Does high tidal volume generate ALI/ARDS in healthy lungs? Intensive Care Med 2005;31(7):893–5.
35. Slutsky AS. Lung injury caused by mechanical ventilation. Chest 1999;116(Suppl 1): 9S–15S.
36. West JB, Tsukimoto K, Mathieu-Costello O, et al. Stress failure in pulmonary capillaries. J Appl Physiol 1991;70(4):1731–42.
37. Duggan M, Kavanagh BP. Pulmonary atelectasis: a pathogenic perioperative entity. Anesthesiology 2005;102(4):838–54.
38. Wolthuis EK, Vlaar AP, Choi G, et al. Mechanical ventilation using non-injurious ventilation settings causes lung injury in the absence of pre-existing lung injury in healthy mice. Crit Care 2009;13(1):R1.
39. Lionetti V, Recchia FA, Ranieri VM. Overview of ventilator-induced lung injury mechanisms. Curr Opin Crit Care 2005;11(1):82–6.
40. Aberle DR, Wiener-Kronish JP, Webb WR, et al. Hydrostatic versus increased permeability pulmonary edema: diagnosis based on radiographic criteria in critically ill patients. Radiology 1988;168(1):73–9.

41. Mäurer J, Kendzia A, Gerlach H, et al. Morphological changes in chest radiographs of patients with acute respiratory distress syndrome (ARDS). Intensive Care Med 1998;24(11):1152–6.
42. Gattinoni L, Pelosi P, Vitale G, et al. Body position changes redistribute lung computed-tomographic density in patients with acute respiratory failure. Anesthesiology 1991;74(1):15–23.
43. Gattinoni L, D'Andrea L, Pelosi P, et al. Regional effects and mechanism of positive end-expiratory pressure in early adult respiratory distress syndrome. JAMA 1993;269(16):2122–7.
44. Pelosi P, Rocco PR, de Abreu MG. Use of computed tomography scanning to guide lung recruitment and adjust positive-end expiratory pressure. Curr Opin Crit Care 2011;17(3):268–74.
45. Tagliabue M, Casella TC, Zincone GE, et al. CT and chest radiography in the evaluation of adult respiratory distress syndrome. Acta Radiol 1994;35(3):230–4.
46. Bellani G, Mauri T, Pesenti A. Imaging in acute lung injury and acute respiratory distress syndrome. Curr Opin Crit Care 2012;18(1):29–34.
47. Constantin JM, Grasso S, Chanques G, et al. Lung morphology predicts response to recruitment maneuver in patients with acute respiratory distress syndrome. Crit Care Med 2010;38(4):1108–17.
48. Bouhemad B, Brisson H, Le-Guen M, et al. Bedside ultrasound assessment of positive end-expiratory pressure-induced lung recruitment. Am J Respir Crit Care Med 2011;183(3):341–7.
49. Xirouchaki N, Magkanas E, Vaporidi K, et al. Lung ultrasound in critically ill patients: comparison with bedside chest radiography. Intensive Care Med 2011;37(9):1488–93.
50. Bellani G, Amigoni M, Pesenti A. Positron emission tomography in ARDS: a new look at an old syndrome. Minerva Anestesiol 2011;77(4):439–47.
51. Musch G. Positron emission tomography: a tool for better understanding of ventilator-induced and acute lung injury. Curr Opin Crit Care 2011;17(1):7–12.
52. Bellani G, Messa C, Guerra L, et al. Lungs of patients with acute respiratory distress syndrome show diffuse inflammation in normally aerated regions: a [18F]-fluoro-2-deoxy-D-glucose PET/CT study. Crit Care Med 2009;37(7):2216–22.
53. Pittet JF, Mackersie RC, Martin TR, et al. Biological markers of acute lung injury: prognostic and pathogenetic significance. Am J Respir Crit Care Med 1997; 155(4):1187–205.
54. Wiener-Kronish JP, Albertine KH, Matthay MA. Differential responses of the endothelial and epithelial barriers of the lung in sheep to Escherichia coli endotoxin. J Clin Invest 1991;88(3):864–75.
55. Pelosi P, D'Onofrio D, Chiumello D, et al. Pulmonary and extrapulmonary acute respiratory distress syndrome are different. Eur Respir J Suppl 2003;42:48s–56s.
56. Plataki M, Hubmayr RD. The physical basis of ventilator-induced lung injury. Expert Rev Respir Med 2010;4(3):373–85.
57. Kurahashi K, Kajikawa O, Sawa T, et al. Pathogenesis of septic shock in Pseudomonas aeruginosa pneumonia. J Clin Invest 1999;104(6):743–50.
58. Sznajder JI. Strategies to increase alveolar epithelial fluid removal in the injured lung. Am J Respir Crit Care Med 1999;160(5 Pt 1):1441–2.
59. Walker MG, Tessolini JM, McCaig L, et al. Elevated endogenous surfactant reduces inflammation in an acute lung injury model. Exp Lung Res 2009;35(7):591–604.
60. Greene KE, Wright JR, Steinberg KP, et al. Serial changes in surfactant-associated proteins in lung and serum before and after onset of ARDS. Am J Respir Crit Care Med 1999;160(6):1843–50.

61. Hillman NH, Kallapur SG, Pillow JJ, et al. Inhibitors of inflammation and endogenous surfactant pool size as modulators of lung injury with initiation of ventilation in preterm sheep. Respir Res 2010;11:151.

62. Baker CS, Evans TW, Randle BJ, et al. Damage to surfactant-specific protein in acute respiratory distress syndrome. Lancet 1999;353(9160):1232–7.

63. Wang HM, Bodenstein M, Duenges B, et al. Ventilator-associated lung injury superposed to oleic acid infusion or surfactant depletion: histopathological characteristics of two porcine models of acute lung injury. Eur Surg Res 2010;45(3–4):121–33.

64. Jaecklin T, Otulakowski G, Kavanagh BP. Do soluble mediators cause ventilator-induced lung injury and multi-organ failure? Intensive Care Med 2010;36(5): 750–7.

65. Mathru M, Rooney MW, Dries DJ, et al. Urine hydrogen peroxide during adult respiratory distress syndrome in patients with and without sepsis. Chest 1994; 105(1):232–6.

66. Muders T, Wrigge H. New insights into experimental evidence on atelectasis and causes of lung injury. Best Pract Res Clin Anaesthesiol 2010;24(2):171–82.

67. Barnett N, Ware LB. Biomarkers in acute lung injury—marking forward progress. Crit Care Clin 2011;27(3):661–83.

68. Cross LJM, Matthay MA. Biomarkers in acute lung injury: insights into the pathogenesis of acute lung injury. Crit Care Clin 2011;27(2):355–77.

69. Pugin J, Verghese G, Widmer MC, et al. The alveolar space is the site of intense inflammatory and profibrotic reactions in the early phase of acute respiratory distress syndrome. Crit Care Med 1999;27(2):304–12.

70. Levitt JE, Gould MK, Ware LB, et al. The pathogenetic and prognostic value of biologic markers in acute lung injury. J Intensive Care Med 2009;24(3):151–67.

71. Gattinoni L, Caironi P, Cressoni M, et al. Lung recruitment in patients with the acute respiratory distress syndrome. N Engl J Med 2006;354(17):1775–86.

72. Prabhakaran P, Ware LB, White KE, et al. Elevated levels of plasminogen activator inhibitor-1 in pulmonary edema fluid are associated with mortality in acute lung injury. Am J Physiol Lung Cell Mol Physiol 2003;285(1):L20–8.

73. Ware LB, Fang X, Matthay MA. Protein C and thrombomodulin in human acute lung injury. Am J Physiol Lung Cell Mol Physiol 2003;285(3):L514–21.

74. Ware LB, Matthay MA, Parsons PE, et al. Pathogenetic and prognostic significance of altered coagulation and fibrinolysis in acute lung injury/acute respiratory distress syndrome. Crit Care Med 2007;35(8):1821–8.

75. Ware LB. Pathophysiology of acute lung injury and the acute respiratory distress syndrome. Semin Respir Crit Care Med 2006;27(4):337–49.

76. Gattinoni L, Bombino M, Pelosi P, et al. Lung structure and function in different stages of severe adult respiratory distress syndrome. JAMA 1994;271(22):1772–9.

77. Matthay MA, Wiener-Kronish JP. Intact epithelial barrier function is critical for the resolution of alveolar edema in humans. Am Rev Respir Dis 1990;142(6 Pt 1): 1250–7.

78. Chesnutt AN, Matthay MA, Tibayan FA, et al. Early detection of type III procollagen peptide in acute lung injury. Pathogenetic and prognostic significance. Am J Respir Crit Care Med 1997;156(3 Pt 1):840–5.

79. Martin C, Papazian L, Payan MJ, et al. Pulmonary fibrosis correlates with outcome in adult respiratory distress syndrome. A study in mechanically ventilated patients. Chest 1995;107(1):196–200.

80. Ware LB, Matthay MA. Alveolar fluid clearance is impaired in the majority of patients with acute lung injury and the acute respiratory distress syndrome. Am J Respir Crit Care Med 2001;163(6):1376–83.

81. Frank JA, Gutierrez JA, Jones KD, et al. Low tidal volume reduces epithelial and endothelial injury in acid-injured rat lungs. Am J Respir Crit Care Med 2002; 165(2):242–9.
82. Folkesson HG, Matthay MA, Weström BR, et al. Alveolar epithelial clearance of protein. J Appl Physiol 1996;80(5):1431–45.
83. Blum JM, Maile M, Park PK, et al. A description of intraoperative ventilator management in patients with acute lung injury and the use of lung protective ventilation strategies. Anesthesiology 2011;115(1):75–82.
84. Adhikari NK, Burns KE, Meade MO, et al. Pharmacologic therapies for adults with acute lung injury and acute respiratory distress syndrome [Internet]. In: The Cochrane Collaboration, Adhikari NK, editors. Cochrane Database of Systematic Reviews. Chichester (United Kingdom): John Wiley & Sons, Ltd; 2004 [cited 2012 Aug 10]. Available at: http://summaries.cochrane.org/CD004477/there-is-little-evidence-to-support-the-use-of-drugs-to-improve-outcomes-in-adults-with-lung-injury. Accessed August 10, 2012.
85. Perkins GD, McAuley DF, Thickett DR, et al. The beta-agonist lung injury trial (BALTI): a randomized placebo-controlled clinical trial. Am J Respir Crit Care Med 2006;173(3):281–7.
86. Gao Smith F, Perkins GD, Gates S, et al. Effect of intravenous β-2 agonist treatment on clinical outcomes in acute respiratory distress syndrome (BALTI-2): a multicentre, randomised controlled trial. Lancet 2012;379(9812):229–35.
87. Geiser T. Mechanisms of alveolar epithelial repair in acute lung injury—a translational approach. Swiss Med Wkly 2003;133(43–44):586–90.
88. Berthiaume Y, Lesur O, Dagenais A. Treatment of adult respiratory distress syndrome: plea for rescue therapy of the alveolar epithelium. Thorax 1999; 54(2):150–60.
89. Zhu YG, Qu JM, Zhang J, et al. Novel interventional approaches for ALI/ARDS: cell-based gene therapy. Mediators Inflamm 2011;2011:560194.
90. Hayes M, Curley G, Ansari B. Clinical review: stem cell therapies for acute lung injury/acute respiratory distress syndrome—hope or hype? Crit Care 2012; 16(2):205.
91. Stripp BR, Shapiro SD. Stem cells in lung disease, repair, and the potential for therapeutic interventions state-of-the-art and future challenges. Am J Respir Cell Mol Biol 2006;34(5):517–22.

Perioperative Oxygen Toxicity

Andrew B. Lumb, MB BS, FRCA[a,b,*], Laura J. Walton, MBChB, FRCA[a]

KEYWORDS

- Oxygen • Hyperoxia • Reactive oxygen species • Antioxidants • Atelectasis
- One-lung ventilation • Chronic obstructive lung disease
- Cardiopulmonary resuscitation

KEY POINTS

- Oxygen molecules can produce reactive oxygen species, which damage cells by reacting with the crucial molecular components.
- Hyperoxia (inspired oxygen of 100%) is commonly used in the perioperative period to prolong the time to hypoxemia if apnea or airway obstruction occurs.
- Other reasons for perioperative hyperoxia include aiding lung collapse during 1-lung ventilation or to improve neurologic function during awake carotid endarterectomy.
- Hyperoxia can disturb normal physiology and produce adverse effects on respiratory control, ventilation/perfusion relationships, and hypoxic pulmonary vasoconstriction, and can also cause vasoconstriction of systemic arterioles.
- The clinical use of hyperoxia can adversely affect outcomes in various acute medical conditions including exacerbations of chronic obstructive pulmonary disease, acute coronary syndromes, and stroke, and following successful cardiopulmonary resuscitation.

In the history of eighteenth century science, the person responsible for discovering oxygen is disputed.[1] Carl Scheele, a pharmacist in Sweden, described a gas named fire air and its role in animal respiration. Joseph Priestley, a church minister in England, described dephlogisticated air and how its production by plants restored its atmospheric loss by animal respiration. In addition, Antoine Lavoisier, a science graduate in Paris, made the same discoveries but extended them into quantitative experiments and named the element oxygene. Joseph Priestley was the first to recognize that an excess of oxygen may be harmful, by writing in 1775 that, "A moralist, at least, may say that the air which nature has provided for us is as good as we deserved."[2]

OXYGEN TOXICITY

Oxygen is a paramagnetic atom containing 2 unpaired electrons in its outer (2P) shell and so reacts rapidly with nearby molecules. Most oxygen atoms exist as dioxygen (O_2) in which the molecules share their unpaired electrons in a stable covalent

[a] Department of Anaesthesia, St James's University Hospital, Leeds LS9 7TF, United Kingdom;
[b] Department of Anaesthesia, University of Leeds, Leeds LS2 9JT, United Kingdom
* Corresponding author.
E-mail address: a.lumb@leeds.ac.uk

Anesthesiology Clin 30 (2012) 591–605
http://dx.doi.org/10.1016/j.anclin.2012.07.009   anesthesiology.theclinics.com

bond. However, in biologic tissues the dioxygen atom can be accidentally or deliberately split, producing reactive oxygen species (ROS) that need to be immediately neutralized by a range of antioxidant systems. Many animals, including mammals, produce ROS to kill invading pathogens.

Direct Toxic Effects of Oxygen

A variety of ROS exist:

- Singlet oxygen, in which the 2 unpaired electrons combine into 1 paired orbital, producing an unstable, high-energy atom.
- Superoxide anion ($O_2^{\cdot-}$) forms when dioxygen gains an electron from elsewhere. Relative to other ROS, superoxide is stable and has few damaging effects, although it does generate other more dangerous ROS.
- Hydroperoxyl ($HO_2^{\cdot}$) forms when superoxide reacts with a hydrogen ion.
- Hydrogen peroxide (H_2O_2) is produced in cells by the action of superoxide dismutase (SOD), which removes an electron from superoxide allowing it to combine with 2 hydrogen ions forming the more stable H_2O_2 (**Fig. 1**).

Sources of ROS in cells include:

- Mitochondrial enzymes that leak electrons to form superoxide anions. It is possible that this accounts for 8% of total cellular oxygen use, indicating the importance of antioxidant systems.
- NADPH (nicotinamide adenine dinucleotide phosphate) oxidase enzymes can produce free electrons, and are involved in the formation of ROS in phagocytic cells.
- Xanthine oxidoreductase is responsible for the metabolism of purines. Under hypoxic conditions the enzyme switches to using a different cofactor (NAD^+ [nicotinamide adenine dinucleotide] instead of NADH [NAD hydrogen]) and so produces ROS. This mechanism is mostly responsible for the ROS damage seen with reperfusion following a period of ischemia.

Cellular toxicity

ROS may damage cells by reacting with any of the crucial molecular components (ie, DNA, lipids, or proteins). Singlet oxygen reacts particularly quickly with fatty acids, inducing a chain reaction of lipid peroxidation that damages nuclear and cellular membranes. Oxidation of DNA is inevitable, but whether this causes damaging

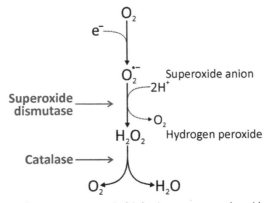

Fig. 1. The reduction of oxygen to water in biologic systems, catalyzed by 2 ubiquitous antioxidant enzymes.

transcription errors is not clear and may depend on the effectiveness of the cell's DNA repair mechanisms. Proteins containing many sulfhydryl groups are particularly susceptible to oxidant damage, with the disruption of sulfhydryl bridges changing their secondary and tertiary structures.

Physiologic antioxidant systems

Three ubiquitous enzymes occur in the cells of all animals that metabolize oxygen (see **Fig. 1**):

1. SOD converts superoxide anion to the slightly less harmful hydrogen peroxide and exists in 3 different forms: extracellular, cytoplasmic (containing manganese), and mitochondrial (containing copper and zinc). Additional SOD can be produced in response to long-term hyperoxia or inflammation and presumably provides some protection from the excess ROS under these conditions. Attempts to artificially boost SOD levels to provide this protection in disease states have been mostly unsuccessful. The prospect of developing molecules that catalyze the same reaction, SOD mimetics, is a potential therapeutic avenue for the future.[3]
2. Catalase has a similar biologic distribution to SOD and converts the H_2O_2 into harmless molecules (see **Fig. 1**).
3. Glutathione (GSH) peroxidase enzymes scavenge many of the ROS and also halt the reactions of lipid peroxidation. Two molecules of GSH are oxidized to 1 molecule of reduced glutathione (GSSG), donating their hydrogen ions to the ROS, normally producing water.

Other molecules with nonspecific antioxidant effects are present in biologic tissue:

- Ascorbic acid is a small molecule that is vital for removal of the hydroxyl ROS, a highly reactive derivative of superoxide anion. Humans, along with guinea-pigs and bats, are unable to produce ascorbate, and so must ingest vitamin C. In those vertebrates able to produce endogenous ascorbate, SOD activity is lower.
- Vitamin E (α-tocopherol) is a fat-soluble molecule found in high concentrations in cell membranes where it has a major antioxidant role in preventing lipid peroxidation.
- Pulmonary surfactant may have antioxidant properties, but the role of this in vivo is unknown.

Symptoms and signs of oxygen toxicity

With increased fraction of inspired oxygen (Fio_2) the lung is inevitably the organ exposed to the highest oxygen partial pressure and so airway lining fluid has high antioxidant activity, mostly from the presence of extracellular SOD. Pulmonary oxygen toxicity is quickly lethal in laboratory animals but humans seem to be less sensitive.

Breathing high concentrations of oxygen initially causes irritation of the tracheobronchial tree and retrosternal tightness, with continued exposure leading to chest pain, cough, and an urge to take deep breaths. After about 24 hours of normobaric 100% oxygen, forced vital capacity is reduced. Continued exposure leads to widespread structural changes in the lung and eventually acute lung injury.

Other direct toxic effects of oxygen include nonspecific neurologic symptoms such as headache and visual disturbances, progressing to convulsions (the Paul Bert effect). This effect only occurs in hyperbaric conditions with Po_2 values of more than 2 atm absolute.

Indirect Adverse Effects of Oxygen: Atelectasis

In the perioperative period, oxygen may exacerbate the effects of general anesthesia on the lungs. As a result of changes in the function of the chest wall muscles and diaphragm, functional residual capacity (FRC) in most patients is reduced by 15% to 20% from their awake supine volumes. This change causes a reduction in airway caliber, and, in some lung regions, airway closure and atelectasis. Ventilation perfusion (V/Q) relationships become abnormal with an increase in areas of both high and low V/Q, impairing pulmonary exchange of both oxygen and carbon dioxide.

In lung regions to which the airway has closed, the rate at which atelectasis forms is related to the gases present in the lung unit when airway closure occurs, referred to as absorption atelectasis. Oxygen is absorbed until the alveolar Po_2 equals that of mixed venous blood, alveolar Pco_2 remains unchanged, and the alveolar PN_2 equilibrates with the PN_2 of blood. Mathematical modeling of this situation indicates that the time from airway occlusion to collapse of the lung unit is more than 100 minutes with 30% oxygen in nitrogen but less than 10 minutes with 100% oxygen.[4] These theoretic considerations translate into perioperative care of patients. Early studies of the effects of preoxygenation indicated that use of 100% compared with 30% oxygen was associated with more atelectasis on computed tomography (CT) and a greater shunt fraction.[5] In a landmark study by the same group in 2003, CT scanning after induction of anesthesia with 3 different preinduction Fio_2 levels (**Table 1**) found a major effect of 100% oxygen on atelectasis formation.[6]

Similar findings have been reported when extubating patients on emergence from anesthesia. Patients receiving 40% oxygen before extubation had less atelectasis on CT scans performed soon after extubation compared with those receiving 100% oxygen, irrespective of whether a reexpansion maneuver was performed.[7] Based on oxygenation in the postanesthesia care unit (PACU), used as an indirect assessment of the amount of atelectasis, the use of continuous positive airway pressure on extubation is ineffective at preventing these changes.[8] In addition, a study of oxygenation in PACU found no differences between patients who breathed 30% or 80% oxygen throughout their anesthesia.[9]

As may be predicted from the mathematical modeling of absorption atelectasis, 100% oxygen seems to cause the worst perioperative disruption of lung function. The presence of even 20% nitrogen seems to be helpful in reducing collapse of lung units (see **Table 1**).

PERIOPERATIVE HYPEROXIA

Why do anesthesiologists use so much oxygen? There are several ways in which this behavior may be justified, some of which are simply dogma.[10]

Table 1
Effect of inspired oxygen before induction of anesthesia on time taken for arterial saturation to reach 90% and the amount of pulmonary atelectasis measured as percentage of cross-sectional area of the lung in a single CT scan slice 10 mm above the right diaphragm

Fio_2 Before Induction	Time (s) to Sao_2 90% Mean (SD)	% Atelectasis Mean (SD)
0.6	213 (69)	0.3 (0.3)
0.8	303 (59)	1.3 (1.2)
1.0	411 (84)	5.6 (3.4)

Abbreviations: Fio_2, fraction of inspired oxygen; Sao_2, arterial oxygen saturation.
Data from Edmark L, Kostova-Aherdan K, Enlund M, et al. Optimal oxygen concentration during induction of general anesthesia. Anesthesiology 2003;98:28–33.

Anxiolysis for Anesthetists

Loss of the ability to deliver oxygen to a patient (the so-called cannot intubate cannot ventilate scenario) is the greatest concern for any anesthetist. This scenario is a rare event on induction of anesthesia: the likelihood of developing a major airway problem on induction of anesthesia is around 1:22,000[11] and needing to do an emergency cricothyroidotomy on induction is about 1:22,600.[12] However, the disastrous consequences for the patient, and potentially the clinician, mean that preoxygenation is thought by some to be mandatory.[13] Delivering 100% oxygen substantially extends the time to arterial desaturation in the event of loss of airway patency following induction (see **Table 1**). The simplest calculation of volume of oxygen in the FRC divided by estimated oxygen consumption reveals an oxygen supply lasting 1.5 minutes if breathing air versus 8 minutes with 100% oxygen. This calculation is an oversimplification, because not all the oxygen reserve can be used before dangerous hypoxemia occurs. Also, the shape of the hemoglobin dissociation curve means that, as alveolar Po_2 reduces, arterial oxygen saturation is maintained for some time before a sudden decrease. For more realistic modeling of arterial saturation following the onset of obstructive apnea, many factors need to be included, such as FRC (affected by obesity), cardiac output, oxygen consumption, the position of the hemoglobin dissociation curve, and shunt fraction.[14,15] Despite these multiple variables, both modeling and clinical studies show that if airway obstruction occurs in a patient breathing air, desaturation occurs in 1 min.[14,16] With preoxygenation this time is increased to 6 minutes.[17] This reassuring duration is substantially reduced in obese patients irrespective of the Fio_2 before induction,[16,17] but can be improved by induction in a 25° head-up position.[18]

These data provide compelling evidence that allowing patients to breathe air on induction of anesthesia is a high-risk strategy, but the data shown in **Table 1** indicate that using 100% oxygen is also potentially harmful. The debate about the wisdom of preoxygenation for all patients is not yet concluded.[10,13,14,19] The authors' opinion is that increased Fio_2 is necessary on induction, but that use of 100% oxygen should be reserved for patients at particularly high risk, and that whenever 100% has been deployed, a recruitment maneuver should follow as soon as feasible.

One-Lung Ventilation

The rapid absorption of oxygen from alveoli can be beneficial in some circumstances, such as when initiating 1-lung ventilation (OLV). In a study comparing ventilation with air, nitrous oxide, and 100% oxygen before commencing OLV, lung collapse was significantly delayed in the air group and fastest in the nitrous oxide group.[20] This strategy may be particularly useful when using bronchial blockers or in patients with profuse secretions in whom gas flow out through the airways and tube is limited. The same study showed that the increase in arterial Po_2 gained by use of 100% oxygen for OLV lasted only a few minutes.[20]

As a result of the frequent occurrence of hypoxemia during OLV, a high Fio_2 is commonly used, both for the ventilated lung and for apneic oxygenation of the nonventilated lung. Both lungs in thoracic surgery are at risk of acute lung injury. The ventilated, dependent lung has a low volume because of the normal changes associated with general anesthesia, exacerbated by the lateral position and open, nondependent chest cavity. As a result, this lung is at high risk of atelectrauma and the requirement to sustain gas exchange on its own means that artificial ventilation may require higher than normal inflation pressure or tidal volume. Both these factors result in the possibility of ventilator-associated lung injury. Improved management of OLV and recognition of the potential harmful effects of oxygen has led to a decline in the use of 100% oxygen. Current recommendations are that Fio_2 should initially be 80%, and then titrated to a target arterial saturation range of 92% to 94%.[21]

The nonventilated lung is particularly susceptible to oxygen toxicity. During surgery, the lung tissue is likely to be hypoxic with no gas in the alveoli and reduced pulmonary blood flow caused by surgical manipulation and hypoxic pulmonary vasoconstriction (HPV). On reexpansion of the lung, an ischemia-reperfusion injury will occur with extensive production of ROS. It is therefore advisable to use the lowest possible amount of oxygen at this stage.[21]

Carotid Endarterectomy

Acute cerebral ischemia can occur during carotid artery surgery, either from clamping of the artery to facilitate surgery or from emboli released because of manipulation and instrumentation of the artery. Recent trends toward earlier surgery for symptomatic carotid stenosis and for performing carotid endarterectomy (CEA) under regional anesthesia have increased the likelihood of acute neurologic events occurring in an awake patient in theater. Management of this situation must follow the Airway, Breathing, Circulation approach, and there is some evidence that increasing blood pressure to supranormal values is beneficial.[22] It has also been shown that breathing 100% oxygen under these circumstances can result in clinical improvements in the neurologic deficit as a result of increased cerebral oxygen saturation in the affected area.[23]

Surgical Site Infection

Perioperative hyperoxia, in the form of an Fio_2 of 80% during and for a few hours following anesthesia, is reported to reduce the incidence of surgical site infections (SSI) after colonic surgery[24,25] or appendicectomy.[26] It is claimed that the high Po_2 facilitates the production of ROS by phagocytes and enhances their bacterial killing abilities.[27] Other studies have failed to reproduce the findings, even in obese patients who are at high risk of SSI.[28] This observation probably relates to improving tissue blood flow by the use of epidural analgesia, more liberal administration of intravenous fluids, and maintenance of normothermia. A recent meta-analysis reached a similar conclusion (ie, that hyperoxia is only beneficial in studies in which patients have colorectal surgery without the benefit of neuraxial analgesia).[29]

Postoperative Nausea and Vomiting

Using hyperoxia to prevent postoperative nausea and vomiting (PONV) has followed a similar pattern to that of preventing SSIs. The first study reporting reduced PONV with hyperoxia involved the same patients as the SSI study and showed PONV incidence to be halved in the 80% compared with the 30% oxygen group.[25] A similar finding was reported by the same group for gynecologic surgery.[30] The purported mechanism was improved Po_2 in the intestinal mucosa. Again, further studies followed that failed to reproduce the initial findings, and a meta-analysis concluded there was no evidence to support the use of hyperoxia for preventing PONV.[31]

PHYSIOLOGIC EFFECTS OF HYPEROXIA

There are numerous ways in which hyperoxia may disturb normal physiology and produce adverse effects.

Respiratory Control

Minute ventilation increases in an exponential fashion with hypoxia, the increase being particularly steep at arterial saturations of less than about 80%,[1] which is a fundamental life-saving response to protect the body from damaging hypoxia, and plays a crucial protective role in sleep disordered breathing and in the perioperative period. For example, in a patient with respiratory depression from opioid overdose, increased Fio_2 is an effective therapy for preventing hypoxemia even with extremely low minute ventilation. Instead, hypercapnia may develop leading to confusion and sedation, and ultimately a vicious cycle is established with inadequate ventilation and hypercapnia despite having normal oxygen saturation. Respiratory rate should always be monitored, even with normal arterial saturation.

Another situation in which respiratory control is affected by oxygen is in some patients with chronic obstructive pulmonary disease (COPD). Long-term hypoxia as part of respiratory failure may be a significant part of the patient's drive to breath, and reversing the hypoxia, particularly acutely, can cause respiratory depression and hypercapnia.

V/Q Relationships

Oxygen therapy is beneficial in patients who have hypoxemia as a result of regions of lung with low V/Q ratios (<1). Increasing the amount of oxygen in the gas in these alveoli allows the blood in these regions to become fully oxygenated. This mechanism is the main way in which oxygen therapy benefits patients with lung disease. However, areas of lung with V/Q = 0 (ie, intrapulmonary shunt) are unaffected by increasing Fio_2 because no gas is reaching alveoli in these regions. For areas with very low V/Q ratio, increasing Fio_2 may still not fully oxygenate the blood because, by definition, blood flow through these lung regions is high. Thus, increasing Fio_2 up to approximately 40% is highly effective, but further increases have a progressively diminishing benefit.[1]

Impaired HPV

HPV is a protective reflex that diverts blood away from regions of inadequately ventilated lung and so improves overall V/Q matching. The reflex is biphasic, phase 1 occurring within a few seconds and a second, more intense, vasoconstriction occurring after approximately 45 minutes.[32] The response is patchy,[33] highly variable between individuals, and occurs in response to low Po_2 in either alveoli or pulmonary arterioles. Overall, HPV is an unpredictable reflex in an individual patient. Increasing Fio_2 impairs HPV in all lung regions where the alveolar Po_2 is increased, and so increases blood flow through these lung regions. This result may not matter, because the additional oxygen in the alveoli may be sufficient to fully oxygenate the blood, but, as discussed earlier, this strategy has a limited effect.

Vascular Effects

Hyperoxia has been known since 1962 to have a vasoconstrictor effect on systemic arteries.[34] The response occurs in arterioles of in-vitro preparations[35] and in regional calf blood flow in humans.[36] There is an increase in systemic vascular resistance in patients with cardiovascular disease, and this can have detrimental effects on cardiac function.[37] Increased production of ROS is causally implicated, the main evidence being that vitamin C infusion abolishes the response.[38] However, some workers have found no vasoconstrictor response in healthy subjects,[39] leading to the hypothesis that the vascular response to hyperoxia is more pronounced in subjects whose vascular systems are already undergoing oxidative stress (ie, their antioxidant defenses are less effective).

Of more concern is a similar response of coronary arteries to hyperoxia in patients with coronary artery disease. Coronary artery resistance was increased by 23% when breathing 100% oxygen, and the effect was also abolished by infusion of vitamin C.[40]

CLINICAL EFFECTS OF HYPEROXIA
COPD Exacerbations

As already described, some patients with COPD may depend on hypoxemia for their respiratory drive. In diseased lungs, abnormal V/Q ratios and potential dependence on HPV for effective oxygenation also make these patients susceptible to the adverse effects of hyperoxia. Despite this physiologic knowledge, and a belief that oxygen was detrimental for some patients with COPD during an exacerbation, no clinical trials addressed this problem for many years. The first to do so was reported in 2010.[41] A total of 214 patients with a presumed acute exacerbation of COPD were randomized to receive either titrated Fio_2 to maintain oxygen saturations between 88% and 92% or conventional high-flow oxygen by paramedics before arrival in hospital. This treatment was continued until arterial blood gases were taken in hospital. Results showed a statistically significantly higher mortality of 9% in the high-flow oxygen group compared with 2% in the titrated oxygen group. Patients in the titrated oxygen group were also less likely to have respiratory acidosis caused by acute hypercapnia.

Another study a year later also showed that the adverse effects of hyperoxia begin before the patient's admission to hospital.[42] This observational study of 250 patients examined whether the use of oxygen by ambulance personnel treating acute exacerbations of COPD were consistent with local and international guidelines. Despite international recommendations to control Fio_2, 72% of patients still received high-flow oxygen and, of the 10 patients who died (4% of the total), all had received high-flow oxygen. The investigators concluded that administration of high-flow oxygen in the ambulance was associated with an increased risk of death, assisted ventilation, or respiratory failure and that the risk of a poor outcome progressively increased as the oxygen flow rate increased. They also found that, when oxygen was analyzed as a continuous variable according to flow rate, there was a statistically significant association between increased flow rates and poor clinical outcomes. The strength of this association increased in the multivariate analysis, which adjusted for independent predictors of poor outcomes, suggesting that the association was not caused by more unwell patients receiving a higher concentration of oxygen therapy.

COPD remains a global challenge because of its high and increasing prevalence. As a result, in 1998, a group of scientists formed the Global Initiative for Chronic Obstructive Lung Disease (GOLD) to improve the diagnosis, management, and prevention of COPD. One of GOLD's major contributions to COPD care is the publication of guidelines. The latest of these[43] includes definitions of an acute exacerbation, and these still consider the use of oxygen to be a key component of hospital treatment, but recommend that supplemental oxygen should be titrated to improve the patient's hypoxemia with a target saturation of 88% to 92%. This recommendation is in keeping with the 2 studies described earlier.

As well as these global guidelines, other international societies publish their own recommendations. The American Thoracic Society and the European Respiratory Society in 2004 produced standards for the diagnosis and management of patients with COPD.[44] Their recommendations were based on the shape of the oxyhemoglobin dissociation curve, concluding that an arterial Po_2 greater than 60 mm Hg confers little added benefit and may increase the risk of carbon dioxide retention.[45,46] Thus, they recommended that the oxygen flow setting should be adjusted to achieve a Po_2 of slightly more than 60 mm Hg or oxygen saturations greater than 90% to prevent tissue hypoxia and preserve cellular oxygenation.

National Institute of Health and Clinical Excellence (NIHCE) guidance from the United Kingdom reiterates that the main aim of treating COPD exacerbation is to prevent life-threatening hypoxia.[47] They go on to say that, if oxygen is necessary, it should be given "to keep the saturations within the individualized target range, ie, according to local protocol." More detailed guidance in the United Kingdom is provided by the British Thoracic Society.[48] They recommend that, in patients with risk factors for hypercapnia (**Table 2**), before the availability of blood gases, Fio_2 should be 28%, which is designed to achieve oxygen saturations of 88% to 92%. The target oxygen saturation can then be adjusted to 94% to 98% if arterial Pco_2 is normal when blood gases are checked, or this range used in all patients who are not at risk of respiratory depression (see **Table 2**). In all other groups, the target saturation should be 94% to 98% from the outset.

Acute Coronary Syndrome Management

The use of oxygen for patients with myocardial ischemia has been recommended since 1900.[49] Evidence from animal experiments showed that oxygen decreased the amount of injury to the ischemic myocardium[50] and, from this work, oxygen was recommended for use in patients.

Subsequent evidence from human subjects suggested that oxygen therapy may not improve clinical outcome and may cause harm. A study in 1976 included 200 consecutive patients thought to have had a myocardial infarct (MI) in a randomized, double-blinded trial comparing oxygen (6 L min^{-1} via mask) versus air for the first 24 hours after admission to hospital.[51] The results showed that there was no significant difference in mortality, incidence of arrhythmias, or use of analgesics between the 2 groups. The investigators therefore concluded that there seems to be no evidence of benefit from routine administration of oxygen for an uncomplicated MI. Another small trial involving 50 patients with acute MI treated with thrombolysis randomized patients (not blinded) to receive either oxygen at 4 L min^{-1} or air via a face-mask.[52] Results were only available for 42 patients, and 1 patient who died within 24 hours was excluded from the trial. Because of this exclusion, the risk of death could not be analyzed but there was no statistical difference in the rate of ventricular tachycardia or use of opiates.

Table 2
Patients at risk of hypercapnic respiratory failure as defined by British Thoracic Society guidelines

Clinical Problem	Comments
Moderate or severe COPD	Particularly if history of: Previous episode of respiratory failure Receiving long-term oxygen therapy
Severe chest wall or spinal disease	eg, Kyphoscoliosis
Neuromuscular disease	eg, Guillain-Barré syndrome
Severe obesity	—
Cystic fibrosis exacerbation	Requires input from specialist center

Data from O'Driscoll BR, Howard LS, Davison AG. British Thoracic Society guideline for emergency oxygen use in adult patients. Thorax 2008;63(Suppl 6):vi1–68.

In 2009, a systematic review of studies investigating the effect of oxygen therapy in MI was performed with the intention of performing a meta-analysis.[53] Studies were excluded if oxygen was used for any other clinical indication (eg, heart failure), as were studies of hyperbaric oxygen or intracoronary oxygen infusion. The primary outcome measure was in-hospital mortality, with secondary outcomes being infarct size by enzyme levels, occurrence of ventricular arrhythmias, and opiate use. Only the 2 trials discussed earlier met these criteria and, because of the small number of available data, a meta-analysis was not possible. The investigators thus concluded that "there is an absence of evidence to support the routine prescription of high-flow oxygen therapy in patients with uncomplicated MI. A pessimistic view of the available evidence is that the use of supplementary oxygen may cause harm when routinely used in this situation."

These conclusions have now been adopted into guidelines. The most recent guideline from the American Heart Association[54] suggests that oxygen should be given in the initial assessment, but there is insufficient evidence to support its routine use in uncomplicated acute coronary syndromes. However, if patients are dyspneic, hypoxic, or there are signs of heart failure, oxygen should be titrated to a target saturation of greater than or equal to 94%. They also advise that, in uncomplicated cases, there is little justification for continuing the routine use of oxygen beyond 6 hours. European Society of Cardiology guidelines also recommend that oxygen at 2 to 4 L min^{-1} should only be administered to those who are breathless or who have any features of heart failure or shock.[55]

Stroke and Transient Ischemic Attack Management

Following cerebral ischemia secondary to a stroke or transient ischemic attack (TIA), it is important to maintain adequate tissue oxygenation. Evidence that hyperoxia is detrimental following cerebral ischemia first came from an animal study, in which gerbils breathing 100% oxygen for 3 to 6 hours after 15 minutes of cerebral ischemia had a 3-fold increase in 14-day mortality compared with those breathing air.[56] Evidence also exists in humans from a study published in 1999 that randomized 550 patients with acute stroke to receive either supplemental oxygen at 3 L min^{-1} for 24 hours or air.[57] One-year survival in the oxygen group was 68.8% compared with 72.9% in the room air group. Although this was not statistically significant ($P = .30$), the investigators hypothesized that oxygen supplementation to nonhypoxic patients with mild or moderate stroke may increase mortality and suggested that nonhypoxic patients with moderate or minor strokes should not routinely receive supplemental oxygen after hospital admission.

Stroke guidelines now suggest that a treatment goal should be to prevent hypoxia and potential worsening of the brain injury.[58] Therefore, in both the out-of-hospital and in-patient management of stroke patients, supplemental oxygen should only be given to hypoxemic patients (oxygen saturations <94%) or those with unknown oxygen saturation.

This advice on oxygen therapy for patients with stroke is at variance with the use of oxygen during CEA as described earlier, but the 2 situations are not comparable because the oxygen use in CEA is for a very short period immediately before the surgery restores much improved cerebral blood flow.

Cardiopulmonary Resuscitation

During cardiopulmonary resuscitation (CPR) 100% oxygen has traditionally been used to maximize oxygen delivery during a period of critically low cardiac output. However, there is some evidence that hyperoxia during CPR may be harmful. In the first animal experiment to show this problem, dogs were resuscitated in normoxic or hyperoxic conditions, or with hyperoxia accompanied by antioxidant treatment (tirilizad mesylate, a lipid peroxidation inhibitor).[59] Hyperoxic resuscitated animals had a significantly worse neurologic deficit at 12 and 24 hours compared with the normoxic and antioxidant pretreated animals. Another study using a canine model found a similarly poor neurologic outcome following resuscitation with 100% oxygen and also showed higher levels of oxidized brain lipids, indicating increased lipid peroxidation, which is thought to cause neurologic damage.[60]

Evidence from animal studies that hyperoxia during CPR is detrimental is therefore inconclusive. As a result, UK Resuscitation Council guidelines continue to recommend high-flow oxygen until return of spontaneous circulation is achieved.[61] The American Heart Association guidelines similarly acknowledge the controversy by stating that "the optimal inspired oxygen concentration during adult CPR has not been established in human or animal studies" and that "it is unknown whether 100% inspired oxygen is beneficial or whether titrated oxygen is better."[62] They thus recommend the empiric use of 100% inspired oxygen as soon as it becomes available during CPR to optimize arterial oxyhemoglobin content and so oxygen delivery.

Post–Cardiac Arrest Care

Following successful CPR, when return of spontaneous circulation (ROSC) occurs, monitoring of oxygen saturation is again possible. Treatment in this period is crucial for minimizing neurologic damage as blood returns to ischemic tissue, potentially causing reperfusion injury. Evidence of detrimental effects of hyperoxia at this time comes from both animal and human studies. In a study of dogs,[63] following 10 minutes of cardiac arrest, animals were randomized to 1 hour of ventilation with either 100% oxygen or a rapid lowering of the arterial oxygen saturations to 94% to 96% with pulse oximetry guidance. Neurologic deficit scores were then recorded (0 = normal, 100 = brain-dead) and were significantly higher (mean of 61) in the hyperoxic animals compared with the normoxic animals (mean of 43). The investigators concluded that reducing postarrest hyperoxia results in significant short-term neuroprotection.

Kuisma and colleagues[64] studied the effects of hyperoxia in 28 patients who had suffered an out-of-hospital ventricular fibrillation arrest. Once ROSC had occurred, patients were randomized by the intensive care unit (ICU) physician to receive either 30% or 100% oxygen and the levels of serum markers of neuronal injury measured. No differences were found between the 2 groups, showing that a lower FiO_2 was not harmful in terms of neuronal injury markers, but the investigators stated that the clinical significance of this finding was difficult to determine because of the small numbers of patients. A larger clinical trial collected data from project IMPACT (a database involving 131 adult ICUs in the United States) analyzing all nontraumatic cardiac arrests admitted to ICUs between 2001 and 2005.[65] Patients included had all received CPR within 24 hours of arrival to the ICU. A total of 6326 patients were included and were retrospectively divided into 3 groups based on their initial arterial PO_2: hyperoxic (>300 mm Hg), hypoxic (<60 mm Hg), and normoxic (cases not classified as either hyperoxic or hypoxic). Mortality was significantly higher in the hyperoxic group, with a mortality of 63% compared with 57% in the hypoxic group and 45% in the normoxia group. Hyperoxia treatment also lowered the likelihood of independent functional status at hospital discharge compared with normoxia. Multivariate analysis went on to show that, after controlling for a predefined set of confounding variables, exposure to hyperoxia was an independent predictor of in-hospital death.

Guidelines on treatment following successful CPR now follow the results of the Kuisma and colleagues[64] study. American Heart Association guidelines state that, once ROSC occurs and there is appropriate equipment available, Fio_2 should be titrated to maintain oxygen saturations greater than or equal to 94%.[66] In the United Kingdom, Resuscitation Council guidelines are similar, stating that, as soon as arterial oxygen saturations can be measured reliably by either blood gas analysis or pulse oximetry, oxygen should be titrated to maintain oxygen saturations of 94% to 98%.[61]

SUMMARY

There are many reasons why oxygen can have direct or indirect adverse effects, particularly at the high levels used under many perioperative situations. However, there is little evidence that this is a clinical problem in the perioperative period, mostly because the studies have not been done. Experience from physiology and clinical studies in many other areas of acute medicine suggests that clinicians may be causing problems for their patients by the indiscriminate use of oxygen. All clinicians have a responsibility to avoid harming their patients, and until more is known about oxygen's effects in the perioperative period, the advice emanating from other disciplines should be followed and oxygen only used to achieve acceptable saturation levels unless there is a convincing reason to use more.

REFERENCES

1. Lumb AB. Nunn's applied respiratory physiology. Edinburgh (United Kingdom): Elsevier; 2010.
2. Priestley J. Experiments and observations on different kinds of air. London: J Johnson; 1775. p. 101.
3. Salvemini D, Riley DP, Cuzzocrea S. SOD mimetics are coming of age. Nat Rev Drug Discov 2002;1:367–74.
4. Joyce CJ, Williams AB. Kinetics of absorption atelectasis during anaesthesia: a mathematical model. J Appl Physiol 1999;86:1116–25.
5. Rothen HU, Sporre B, Engberg G, et al. Prevention of atelectasis during general anaesthesia. Lancet 1996;345:1387–91.
6. Edmark L, Kostova-Aherdan K, Enlund M, et al. Optimal oxygen concentration during induction of general anesthesia. Anesthesiology 2003;98:28–33.
7. Benoit Z, Wicky S, Fischer JF, et al. The effect of increased FIO_2 before tracheal extubation on postoperative atelectasis. Anesth Analg 2002;95:1777–81.
8. Lumb AB, Greenhill SJ, Simpson MP, et al. Lung recruitment and positive airway pressure before extubation does not improve oxygenation in the post-anaesthesia care unit: a randomized clinical trial. Br J Anaesth 2010;104:643–7.
9. Akça O, Podolsky A, Eisenhuber E, et al. Comparable postoperative pulmonary atelectasis in patients given 30% or 80% oxygen during and 2 hours after colon resection. Anesthesiology 1999;91:991–8.
10. Gordon RJ. Anesthesia dogmas and shibboleths: barriers to patient safety? Anesth Analg 2012;114:694–9.
11. Cook TM, Woodall N, Frerk C. Major complications of airway management in the UK: results of the Fourth National Audit Project of the Royal College of Anaesthetists and the difficult airway society. Part 1: anaesthesia. Br J Anaesth 2011;106: 617–31.
12. Kheterpal S, Han R, Tremper KK, et al. Incidence and predictors of difficult and impossible mask ventilation. Anesthesiology 2006;105:885–91.
13. Bell MDD. Routine pre-oxygenation – a new 'minimum standard' of care? Anaesthesia 2004;59:943–5.

14. Farmery AD. Simulating hypoxia and modelling the airway. Anaesthesia 2011; 66(Suppl 2):11–8.
15. Farmery AD, Roe PG. A model to describe the rate of oxyhaemoglobin desaturation during apnoea. Anaesthesia 1996;76:284–91.
16. Drummond GB, Park GR. Arterial oxygen saturation before intubation of the trachea. An assessment of oxygenation techniques. Br J Anaesth 1984;56:987–92.
17. Jense HG, Dubin SA, Silverstein PI, et al. Effect of obesity on safe duration of apnoea in anesthetized humans. Anesth Analg 1991;72:89–93.
18. Dixon BJ, Dixon JB, Carden JR, et al. Preoxygenation is more effective in the 25° head-up position than in the supine position in severely obese patients. Anesthesiology 2005;102:1110–5.
19. Lumb AB. Just a little oxygen to breathe as you go off to sleep...is it always a good idea? Br J Anaesth 2007;99:769–71.
20. Ko R, McRae K, Darling G, et al. The use of air in the inspired gas mixture during two-lung ventilation delays lung collapse during one-lung ventilation. Anesth Analg 2009;108:1092–6.
21. Slinger PD, editor. Principles and practice of anesthesia for thoracic surgery. London: Springer; 2011. p. 89.
22. Stoneham MD, Thompson JP. Arterial pressure management and carotid endarterectomy. Br J Anaesth 2009;102:442–52.
23. Stoneham MD, Lodi O, de Beer TCD, et al. Increased oxygen administration improves cerebral oxygenation in patients undergoing awake carotid surgery. Anesth Analg 2008;107:1670–5.
24. Belda FJ, Aguilera L, de la Asuncion JG, et al. Supplemental perioperative oxygen and the risk of surgical wound infection. JAMA 2005;294:2035–42.
25. Greif R, Laciny S, Rapf B, et al. Supplemental oxygen reduces the incidence of postoperative nausea and vomiting. Anesthesiology 1999;91:1246–52.
26. Bickel A, Gurevits M, Vamos R, et al. Perioperative hyperoxygenation and wound site infection following surgery for acute appendicitis: a randomized, prospective, controlled trial. Arch Surg 2011;146:464–70.
27. Govinda R, Kasuya Y, Bala E, et al. Early postoperative subcutaneous tissue oxygen predicts surgical site infection. Anesth Analg 2010;111:946–52.
28. Staehr AK, Meyhoff CS, Rasmussen LS, PROXI Trial Group. Inspiratory oxygen fraction and postoperative complications in obese patients: a subgroup analysis of the PROXI Trial. Anesthesiology 2011;114:1313–9.
29. Togioka B, Galvagno S, Sumida S, et al. The role of perioperative high inspired oxygen therapy in reducing surgical site infection: a meta-analysis. Anesth Analg 2012;114:334–42.
30. Goll V, Akça O, Greif R, et al. Ondansetron is no more effective than supplemental intraoperative oxygen for prevention of postoperative nausea and vomiting. Anesth Analg 2001;92:112–7.
31. Orhan-Sungur M, Kranke P, Sessler D, et al. Does supplemental oxygen reduce postoperative nausea and vomiting? a meta-analysis of randomized controlled trials. Anesth Analg 2008;106:1733–8.
32. Talbot NP, Balanos GM, Dorrington KL, et al. Two temporal components within the human pulmonary vascular response to ~2 h of isocapnic hypoxia. J Appl Physiol 2005;98:1125–39.
33. Dehnert C, Risse F, Ley S, et al. Magnetic resonance imaging of uneven pulmonary perfusion in hypoxia in humans. Am J Respir Crit Care Med 2006;174:1132–8.
34. Eggers GW, Paley HW, Leonard JJ, et al. Hemodynamic responses to oxygen breathing in man. J Appl Physiol 1962;17:75–9.

35. Messina EJ, Sun D, Koller A, et al. Increases in oxygen tension evoke arteriolar constriction by inhibiting endothelial prostaglandin synthesis. Microvasc Res 1994;48:151–60.

36. Rousseau A, Bak Z, Janerot-Sjöberg B, et al. Acute hyperoxaemia-induced effects on regional blood flow, oxygen consumption and central circulation in man. Acta Physiol Scand 2005;183:231–40.

37. Park JH, Balmain S, Berry C, et al. Potentially detrimental cardiovascular effects of oxygen in patients with chronic left ventricular systolic dysfunction. Heart 2010; 96:533–8.

38. Mak S, Egri Z, Tanna G, et al. Vitamin C prevents hyperoxia-mediated vasoconstriction and impairment of endothelium-dependent vasodilation. Am J Physiol Heart Circ Physiol 2002;282:H2414–21.

39. Thomson AJ, Drummond GB, Waring WS, et al. Effects of short-term isocapnic hyperoxia and hypoxia on cardiovascular function. J Appl Physiol 2006;101: 809–16.

40. McNulty PH, Robertson BJ, Tulli MA, et al. Effect of hyperoxia and vitamin C on coronary blood flow in patients with ischemic heart disease. J Appl Physiol 2007;102:2040–5.

41. Austin MA, Wills KE, Blizzard L, et al. Effect of high-flow oxygen on mortality in chronic obstructive pulmonary disease patients in pre-hospital setting: randomized controlled trial. BMJ 2010;341:c5462.

42. Wijesinghe M, Perrin K, Healy B, et al. Pre-hospital oxygen therapy in acute exacerbations of chronic obstructive pulmonary disease. Intern Med J 2011;41: 618–22.

43. Global strategy for the diagnosis, management and prevention of COPD, Global Initiative for Chronic Obstructive Lung Disease (GOLD) 2011. Available at: http://www.goldcopd.org/. Accessed July 11, 2012.

44. Celli BR, MacNee W, Agusti A, et al. Standards for the diagnosis and treatment of patients with COPD: a summary of the ATS/ERS position paper. Eur Respir J 2004;23:932–46.

45. Aubier M, Murciano D, Milic-Emili M, et al. Effects of the administration of oxygen therapy on ventilation and blood gases in patients with chronic obstructive pulmonary disease during acute respiratory failure. Am Rev Respir Dis 1980; 122:747–54.

46. Dumont CP, Tiep BL. Using a reservoir nasal cannula in acute care. Crit Care Nurse 2002;22:41–6.

47. National Institute for Health and Clinical Excellence. Chronic obstructive pulmonary disease. Management of chronic obstructive pulmonary disease in adults in primary and secondary care: NICE clinical guideline 101. London: NICE; 2010.

48. O'Driscoll BR, Howard LS, Davison AG. British Thoracic Society guideline for emergency oxygen use in adult patients. Thorax 2008;63(Suppl 6):vi1–68.

49. Steele C. Severe angina pectoris relieved by oxygen inhalations. BMJ 1900;2: 1568.

50. Kelly RF, Hursey TL, Parrillo JE, et al. Effect of 100% oxygen administration on infarct size and left ventricular function in a canine model of myocardial infarction and reperfusion. Am Heart J 1995;130:957–65.

51. Rawles JM, Kenmure AC. Controlled trial of oxygen in uncomplicated myocardial infarction. BMJ 1976;1(6018):1121–3.

52. Wilson AT, Channer KS. Hypoxaemia and supplemental oxygen therapy in the first 24 hours after myocardial infarction: the role of pulse oximetry. J R Coll Physicians Lond 1997;31:657–61.

53. Wijesinghe M, Perrin K, Ranchord A, et al. Routine use of oxygen in the treatment of myocardial infarction: systematic review. Heart 2009;95:198–202.

54. O'Connor RE, Brady W, Brooks SC, et al. Acute coronary syndromes: 2010 American Heart Association Guidelines for cardiopulmonary resuscitation and emergency cardiovascular care. Circulation 2010;122:S787–817.

55. The task force on the management of ST-segment elevation acute myocardial infarction of the European Society of Cardiology. Management of acute myocardial infarction in patients presenting with persistent ST-segment elevation. Eur Heart J 2008;29:2909–45.

56. Mickel HS, Vaishnav YN, Kempski O, et al. Breathing 100% oxygen after global brain ischaemia in Mongolian gerbils results in increased lipid peroxidase and increased mortality. Stroke 1987;18:426–30.

57. Rønning OM, Guldvog B. Should stroke victims routinely receive supplemental oxygen? A quasi-randomized controlled trial. Stroke 1999;30:2033–7.

58. Jauch EC, Cucchiara B, Adeoye O, et al. Adult Stroke: 2010 American Heart Association Guidelines for cardiopulmonary resuscitation and emergency cardiovascular care. Circulation 2010;122:S818–28.

59. Zwemer CF, Whitesall SE, D'Alecy LG, et al. Cardiopulmonary resuscitation with 100% oxygen exacerbates neurological dysfunction following nine minutes of normothermic cardiac arrest in dogs. Resuscitation 1994;27:159–70.

60. Liu Y, Rosenthal RE, Haywood Y, et al. Normoxic ventilation after cardiac arrest reduces oxidation of brain lipids and improves neurological outcome. Stroke 1998;29:1679–86.

61. Resuscitation Council (UK). The resuscitation guidelines 2010. London: Resuscitation Council; 2010.

62. Neumer RW, Otto CW, Link MS, et al. Adult advanced cardiovascular life support: 2010 American Heart Association Guidelines for cardiopulmonary resuscitation and emergency cardiovascular care. Circulation 2010;122:S729–67.

63. Balan IS, Fiskum G, Hazelton J, et al. Oximetry-guided reoxygenation improves neurological outcome after experimental cardiac arrest. Stroke 2006;37:3008–13.

64. Kuisma M, Boyd J, Voipio V, et al. Comparison of 30 and the 100% inspired oxygen concentrations during early post-resuscitation period: a randomised controlled pilot study. Resuscitation 2006;69:199–206.

65. Kilgannon JH, Jones AE, Shapiro NI, et al. Association between arterial hyperoxia following resuscitation from cardiac arrest and in-hospital mortality. JAMA 2010;303:2165–71.

66. Peberdy MA, Callaway CW, Neumar RW, et al. Post-cardiac arrest care: 2010 American Heart Association Guidelines for cardiopulmonary resuscitation and emergency cardiovascular care. Circulation 2010;122:S768–86.

Perioperative Lung Protection Strategies in Cardiothoracic Anesthesia: Are They Useful?

Peter Slinger, MD, FRCPC[a],*, Bruce Kilpatrick, MBBCh, FCA(SA)[b]

KEYWORDS

- Thoracic anesthesia • Cardiac anesthesia • Thoracic surgery • Cardiac surgery
- Acute lung injury

KEY POINTS

- The use of nonphysiologic ventilation strategies, such as large tidal volumes (VTs) and high airway pressures, can contribute to acute lung injury (ALI) in normal lungs.
- These strategies are particularly harmful in patients who undergo a subclinical lung injury during surgery, which involves a large pulmonary resection or cardiopulmonary bypass (CPB).
- Acute perioperative lung injury is associated with injury of remote organ systems.
- Volatile anesthetics may have some lung-protective effect in this context.

INTRODUCTION

Patients are at risk for several types of lung injury in the perioperative period. These injuries include atelectasis, pneumonia, pneumothorax, bronchopleural fistula, ALI, and acute respiratory distress syndrome (ARDS). Anesthetic management can cause, exacerbate, or ameliorate most of these injuries. Lung-protective ventilation strategies using more physiologic VTs and appropriate levels of positive end-expiratory pressure (PEEP) can decrease the extent of this injury.[1] This review discusses the effects of mechanical ventilation and its role in ventilator-induced lung injury (VILI) with specific reference to cardiothoracic anesthesia. The specific clinical scenarios of chronic obstructive pulmonary disease (COPD), one-lung ventilation (OLV), CPB, and transfusion-related acute lung injury (TRALI) are examined. Newer

No disclosures.

[a] Department of Anesthesia, Toronto General Hospital, University of Toronto, 3 Eaton North, 200 Elizabeth Street, Toronto, Ontario M5G 2C4, Canada; [b] Department of Anaesthesia, Royal Inland Hospital, 311 Columbia Street, Kamloops, British Columbia V2C 2T1, Canada
* Corresponding author.
E-mail address: peter.slinger@uhn.on.ca

work addressing lung protection strategies, including the relevance of fluid restriction and inflammation, is discussed. The terms, *ARDS* and *ALI*, are used in this review. A recent recommendation by the ARDS Definition Task Force has suggested that the term, *ALI*, be replaced with *mild ARDS* (200 mm Hg < Pao_2/fraction of inspired oxygen [Fio_2] ≤ 300 mm Hg) and that ARDS be subdivided into *moderate ARDS* (100 mm Hg < Pao_2/Fio_2 ≤ 200 mm Hg) and *severe ARDS* (Pao_2/Fio_2 ≤100 mm Hg).[2]

MECHANICAL VENTILATION

Historically, anesthesiologists have been taught to ventilate patients in the perioperative period with large V_{TS}. Volumes as high as 15 mL/kg^{-1} ideal body weight (IBW) have been suggested to avoid intraoperative atelectasis.[3] This far exceeds the normal spontaneous V_{TS} (6 mL/kg^{-1}) common to most mammals. Recent studies have identified the use of large V_{TS} as a major risk factor for development of lung injury in mechanically ventilated patients without ALI. Gajic and colleagues[4] reported that 25% of patients with normal lungs ventilated in an ICU setting for 2 days or longer developed ALI or ARDS. The main risk factors for ALI were use of large V_{TS}, restrictive lung disease, and blood product transfusion. A prospective study from the same group found that V_{TS} greater than 700 mL and peak airway pressures greater than 30 cm H_2O were independently associated with the development of ARDS.[5] An intraoperative study of patients having esophageal surgery compared the use of V_{TS} of 9 mL/kg^{-1} without PEEP during two-lung ventilation and OLV versus 9 mL/kg^{-1} during two-lung ventilation and 5 mL/kg^{-1} during OLV with PEEP 5 cm H_2O throughout.[6] The investigators found significantly lower serum makers of inflammation (cytokines, interleukin [IL]-1β, IL-6, and IL-8) in the lower V_T plus PEEP group. The study did not find any major difference in postoperative outcome between the 2 groups; however, it was not powered to do this. The study demonstrated better oxygenation in the lower V_T group during and immediately after OLV but not after 18 hours. In a study of conventional versus protective ventilation in critically ill patients without lung injury, de Oliveira and colleagues[7] randomized patients to ventilation with either 10 mL/kg^{-1} to 12 mL/kg^{-1} or 6 mL/kg^{-1} to 8 mL/kg^{-1} predicted body weight. In both groups, PEEP of 5 was applied and the Fio_2 titrated to keep oxygen saturation as measured by pulse oximetry (SpO_2) greater than 90%. At 12 hours' postventilation, inflammatory markers in bronchoalveolar lavage fluid (tumor necrosis factor [TNF]-α and IL-8) were significantly higher in the larger V_T group. Choi and colleagues[8] compared 12 mL/kg^{-1} without PEEP with 6 mL/kg^{-1} with 10-cm PEEP and showed procoagulant changes in lavage fluid of the larger V_T group after 5 hours of mechanical ventilation. A recent randomized controlled trial in 150 critically ill patients without ALI compared V_{TS} of 10 mL/kg^{-1} versus 6 mL/kg^{-1} predicted body weight.[9] The conventional V_{TS} were associated with a sustained plasma increase in inflammatory cytokines.

Of importance is recent work suggesting that noninjurious or so-called protective ventilatory settings can induce lung injury in previously healthy lungs. An animal study using an elegant murine 1-hit VILI model showed that even least injurious lung settings induced biochemical and histologic changes consistent with lung injury.[10] Work with rodents undergoing mechanical ventilation showed significant gene expression (including genes involved in immunity and inflammation) after only 90 minutes of protective ventilation.[11] Whether this has an impact on clinical outcome is unknown at this time.

ALI is the most common cause of postoperative respiratory failure and is associated with a markedly decreased postoperative survival.[12] A prospective case-controlled study by Fernandez-Perez and colleagues of intraoperative ventilator settings and ALI after elective surgery in more than 4000 patients showed a 3% incidence of ALI in high-risk elective surgeries. Compared with controls, patients with ALI had significantly lower postoperative survival and increased length of hospital stay. In this study, intraoperative peak airway pressure, but not V_T, PEEP, or Fio_2, was associated with ALI.

VENTILATOR-INDUCED LUNG INJURY

The phenomenon of VILI is well recognized and can be particularly significant in surgical specialties that require large transfusions, CPB, and associated lung ischemia-reperfusion injury. The deleterious effects of mechanical ventilation may be mediated by localized inflammation and the systemic release of inflammatory cytokines (biotrauma). Mechanical stretch from cyclical alveolar opening and closing sets up an inflammatory response in the alveolar epithelial cells and the vascular endothelial cells. Hyperinflation causes nuclear translocation of nuclear factor κB (a key regulator of the expression of multiple genes involved in inflammatory response) and upregulation of other proinflammatory cytokines. Polymorphonuclear leukocyte recruitment and activation seem to be key components of the mechanical stretch-induced inflammatory response. The balance between apoptosis and necrosis is unfavorably altered by both ischemia-reperfusion and mechanical stretch.[13]

Biotrauma not only aggravates ongoing lung injury but also has important systemic consequences due to the spillover of these inflammatory mediators into the systemic circulation, inducing remote organ dysfunction. A study of novel mechanisms of remote organ injury resulting from VILI showed that mechanical ventilation can lead to epithelial cell apoptosis in the kidney and the small intestine with accompanying biochemical evidence of organ dysfunction.[14] In mice undergoing injurious mechanical ventilation, alveolar stretch induced adhesion molecules not only in the lung but also in the liver and kidney. In addition, cytokine and chemokine expression in pulmonary, hepatic, and renal tissue after mechanical ventilation was accompanied by enhanced recruitment of granulocytes to these organs.[15] These studies go some way to explain the remote organ dysfunction seen with ALI/ARDS and the role optimizing ventilatory strategies play in ameliorating this.

This leads to the question, Are the lung-protective strategies in ARDS[16] applicable to the perioperative environment, specifically in patients with healthy lungs? A recent article addressing this question highlights the lack of randomized controlled trials of best intraoperative V_T, PEEP, and use of intraoperative lung recruitment.[17] Although outcome studies are lacking, based on what is known about the effects of mechanical ventilation, it seems reasonable to aim toward protective ventilatory strategies in perioperative practice.

PERIOPERATIVE SURGICAL ENVIRONMENT FACTORS

There are many factors in the surgical environment that can contribute to lung injury; the most obvious is the surgical approach. Site of operation is an important predictor of pulmonary complications, with upper abdominal and thoracic incisions the most important (any surgery approaching the diaphragm).[18] A decrease in respiratory complications has been documented if major cavity procedures can be done with minimally invasive versus open techniques.[19,20] Atelectasis occurs frequently after open surgical procedures and in up to 90% of patients undergoing general anesthesia.[21] It is a pathologic state that can contribute to or exacerbate lung injury. Thus, anesthesiologists must be aware of techniques to avoid or treat it.[22] Although open to debate, retrospective[23,24] and prospective[25] studies have shown that appropriate thoracic epidural analgesia reduces the incidence of respiratory complications (atelectasis, pneumonia, and respiratory failure) after major abdominal and thoracic surgery. The benefits of epidural analgesia seem to be in direct proportion to the severity of the patients underlying lung disease. Patients with COPD seem to derive the most benefit from epidural analgesia.[26] Reviews comparing paravertebral block versus epidural analgesia in patients undergoing thoracic surgery showed equivalent analgesia efficacy but a better side-effect profile and lower complication rate with paravertebral block.[27,28] Aggressive physiotherapy with CPAP in the postoperative period in patients after major abdominal surgery who develop early desaturation leads to lower rates of major respiratory complications.[29]

PATIENTS WITH CHRONIC OBSTRUCTIVE PULMONARY DISEASE

COPD patients are at an increased risk of lung injury in the perioperative period.[30] Key concepts that are relevant to anesthetic management and lung protection include the following.

Dynamic Hyperinflation

Emphysema is almost exclusively an expiratory disease; thus, during positive pressure ventilation, moving gas into the patient's lungs is easy, but due to intrinsic PEEP (auto-PEEP) it is difficult to move the gas out. This intrathoracic gas trapping is called dynamic hyperinflation.[31] Severe hyperinflation impairs cardiac venous return, leading to hypotension and, in severe cases, cardiac arrest.[32] This can occur during seemingly low levels of positive airway pressure, such as during bag-mask ventilation at induction. Anaesthesiologists must be alert to this entity. Thorough preoxygenation before induction, use of small Vts, slow respiratory rates with long expiratory times, tolerance of hypercarbia, and hemodynamic support are key to avoiding hemodynamic collapse in these patients. Acute decompensation during positive pressure ventilation of these patients presents a challenging differential diagnosis between dynamic hyperinflation and tension pneumothorax. Unilateral breath sounds, tracheal shift, and presence of bullae favor pneumothorax and the need for urgent decompression. In the absence of these clues it is reasonable to disconnect patients from the ventilatory circuit and allow passive exhalation to the atmosphere. If there is no improvement with a period of apnea, then treatment measures for pneumothorax should be instituted.

Bullae

Many patients with moderate to severe COPD develop cystic air spaces in the lung parenchyma. These bullae tend to be asymptomatic unless occupying more than 50% of the hemithorax, in which case patients have features of restrictive and obstructive lung disease. These bullae are localized areas of loss of structural support tissue in the lung with elastic recoil of surrounding parenchyma. The pressure in the bullae is the mean pressure in the surrounding alveoli averaged over the respiratory cycle. This means that during normal spontaneous ventilation, the intrabulla pressure is slightly negative in comparison to the surrounding parenchyma.[33] When positive pressure ventilation is instituted, the pressure in the bulla becomes positive in relation to adjacent structures and the bulla expand, with the attendant risk of rupture, tension pneumothorax, and bronchopleural fistula. Positive pressure ventilation can be safely used if airway pressures are kept low and there is the expertise and equipment available for chest drain insertion and lung isolation.

Respiratory Drive

Determining a COPD patient's $Paco_2$ baseline with preoperative arterial blood gases is important in setting goals for intraventilation and postventilation. It is not possible to predict which patients are CO_2 retainers based on severity of their disease.[34] CO_2 retention seems primarily related not to an alteration of respiratory control mechanisms but an inability to maintain the increased work of respiration.[35] In patients receiving supplemental oxygenation, the $Paco_2$ rises primarily not because of decreased minute ventilation[36] but mostly due to a relative increase in alveolar dead space by the redistribution of lung perfusion and the Haldane effect.[37] Postoperative hypoxemia must be prevented, however, with supplemental oxygen; the attendant rise in $Paco_2$ must be anticipated and monitored. Arterial blood gases and level of consciousness are the best monitors, with $Paco_2$ levels of greater than 90 mm Hg having sedative and anesthetic effects.

Nocturnal Hypoxemia

COPD patients desaturate more frequently and more severely than normal patients during sleep. This is related to the rapid shallow pattern of ventilation, which occurs in all patients during rapid eye movement sleep.[38] This tendency to desaturate combined with the postoperative fall in functional residual capacity (FRC) and opioid analgesia places these patients at high risk for severe hypoxemia postoperatively during sleep.

Right Ventricular Dysfunction

Right ventricular dysfunction occurs in up to 50% of COPD patients.[39] A dysfunctional right ventricle is intolerant of the sudden changes in afterload associated with switching from spontaneous to controlled ventilation or large pulmonary resections.[40]

PERIOPERATIVE THERAPY OF COPD TO DECREASE LUNG INJURY
Physiotherapy

It has been shown that patients with COPD benefit from an intensive program of preoperative chest physiotherapy, with fewer postoperative pulmonary complications.[41] It is possible to improve exercise tolerance in even the most severe COPD patients.[42] Little improvement is seen before 1 month, however. Those COPD patients with excessive sputum production benefit the most from chest physiotherapy.[43]

Smoking Cessation

A preoperative smoking cessation program can significantly decrease the incidence of respiratory complications (after 4–8 weeks' abstinence), wound complications (4 weeks' abstinence), and intraoperative myocardial ischemia (48 hours' abstinence).[44]

Bronchodilation

Bronchoconstriction is assessed by history, physical examination, and evaluation of pulmonary function response to bronchodilators. Patients should receive maximal bronchodilator therapy as guided by their symptoms. It is not clear if corticosteroids are as beneficial as they are in asthma, but in patients poorly controlled on sympathomimetic and anticholinergic bronchodilators, a trial of corticosteroids may be beneficial.[45] Pulmonary function tests are not useful screening tools for all patients but are valuable in assessing flow rates in symptomatic patients, to confirm the diagnosis and to assess adequacy of treatment. The incidence of intraoperative, life-threatening bronchospasm has become low.[46] The principles for managing patients with reactive airways remains the same, however: preoperative optimizing of bronchodilation, avoiding instrumentation of the airway, airway instrumentation at an adequate depth of anesthesia, use of bronchodilating anaesthetics (volatiles, propofol, and ketamine), and appropriate warming and humidification of gases.[47] In patients with bronchial hyperactivity on regular bronchodilator therapy, postintubation wheezing can be significantly reduced by a 5-day preoperative course of corticosteroids.[48]

ONE-LUNG VENTILATION

Anesthesiologists are faced with a heterogeneous patient group, in terms of underlying pathology and surgical procedure, requiring OLV. Both a patient's pathology and the surgical procedure can predispose to or cause ALI. ALI after pulmonary resection has been described since the beginning of OLV use for thoracic surgery. The most publicized report is a compilation of 10 pneumonectomy cases published in 1984,[49] which focused on the role of intravenous overhydration as a cause of postpneumonectomy pulmonary edema. Much work has subsequently followed and understanding of risk factors, mechanisms of injury, and management strategies for what is now termed *post-thoracotomy ALI* has greatly advanced.

A thorough retrospective study of 806 pneumonectomies found a 2.5% incidence of postpneumonectomy pulmonary edema with 100% mortality in affected patients.[50] There was no difference in perioperative fluid balance between postpneumonectomy ALI cases (24-h fluid balance 10 mL/kg^{-1}) and matched pneumonectomy controls (13 mL/kg^{-1}). The investigators used rigorous fluid restriction compared with other studies,[51] suggesting that limiting intraoperative fluids might decrease but not eliminate ALI. Postpneumonectomy ALI has been shown to have a bimodal distribution of onset.[52] Late cases presented 3 days to 10 days postoperatively and were secondary to obvious causes, such as bronchopneumonia, aspiration, and so forth. Early, or primary, ALI presented on postoperative days 0 to 3. Four factors were independent significant predictors of primary ALI: high intraoperative ventilation pressures, excessive intravenous volume replacement, pneumonectomy, and preoperative alcohol abuse. Studying specifically ventilation pressures, Licker and colleagues[52] used a barotrauma index taking into account both duration of OLV and increased inspiratory pressure. This index represented the strongest risk factor for ALI (approximately 3-fold increase risk if PIP $\geq$25 cm H_2O vs PIP = 15 cm H_2O).

The known facts about ALI after lung surgery include an incidence after pneumonectomy of 2% to 4%, greater frequency after right versus left pneumonectomy, symptom onset 1 to 3 days postsurgery, high associated mortality (25%–50%), and resistance to standard therapies. Although ALI occurs after lesser resections (eg, lobectomy), it has a much lower mortality rate. In 8 of 9 cases in which patients developed unilateral ALI after lobectomy, the ALI was in the nonoperated (ie, the ventilated) lung.[53] Although there is an association between postoperative ALI and fluid overload, the noncardiogenic nature of the pulmonary edema (low/normal pulmonary occlusion pressures) and the protein-rich edema fluid is more in keeping with an ARDS-type picture, with endothelial damage playing a key role.

Postoperative increases in lung permeability of the nonoperated lung have been demonstrated after pneumonectomy but not lobectomy.[54] This capillary-leak injury may be due to an inflammatory cascade affecting even the nonoperative lung that is triggered by lung resection and is proportional to the amount of lung resected.[55,56] Free oxygen radical generation in lung cancer patients is related to the duration of OLV.[57] Although there is no single mechanism to explain ALI post–lung resection, a unifying hypothesis is that there is a spectrum of ALI that occurs during all lung resections; the more extensive the resection, the more likely there is postoperative injury.

End-inspiratory lung volume is a key factor in VILI.[58] Many patients, especially emphysema patients, develop auto-PEEP with OLV[59]; thus, inspiration begins at a lung volume above FRC. Using large V_{TS} (10–12 mL/kg^{-1}) during OLV in such patients produces end-inspiratory levels that may cause or contribute to ALI. The effects of PEEP during OLV are variable and dependant on the lung mechanics of the individual patient, with initial studies suggesting that it leads to a deterioration of arterial oxygenation.[60] Most COPD patients develop auto-PEEP during OLV, leading to hyperinflation and increased shunt (**Fig 1**A).[61] Patients with normal lung parenchyma or those with restrictive lung diseases, however, tend to fall below their FRC at end expiration during OLV and benefit from external PEEP (see **Fig. 1**B). Avoiding atelectasis is important to avoid setting up a preinflammatory state leading to injury in both

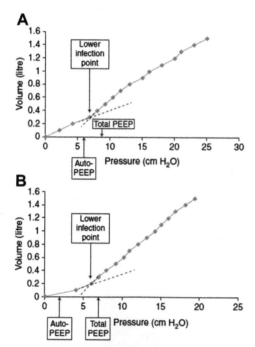

Fig. 1. (A) An inspiratory compliance curve (lung volume vs airway pressure) during OLV as the lung is slowly inflated in 100-mL increments in a patient with COPD. The lower inflection point of the curve (thought to represent FRC) is at 7 cm H_2O. During OLV, this patient developed intrinsic PEEP (also called auto-PEEP) of 6 cm H_2O (measured as the end-expiratory airway occlusion plateau pressure). The addition of 5 cm H_2O PEEP from the ventilator raised the total PEEP in the circuit to 9 cm H_2O, thus raising the end-expiratory lung volume above FRC, which in turn raised pulmonary vascular resistance in the ventilated lung and caused a deterioration of oxygenation. (B) The inspiratory compliance curve during OLV from a patient with normal pulmonary function. The lower inflection point is at 6 cm H_2O. During OLV, this patient developed intrinsic PEEP of 2 cm H_2O. The addition of 5 cm H_2O via the ventilator raised the end-expiratory lung volume closer to FRC, thus decreasing pulmonary vascular resistance in the ventilated lung, and oxygenation improved. ([B] Data from Slinger PD, Kruger M, McRae K, et al. Relation of the static compliance curve and positive end-expiratory pressure to oxygenation during one-lung ventilation. Anesthesiology 2001;95:1096–102.)

the atelectatic lung and the ventilated portions of the lung, which become hyperinflated.[62] Just as in two-lung ventilation, high Vтs in OLV cause or contribute to ALI.

In an animal model of thoracic surgery, sheep ventilated with a Vт of 6 mL/kg and 5 cm H_2O for 4 hours after a pneumonectomy had no increase in extravascular lung water compared with the lungs of control animals. Sheep ventilated with 12 mL/kg without PEEP for 4 hours, however, had a greater than 100% increase in extravascular lung water (**Fig. 2**).[63]

Large pulmonary resections (pneumonectomy or bilobectomy) should be considered associated with some degree of ALI: 42% of pneumonectomy patients who had been ventilated with peak airway pressures greater than 40 cm H_2O had ALI diagnosed radiographically.[64] A retrospective study found that postpneumonectomy respiratory failure was associated with the use of higher intraoperative Vтs (8.3 mL/kg^{-1} vs 6.7 mL/kg^{-1} in those patients who did not develop respiratory failure).[65] Thus, current understanding of post-thoracotomy ALI supports applying the management strategies of least injurious lung ventilation: Fio$_2$ as low as acceptable, variable Vтs,[66] beginning inspiration at FRC, and avoiding atelectasis with frequent recruitment maneuvers.[67] An observational study in patients undergoing lung cancer surgery by Licker and workers[68] seems to confirm this. Using a protective lung ventilation strategy (Vт <8 mL/kg^{-1} predicted body weight, pressure control ventilation, peak inspiratory pressure <35 cm H_2O, external PEEP 4 cm to 10 cm, and frequent recruitment maneuvers) in a protocol group (558 patients) versus conventional ventilation in a historical group (533 patients), they showed a decreased incidence of ALI (3.7%–0.9%, $P<.01$) and atelectasis (8.8–5.0, $P = .018$), fewer ICU admissions (9.4% vs 2.5% $P<.001$), and shorter hospital stay (**Fig. 3**).

Mild hypercapnia (Paco$_2$ 45–60 mm Hg) resulting from smaller minute volumes should be accepted during OLV. Permissive hypercapnia has become a central component of protective ventilatory strategies and humans have been shown remarkably tolerant of even extreme hypercapnia.[69] Minimizing pulmonary capillary pressure by avoiding overhydration for patients undergoing pneumonectomy is reasonable

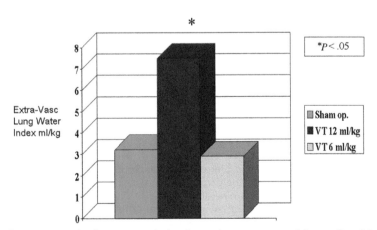

Fig. 2. The extravascular lung water index from the nonoperated lung after 4 hours of ventilation during thoracic surgery in 3 groups of sheep. The Sham op. group had a thoracotomy and two-lung ventilation with 12 mL/kg. The Vт 12 mL/kg group was ventilated with a large Vт during OLV. The Vт 6 mL/kg group received a smaller Vт with 5 cm H_2O PEEP. (*Data from* Kuzkov V, Subarov E, Kirov M. Extravascular lung water after pneumonectomy and one-lung ventilation in sheep. Crit Care Med 2007;35:1550–9.)

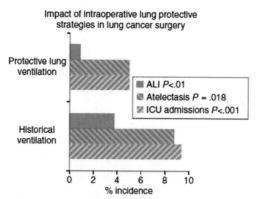

Impact of intraoperative lung protective
strategies in lung cancer surgery

Protective lung
ventilation

- ALI $P<.01$
- Atelectasis $P = .018$
- ICU admissions $P<.001$

Historical
ventilation

% incidence

Fig. 3. The impact of intraoperative ventilation strategies in lung cancer surgery. Comparison of a historical large VT ventilation group with a smaller VT lung-protective ventilation group. Patients undergoing OLV with smaller VTs had fewer complications, such as postoperative ALI, atelectasis, and admission to the ICU. (*Data from* Licker M, Diaper J, Villiger Y, et al. Impact of intraoperative lung-protective interventions in patients undergoing lung cancer surgery. Crit Care 2009;13:R41.)

while acknowledging that not all perioperative increases in pulmonary artery pressures are due to intravascular volume replacement. Finally it must be appreciated that not all hyperinflation of the residual lung occurs in the operating room. The use of a balanced chest drainage system after pneumonectomy to keep the mediastinum in neutral position and avoid hyperinflation of the residual lung has been suggested as contributing to a decrease in ALI in some centers.[70]

ROLE OF VOLATILE ANESTHETIC AGENTS IN LUNG PROTECTION

Volatile agents have immunomodulatory effects. Much work has been done, especially in the cardiac setting, on the role of volatiles in ischemia-reperfusion injury and in preconditioning and postconditioning. Recent studies in models of ALI, during OLV and in cases of lung ischemia-reperfusion,[71] suggest that volatiles may act as preconditioning and postconditioning agents inducing lung protection by inhibition of the expression of proinflammatory mediators. Isoflurane pretreatment in an endotoxin-mediated animal model of lung injury exerted protective effects, as evidenced by reduction of polymorphonulcear recruitment and microvascular protein leakage.[72] Postconditioning with sevoflurane attenuated lung damage and preserved lung function in an in vivo rat ALI model.[73] In a prospective study, patients undergoing thoracic surgery with OLV were randomized to either propofol or sevoflurane anesthesia.[74] Studying inflammatory markers in the nonventilated lung, they showed an attenuated inflammatory reaction in the sevoflurane group. Significantly, the sevoflurane group had an improved outcome and significantly lower overall number of adverse events. A study comparing OLV (VT 10 mL/kg^{-1}) with desflurane versus propofol anesthesia addressed the inflammatory response in the ventilated lung.[75] The inflammatory markers IL-8, IL-10, polymorphonuclear granulocyte elastase, and TNF-α were significantly lower in the desflurane group (**Fig. 4**). Sevoflurane has been shown to be lung protective in a pig lung autotransplant model.[76] Although much work remains to be done, this exciting work points toward a role for volatiles in attenuating the proinflammatory response in the lungs to a host of insults, whether this is preinsult, during insult, or postinsult.

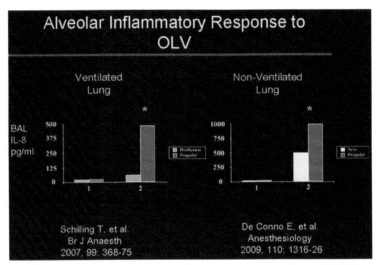

Fig. 4. The inflammatory response, measured as bronchoalveolar lavage (BAL) levels of the cytokine IL-8 before and after OLV with either intravenous or volatile anesthesia. (*Left*) Patients were anesthetized with propofol or desflurane and cytokines were significantly (* = P<.01) increased in the ventilated lung after OLV. (*Right*) Patients received either pro-pofol or sevoflurane and cytokines were higher in the nonventilated lung after OLV in the propofol group. ([*Left*] *Data from* Schilling T, Kozian A, Kretzschmar M, et al. Effects of pro-pofol and desflurane anesthesia on the alveolar inflammatory response to one-lung venti-lation. Br J Anaesth 2007;99:368–75; and [*Right*] De Conno E, Steurer MP, Wittlinger M, et al. Anesthetic-induced improvement of the inflammatory response to one-lung ventila-tion. Anesthesiology 2009;110:1316–26.)

TRANSFUSION-RELATED LUNG INJURY

TRALI jury has emerged as a leading cause of transfusion morbidity and mortality,[77] with a disproportionate number of cases occurring in the perioperative period.[78] Anesthesiologists are routinely involved in transfusion decisions and are well placed to both decrease the incidence and the morbidity and mortality of TRALI. Diagnostic criteria consist of hypoxia or bilateral pulmonary edema during or within 6 hours of transfusion, in the absence of circulatory overload.[79] Difficulties lie in patients with other risk factors for ALI, pre-existing ALI, and subtle cases that may not meet current criteria. The exact pathogenesis is not completely understood.[80,81] Although an immune antibody-mediated mechanism is implicated in most cases (with good supporting experimental and clinical evidence), supporting antibodies are not found in 15% or more of cases. Thus, an antibody-independent 2-hit model has been proposed. The antibody-mediated mechanism is primarily due to leuko-agglutinating antibodies in the transfused plasma binding to recipient neutrophils. These antibody-bound neutrophils are activated and sequestered in the lung, where complement activation and release of neutrophil bioactive products results in endo-thelial damage, capillary leak, and ALI. Antibodies implicated are human leukocyte antigens class I and II and neutrophil-specific antibodies. The 2-hit model postulates that an initial insult (eg, sepsis, surgery, or injurious ventilation) to the vascular endo-thelium results in endothelial activation, resulting in release of cytokines and adhesion molecules. Neutrophils are then attracted, primed, and sequestered in the lung in this proinflammatory milieu.

A second hit, by transfusion of biologic response modifiers, activates these sequestered neutrophils, resulting in the release of oxidases and proteases, resulting in endothelial damage and subsequent ALI. Both mechanisms have their limitations, but it seems reasonable that both may occur and that TRALI may represent the final common pathway of neutrophil activation and subsequent endothelial injury. True incidence is unknown because standardized definitions have only recently been developed, but a prospective cohort study of an ICU population using current definitions reported an 8% incidence (901 patients), with plasma and platelets having the highest associations.[82] Mortality is estimated at 5% to 10%. All blood products have been implicated, with most of the products containing more than 50 mL of plasma. Data suggest plasma and apheresis platelets have the highest component risk.[83]

Strategies for prevention for transfusion services include, but are not limited to, fresher products, washed components, and plasma primarily or exclusively from male donors (avoiding multiparous women). More importantly for anesthesiologists is the appropriate use of blood products and to avoid further lung injury. Transfusion triggers must be individualized for each patient and aimed at clinical endpoints. Prothrombin complex concentrates may have a future role in place of FFP and there is a sound theoretic basis for this.

CARDIOPULMONARY BYPASS

Pulmonary dysfunction post-CPB is a well described but poorly understood phenomenon.[84] Although the incidence of ARDS post-CPB is low (<2%) the mortality associ­ated with it is high (>50%).[85] Although the systemic inflammatory response syndrome initiated by CPB plays a major role, the pulmonary insult is multifactorial and not all related to the bypass itself. Extra-CPB factors are general anesthesia, sternotomy, and breaching of the pleura. Intra-CPB factors include but are not limited to hypothermia, blood contact with artificial surfaces, ischemia-reperfusion injury, administration of blood products, and ventilatory arrest.

It must be emphasized that intraoperative, lung-protective strategies, although having good theoretic basis, have shown inconsistent results in the literature in terms of improving pulmonary outcome. Protective postoperative ventilatory strategies of these at-risk lungs is key. A randomized controlled trial compared the use of nonprotective high V_{TS} (10–12 mL/kg^{-1}) versus lung-protective low V_{TS} (8 mL/kg^{-1}) plus PEEP (10 cm H_2O) in patients ventilated for 6 hours after CPB for coronary artery bypass surgery.[86] Serum and bronchiolar lavage levels of the inflammatory cytokines IL-6 and IL-8 were significantly increased at 6 hours only in the nonprotective ventilation group (**Fig. 5**). A study of more than 3000 patients after cardiac surgery found that patients ventilated with V_{TS} less than 10 mL/kg^{-1} IBW had significantly lower rates of failure of any organ system (11%) versus patients ventilated with 10 mL/kg^{-1} to 12 mL/kg^{-1} (15%) and greater than 12 mL/kg^{-1} (18%).[87]

ULTRAPROTECTIVE LUNG VENTILATION

On the continuum of lung-protective ventilation in ALI/ARDS is the concept of ultraprotective ventilation. This concept uses extracorporeal lung assist, such as the pumpless Novalung interventional lung-assist (iLA) device and near static ventilation. An iLA is a membrane ventilator that allows O_2 and CO_2 gas exchange via simple diffusion.[88] The membranes are biocompatible and provide a nonthrombogenic surface. It is designed to work without a mechanical pump in an arteriovenous configuration (**Fig. 6**), thus requiring an adequate mean arterial pressure to drive flow. Flow rates are typically 1 L/min^{-1} to 2 L/min^{-1}, or approximately 15% of cardiac output. CO_2

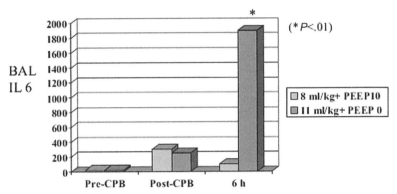

Fig. 5. Bronchoalveolar lavage (BAL) levels of cytokines, such as IL-6, were significantly increased 6 hours after CPB for cardiac surgery in patient's ventilated post-CPB with larger V$_T$s and lower levels of PEEP. (*Data from* Zupancich E, Paparella D, Turani F, et al. Mechanical ventilation affects inflammatory mediators in patients undergoing cardiopulmonary bypass for cardiac surgery: a randomized clinical trial. J Thorac Cardiovasc Surg 2005;130:378–83.)

clearance is controlled by varying the oxygen flow rate. Oxygenation may be variable and may not be sufficient in severe hypoxic disorders. Compared with conventional extracorporeal membrane oxygenation, the Novalung is a portable device. Anticoagulation requirements are much reduced with an activated partial thromboplastin time (aPPT) target of 55 seconds. Bleeding complications and blood product requirements are significantly less.

ARDS Clinical Network (ARDSnet) and animal data demonstrate that lower V$_T$s (3 mL/kg^{-1}) compared with 6 mL/kg^{-1} to 12 mL/kg^{-1} significantly reduces endothelial and epithelial injury.[89,90] In other words, "protective" V$_T$s can still induce VILI. Clearance of CO_2 and oxygenation, however, become an issue at these lower minute volumes. An iLA allows for this marked reduction in MV and the simultaneous correction of PaCO_2 and pH. An animal model of postpneumonectomy ARDS using the Novalung and V$_T$s of 2.2 mL/kg^{-1} and respiratory rate of 6 showed significantly better outcomes compared with conventional lung-protective strategies.[91] Several case reports in humans in a variety of clinical scenarios have been encouraging.[92–95] V$_T$s

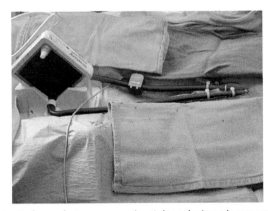

Fig. 6. An iLA device is shown between a patient's legs during placement with femoral cannulations. The patient's body is to the right, out of the photograph. The inflow to the device is from the femoral artery (near cannula) and the return is via the femoral vein (far cannula).

less than or equal to 3 mL/kg^{-1}, low inspiratory plateau pressure, high PEEP, and low respiratory rates are all possible with an iLA, causing less VILI and subsequent remote secondary organ failure. It is possible that a plateau has been achieved in therapy for ALI with different modifications of mechanical ventilation and the next advances in therapy will be in the form of extracorporeal devices, such as iLA and extracorporeal membrane oxygenation.

FLUIDS, INFLAMMATION, AND THE GLYCOCALYX

A retrospective cohort study of specifically intraoperative risk factors for ARDS in critically ill patients found that for patients receiving fluid resuscitation greater than 20 mL/kg^{-1}/h^{-1} the odds of developing ARDS were 3 times greater than if less than 10 mL/kg^{-1}/h^{-1} was given (odds ratio 3.1; 95% CI, 1.0–9.9; P = .05).[96] V$_T$/ IBW^{-1} (mL/kg^{-1}) and number of blood products were not associated with ARDS in this study. The majority of patients were ventilated with a V$_T$/IBW^{-1} of 8 mL/kg^{-1} to 10 mL/kg^{-1} and an intraoperative PEEP of 0. It has long been a concern that excess amounts of intravenous fluids predispose patients to develop ALI.

It is a conflicting concern for anesthesiologists, however, that fluid restriction in thoracic surgery may contribute to postoperative renal dysfunction, which previously was reported associated with a high (19%) mortality rate.[97] In a recent review of greater than 100 pneumonectomies at the authors' institution, acute kidney injury (AKI), as defined by the renal injury, failure, loss, end-stage kidney disease (RIFLE) classification,[98] occurred in 22% of patients (**Table 1**).[99] There was no association, however, of AKI with fluid balance and no increased 30-day mortality in the AKI patients. AKI was associated with preoperative hypertension and complex surgical procedures, such as extrapleural pneumonectomy. A similar retrospective study of all pulmonary resection patients found that AKI, as defined by the Acute Kidney Injury Network criteria, which occurred in 67 of 1129 (6%) patients, was not associated with a statistically significant increase in mortality versus non-AKI patients (3% vs 1%).[100]

Fluid requirements vary widely between patients and procedures and ultimately represent the sum of preoperative deficits, maintenance requirements, and ongoing losses. Fluid management for major esophageal surgery is particularly challenging. Preoperative fluid deficits in patients with severe esophageal disease may be substantial, although they have not been well defined.[101] Fluid requirements in patients undergoing esophageal procedures may be complicated by patients possibly being hypovolemic after long preoperative fasts, particularly if esophageal obstruction or dysphagia limits fluid intake. Perioperative losses occur via several mechanisms,

Table 1 Renal injury in pneumonectomy patients		
	RIFLE −ve (n = 83)	**RIFLE +ve (n = 24)**
Intraoperative fluids (mL/h)	562	632
24-h fluid balance (mL)	2361	3922
Respiratory failure	6%	21% (P = .03)
Atrial fibrillation	17%	38% (P = .03)
30-d mortality	5%	4%

Mean values for fluid balances, 2004–2008.
   Abbreviations: RIFLE, renal risk, injury, and failure score; −ve, negative; +ve, positive.
   Data from Reimer C, McRae K, Seitz D, et al. Perioperative acute kidney injury in pneumonectomy: a retrospective cohort study. Can J Anaesth 2010:A802743.

including urinary, gastrointestinal, and evaporative losses; bleeding; and interstitial fluid shifting. This shift of fluid from the vascular compartment into the interstitial space accompanies surgical trauma and is likely to reflect vascular injury and loss of endothelial integrity. So-called third-space losses describe fluid loss into noninterstitial extracellular spaces, which are not in equilibrium with the vascular compartment and thus considered a nonfunctional extracellular fluid compartment. It is possible, however, that the third space does not exist and was described as a result of measurement errors in early studies of the fluid compartments in the body.[102]

One of the factors complicating fluid management for esophageal resection is that thoracic epidural analgesia has been shown to improve outcome for these patients[103] but its use tends to contribute to hypotension. Hypotension is well known to contribute to ischemia of the gut anastomosis[104] and treatment with excessive fluids likely exacerbates the problem.[105] Many surgeons are concerned about the effects of vasopressors on the anastomotic gut blood flow.[106] Several recent animal studies suggest, however, that treatment of intraoperative hypotension with norepinephrine does not cause any reduction of gut blood flow.[107,108]

An ideal fluid regimen for major surgeries, including esophageal surgery, is individualized and optimizes cardiac output and oxygen delivery while avoiding excessive fluid administration. There is some evidence that fluid therapies that are designed to achieve individualized and specific flow-related hemodynamic endpoints, such as stroke volume, cardiac output, or measures of fluid responsiveness, such as stroke volume variation (collectively referred to as goal-directed fluid therapy), may provide a superior alternative to fixed regimens or those based on static measures of cardiac filling, such as central venous pressure, which does not predict fluid responsiveness or correlate with circulating blood volume after transthoracic esophagectomy.[109,110]

In addition to the potential importance of the amount and timing of fluid administration, there is some clinical evidence that the choice of fluid type may be important in affecting clinical outcomes.[111] Intravascular colloid retention during treatment of hypovolemia may approach 90% versus 40% when administered during normovolemia.[102]

The relationship of hydrostatic and oncotic pressure for determining fluid flux across a semipermeable membrane was described in a classic equation developed in 1896 by Starling[112]:

$$J_v = K_f([P_c - P_i] - \sigma[\pi_c - \pi_i])$$

where

- J_v is the net fluid movement between compartments
- K_f is the proportionality constant
- $P_c–P_i$ is the balance of capillary and interstitial hydrostatic pressures
- σ is the reflection coefficient
- $\pi_c–\pi_i$ is the difference between capillary and interstitial oncotic pressures

Several clinical observations, such as the relative resistance of the intact organism to develop edema and the inability of therapy with hyperoncotic agents to draw fluid from the pulmonary interstitium into the vascular compartment, are not explained by the Starling formula (**Fig. 7**).[113] This discrepancy is now attributed to the glycocalyx, a microcilial layer that lines the endothelium and acts as a molecular sieve (**Fig. 8**). This layer tends to increase the oncotic pressure on the inner surface of the endothelium and decrease leukocyte and platelet adhesion to the endothelium. The glycocalyx deteriorates during ischemia-reperfusion injury and in the presence of a wide variety of inflammatory mediators, such as cytokines, and probably contributes to the increased

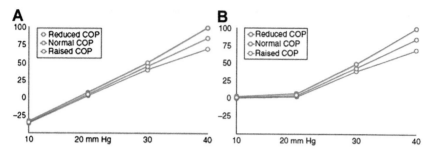

Fig. 7. (*A*) The rate of fluid flux (vertical axis) across the endothelium plotted against the hydrostatic pressure difference between the capillary lumen and the interstitial space (horizontal axis) as predicted by the classic Starling equation for various levels of plasma colloid oncotic pressure (COP). Capillary pressure is normally approximately 20 mm Hg and the Starling equation predicts that at lower capillary pressures fluid is absorbed from the interstitium into the intravascular space. (*B*) The observed pattern of fluid exchange across semipermeable membranes. The loss of fluid to the interstitial compartment can be reduced to essentially zero at capillary pressures below 20 mm Hg. There is never a net absorption of fluid into the intravascular space, however. Excess fluid must be removed from the interstitial space by lymphatics. ([*B*] *Reproduced from* Woodcock TE, Woodcock TM. Revised Starling equation and the glycocalyx model of transvascular fluid exchange. Br J Anaesth 2012;108:384–94; with permission.)

vascular permeability seen in these situations. Also, the glycocalyx deteriorates in the presence of atrial natriuretic peptide and may explain the increase in plasma protein filtration seen with colloid boluses. Protecting the glycocalyx may be among anesthesiologists' most important duties perioperatively.

OTHER THERAPIES FOR LUNG PROTECTION

Beyond those already discussed, there are several therapies that may play a future role in lung protection. Permissive hypercapnia's place in protective ventilation has

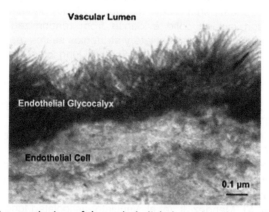

Fig. 8. Electron microscopic view of the endothelial glycocalyx. The glycocalyx is a carpet of microtubules that lines the inner surface of the endothelium and in combination with the capillary pores is responsible for the normal observed patterns of fluid fluxes across semipermeable membranes. (*Reproduced from* Chappell D, Jacob M, Hofmann-Kiefer K, et al. A rational approach to perioperative fluid management. Anesthesiology 2008;109 [4]:723–40; with permission.)

been alluded to previously but, as found in the original ARDsnet data, may be protective in the presence of higher V_T.[114] Hypercapnic acidosis is protective in a variety of models of ALI. Beneficial effects include attenuation of lung neutrophil recruitment, pulmonary and systemic cytokine concentrations, cell apoptosis, and free radical injury.[115] Inhaled hydrogen sulfide shows beneficial effects in a model of VILI via the inhibition of inflammatory and apoptotic responses, independent of its effects on body temperature.[116] Inhaled aerosolized activated protein C in a sheep model of ALI demonstrated improved oxygenation as well as lung aeration (as assessed by CT scan)[117] β-Adrenergic agonists have potential benefits by increasing the rate of alveolar fluid clearance by increasing cellular cyclic adenosine monophosphate, and they have anti-inflammatory properties.[118] A randomized controlled trial in 40 patients with ALI showed a decrease in extravascular lung water and plateau airway pressure with intravenous salbutamol, although it showed no differences in outcome.[119] Randomized placebo-controlled trials of several different therapies, including surfactant, prone positioning, inhaled nitric oxide, and anti-inflammatories, have not shown significant clinical benefits in patients with established ALI.[120] Although it is unreasonable to expect a single therapy (or magic bullet) that will prevent ALI, the exciting research does hold promise in both furthering understanding and management of injured or at risk lungs.

SUMMARY

To summarize what is known: (1) nonphysiologic ventilation in healthy lungs induces ALI; (2) protective lung ventilation in patients with ALI/ARDS improves outcome; (3) protective lung ventilation in noninjured lungs and in the absence of a primary pulmonary insult may initiate subclinical VILI (as evidenced by inflammatory markers); (4) VILI has important implications for organs remote to the lungs and is associated with significant morbidity and mortality; (5) volatile anesthetics may have a lung-protective effect; and (5) the glycocalyx is vital to normal intact endothelial function.

Anesthesiologists manage a heterogeneous group of patients in the perioperative period; from patients with healthy lungs, to patients with at risk lungs, to patients with established ALI/ARDS. More patients are at risk for ALI during surgery than previously thought. Appropriate perioperative management may prevent or ameliorate this lung injury. Although lacking solid evidence from randomized controlled trials, applying intraoperative protective ventilatory strategies seems reasonable based on current understanding of mechanical ventilation and lung injury.

REFERENCES

1. Kilpatrick B, Slinger P. Lung protective strategies in anaesthesia. Br J Anaesth 2010;105(S1):i108–16.
2. ARDS Definition Task Force. Acute respiratory distress syndrome: the Berlin definition. JAMA May 21, 2012 [Online].
3. Bendixen HH, Hedley-White J, Laver MB. Impaired oxygenation in surgical patients during general anesthesia with controlled ventilation: a concept of atelectasis. N Engl J Med 1963;96:156–66.
4. Gajic O, Dara SI, Mendez JL, et al. Ventilator-associated lung injury in patients with out acute lung injury at the onset of mechanical ventilation. Crit Care Med 2004;32:1817–24.
5. Gajic O, Frutos-Vivar F, Esteban A, et al. Ventilator settings as a risk factor for acute respiratory distress syndrome in mechanically ventilated patients. Intensive Care Med 2005;31:922–6.

6. Michelet P, D'Journo XB, Roch A, et al. Protective ventilation influences systemic inflammation after esophagectomy: a randomized controlled study. Anesthesiology 2006;105:911–9.

7. de Oliveira RP, Hetzel MP, Silva M, et al. Mechanical ventilation with high tidal volume induces inflammation in patients without lung disease. Crit Care 2010; 14:R39.

8. Choi G, Wolthuis EK, Bresser P, et al. Mechanical ventilation with lower tidal volumes and positive end-expiratory pressure prevents alveolar coagulation in patients without lung injury. Anesthesiology 2006;105:689–95.

9. Determann R, Royakkers A, Wolthuis EK, et al. Ventilation with lower tidal volumes as compared with conventional tidal volumes for patients without acute lung injury: a preventive randomized controlled trial. Crit Care 2010;14:R1.

10. Wolthuis EK, Vlaar AP, Choi G, et al. Mechanical ventilation using non-injurious ventilation settings causes lung injury in the absence of pre-existing lung injury in healthy mice. Crit Care 2009;13:R1.

11. Ng CS, Wan S, Ho AM, et al. Gene expression changes with a "non-injurious" ventilation strategy. Crit Care 2009;13:403.

12. Fernandez-Perez ER, Sprung J, Alessa B, et al. Intraoperative ventilator settings and acute lung injury after elective surgery: a nested case control study. Thorax 2009;64:121–7.

13. Lionetti V, Recchia FA, Ranieri VM. Overview of ventilator-induced lung injury mechanisms. Curr Opin Crit Care 2005;11:82–6.

14. Imai Y, Parodo J, Kajikawa O, et al. Injurious mechanical ventilation and end-organ epithelial cell apoptosis and organ dysfunction in an experimental model of acute respiratory distress syndrome. JAMA 2003;280:2104–12.

15. Hegeman MA, Henmus MP, Heijnen CJ, et al. Ventilator-induced endothelial activation and inflammation in the lung and distal organs. Crit Care 2009;13: R182.

16. The Acute Respiratory Distress Syndrome Network. Ventilation with lower tidal volumes as compared with traditional tidal volumes for acute lung injury and the acute respiratory distress syndrome. N Engl J Med 2000;342:1301–8.

17. Beck-Schimmer B, Schimmer RC. Perioperative tidal volume and intraoperative open lung strategy in healthy lungs: where are we going? Best Pract Res Clin Anaesthesiol 2010;24:199–210.

18. Smetana GW. Postoperative pulmonary complications: an update on risk assessment and reduction. Cleve Clin J Med 2009;76:S60–5.

19. Weller WE, Rosati C. Comparing outcomes of laparoscopic versus open bariatric surgery. Ann Surg 2008;248:10–5.

20. Ramivohan SM, Kaman L, Jindal R, et al. Postoperative pulmonary function in laparoscopic versus open cholecystectomy: prospective, comparative study. Indian J Gastroenterol 2005;24:6–8.

21. Duggan M, Kavanagh B. Pulmonary atelectasis: a pathogenic perioperative entity. Anesthesiology 2005;102:834–54.

22. Tusman G, Bohm SH, Suarez-Shipman F. Alveolar recruitment improves ventilatory efficiency of the lungs during anesthesia. Can J Anaesth 2004;51:723–7.

23. Ballantyne JC, Carr DB, de Ferranti S. The comparative effects of postoperative analgesic therapies on pulmonary outcome: cumulative meta-analysis of randomized, controlled trials. Anesth Analg 1998;86:598–612.

24. Liu SS, Wu CL. Effect of postoperative analgesia on major postoperative complications: a systematic update of the evidence. Anesth Analg 2007;3: 689–702.

25. Rigg J, Jamrozik K, Myles P, et al. Epidural anaesthesia and analgesia and outcome after major surgery: a randomized trial. Lancet 2002;359:1276–82.
26. Licker MJ, Widikker I, Robert J, et al. Operative mortality and respiratory complications after lung resection for cancer: impact of chronic obstructive pulmonary disease and time trends. Ann Thorac Surg 2006;81:1830–8.
27. Scarci M, Joshi A, Attia R. In patients undergoing thoracic surgery is paravertebral block as effective as epidural analgesia for pain management. Interact Cardiovasc Thorac Surg 2010;10:92–6.
28. Davies RG, Myles PS, Graham JM. A comparison of the analgesic efficacy and side effects of paravertebral vs. epidural blockade for thoracotomy—a systematic review and meta-analysis of randomized trials. Br J Anaesth 2006;96:418–26.
29. Squadrone V, Coha M, Cerutti E, et al. Continuous positive airway pressure for the treatment of postoperative hypoxemia: a randomized controlled trial. JAMA 2005;293:589–95.
30. Edrich T, Sadovnikoff N. Anesthesia for patients with severe chronic obstructive pulmonary disease. Curr Opin Anaesthesiol 2010;23:18–24.
31. Myles PE, Madder H, Morgan EB. Intraoperative cardiac arrest after unrecognized dynamic hyperinflation. Br J Anaesth 1995;74:340–1.
32. Ben-David B, Stonebaker VC, Hersham R, et al. Survival after failed intraoperative resuscitation: a case of "Lazarus syndrome". Anesth Analg 2001;92:690–1.
33. Morgan MD, Edwards CW, Morris J, et al. Origin and behavior of emphysematous bullae. Thorax 1989;44:533–6.
34. Parot S, Saunier C, Gauthier H, et al. Breathing pattern and hypercapnia in patients with obstructive pulmonary disease. Am Rev Respir Dis 1980;121:985–91.
35. Levetown M. Oxygen-induced hypercapnia in chronic obstructive pulmonary disease: what's the problem? Crit Care Med 2002;30:258–9.
36. Aubier M, Murciano D, Milic-Emili J, et al. Effects of the administration of O_2 on ventilation and blood gases in patients with chronic obstructive pulmonary disease during acute respiratory failure. Am Rev Respir Dis 1980;122:747–54.
37. Hanson CW III, Marshall BE, Frasch HF, et al. Causes of hypercarbia in patients with chronic obstructive pulmonary disease. Crit Care Med 1996;24:23–8.
38. Douglas NJ, Flenley DC. Breathing during sleep in patients with obstructive lung disease. Am Rev Respir Dis 1990;141:1055–70.
39. Klinger JR, Hill NS. Right ventricular dysfunction in chronic obstructive pulmonary disease. Chest 1991;99:715–23.
40. Schulman DS, Mathony RA. The right ventricle in pulmonary disease. Cardiol Clin 1992;10:111–35.
41. Warner DO. Preventing postoperative pulmonary complications. Anesthesiology 2000;92:1467–72.
42. Niederman MS, Clemente P, Fein AM, et al. Benefits of a multidisciplinary pulmonary rehabilitation program. Chest 1991;99:798–801.
43. Selsby D, Jones JG. Some physiological and clinical aspects of chest physiotherapy. Br J Anaesth 1990;64:621–6.
44. Warner DO. Helping surgical patients quit smoking: why, when and how. Anesth Analg 2005;101:481–7.
45. Nisar M, Eoris JE, Pearson MG, et al. Acute broncho-dilator trials in chronic obstructive pulmonary disease. Am Rev Respir Dis 1992;146:555–9.
46. Bishop M, Cheny F. Anesthesia for patients with asthma: low risk but not no risk. Anesthesiology 1996;85:455–6.

47. Hurford W. The bronchospastic patient. Int Anesthesiol Clin 2000;38:77–90.
48. Silvanus MT, Groeben H, Peters J. Corticosteriods and inhaled salbutamol in patients with reversible airway obstruction markedly decrease the incidence of bronchospasm after tracheal intubation. Anesthesiology 2004;100:1052–7.
49. Zeldin RA, Normadin D, Landtwing BS, et al. Postpneumonectomy pulmonary edema. J Thorac Cardiovasc Surg 1984;87:359–65.
50. Turnage WS, Lunn JL. Postpneumonectomy pulmonary edema. A retrospective analysis of associated variables. Chest 1993;103:1646–50.
51. Waller DA, Gebitekin C, Saundres NR, et al. Noncardiogenic pulmonary edema complicating lung resection. Ann Thorac Surg 1993;55:140–3.
52. Licker M, de Perrot M, Spiliopoulos A, et al. Risk factors for acute lung injury after thoracic surgery for lung cancer. Anesth Analg 2003;97:1558–65.
53. Padley SP, Jordan SJ, Goldstraw P, et al. Asymmetric ARDS following pulmonary resection: CT findings initial observations. Radiology 2002;223:468–73.
54. Waller DA, Keavey P, Woodfine L, et al. Pulmonary endothelial permeability changes after major resection. Ann Thorac Surg 1996;61:1435–40.
55. Williams EA, Quinlan GJ, Goldstraw P, et al. Postoperative lung injury and oxidative damage in patients undergoing pulmonary resection. Eur Respir J 1998;11: 1028–34.
56. Tayama K, Takamori S, Mitsuoka M, et al. Natriuretic peptides after pulmonary resection. Ann Thorac Surg 2002;73:1582–6.
57. Misthos P, Katsaragakis S, Milingos N, et al. Postresectional pulmonary oxidative stress in lung cancer patients. The role of one-lung ventilation. Eur J Cardiothorac Surg 2005;27:370–83.
58. Dreyfuss D, Soler P, Basset G, et al. High inflation pressure pulmonary edema. Respective effects of high airway pressure, high tidal volume, and positive endexpiratory pressure. Am Rev Respir Dis 1988;137:1159–64.
59. Slinger P, Hickey DR. The interaction between applied PEEP and Auto-PEEP during One-Lung Ventilation. J Cardiothorac Vasc Anesth 1998;12:133–6.
60. Capan LM, Turndorf H, Patel C, et al. Optimization of arterial oxygenation during one-lung anesthesia. Anesth Analg 1980;59:847–51.
61. Slinger PD, Kruger M, McRae K, et al. Relation of the static compliance curve and positive end-expiratory pressure to oxygenation during one-lung ventilation. Anesthesiology 2001;95:1096–102.
62. Muders T, Wrigge H. New insights into experimental evidence on atelectasis and causes of lung injury. Best Pract Res Clin Anaesthesiol 2010;24:171–82.
63. Kuzkov V, Subarov E, Kirov M. Extravascular lung water after pneumonectomy and one-lung ventilation in sheep. Crit Care Med 2007;35:1550–9.
64. van der Werff YD, van der Houwen HK, Heijmans PJ, et al. Postpneumonectomy pulmonary edema. A retrospective analysis of incidence and possible risk factors. Chest 1997;111:1278–84.
65. Fernández-Pérez ER, Keegan MT, Brown DR, et al. Intraoperative tidal volume as a risk factor for respiratory failure after pneumonectomy. Anesthesiology 2006;105:14–8.
66. Boker A, Haberman CJ, Girling L, et al. Variable ventilation improves perioperative lung function in patients undergoing abdominal aortic aneurysmectomy. Anesthesiology 2004;100:608–16.
67. Mols G, Priebe HJ, Guttmann J. Alveolar recruitment in acute lung injury. Br J Anaesth 2006;96:156–66.
68. Licker M, Diaper J, Villiger Y, et al. Impact of intraoperative lung-protective interventions in patients undergoing lung cancer surgery. Crit Care 2009;13:R41.

69. Ni Chonghaile M, Higgins B, Laffey JG. Permissive hypercapnia: role in protective lung ventilatory strategies. Curr Opin Crit Care 2005;11:56–62.
70. Alvarez JM, Panda RK, Newman MA, et al. Postpneumonectomy pulmonary edema. J Cardiothorac Vasc Anesth 2003;17:388–95.
71. Fujinaga T, Nakamura T, Fukuse T, et al. Isoflurane inhalation after circulatory arrest protects against warm ischemia reperfusion injury of the lungs. Transplantation 2006;82:1168–74.
72. Reutershan J, Chang D, Hayes JK, et al. Protective effects of isoflurane pretreatment in endotoxin-induced lung injury. Anesthesiology 2006;104:511–7.
73. Voigtsberger S, Lachmann RA, Leutert AC, et al. Sevoflurane ameliorates gas exchange and attenuates lung damage in experimental lipopolysaccharide-induced lung injury. Anesthesiology 2009;111:1238–48.
74. De Conno E, Steurer MP, Wittlinger M, et al. Anesthetic-induced improvement of the inflammatory response to one-lung ventilation. Anesthesiology 2009;110:1316–26.
75. Schilling T, Kozian A, Kretzschmar M, et al. Effects of propofol and desflurane anaesthesia on the alveolar inflammatory response to one-lung ventilation. Br J Anaesth 2007;99:368–75.
76. Casanova J, Garutti I, Simon C, et al. The effects of anesthetic preconditioning with sevoflurane in an experimental lung autotransplant model in pigs. Anesth Analg 2011;113:742–8.
77. Goldman M, Webert KE, Arnold DM, et al. Proceedings of a consensus conference: towards an understanding of TRALI. Transfus Med Rev 2005;19:2–31.
78. Popovsky MA, Moore SB. Diagnostic and pathogenetic considerations in transfusion-related acute lung injury. Transfusion 1985;25:573–7.
79. Toy P, Popovsky MA, Abraham E, et al, National Heart, Lung and Blood Institute Working Group on TRALI. Transfusion-related acute lung injury: definition and review. Crit Care Med 2005;33:721–6.
80. Triulzi DJ. Transfusion-related acute lung injury: current concepts for the clinician. Anesth Analg 2009;108:770–6.
81. Marik PE, Corwin HL. Acute lung injury following blood transfusion: expanding the definition. Crit Care Med 2008;36:3080–4.
82. Gajic O, Rana R, Winters JL, et al. Transfusion-related acute lung injury in the critically ill: prospective nested case-control study. Am J Respir Crit Care Med 2007;176:886–91.
83. Eder AF, Herron R, Strupp A, et al. Transfusion-related acute lung injury surveillance (2003-2005) and the potential impact of the selective use of plasma from male donors in the American Red Cross. Transfusion 2007;47:599–607.
84. Apostolakis EE, Koletsis EN, Baikoussis NG, et al. Strategies to prevent intraoperative lung injury during cardiopulmonary bypass. J Cardiothorac Surg 2010;5:1.
85. Ng CS, Wan S, Yim AP, et al. Pulmonary dysfunction after cardiac surgery. Chest 2002;121:1269–77.
86. Zupancich E, Paparella D, Turani F, et al. Mechanical ventilation affects inflammatory mediators in patients undergoing cardiopulmonary bypass for cardiac surgery: a randomized clinical trial. J Thorac Cardiovasc Surg 2005;130:378–83.
87. Lellouche F, Dionne S, Simard S, et al. High tidal volumes in mechanically ventilated patients increase organ dysfunction after cardiac surgery. Anesthesiology 2012;116:1072–82.
88. The Cardiothoracic Surgery Network website. Available at: http://www.ctsnet.org. Accessed July 26, 2012.

89. Hager DN, Krishnan JA, Hayden DL, et al, ARDS Clinical Trials Network. Tidal volume reduction in patients with acute lung injury when plateau pressures are not high. Am J Respir Crit Care Med 2005;10:1241–5.

90. Frank JA, Gutierrez JA, Jones KD, et al. Low tidal volume reduces epithelial and endothelial injury in acid-injured rat lungs. Am J Respir Crit Care Med 2002;165: 242–9.

91. Iglesias M, Jungebluth P, Petit C, et al. Extracorporeal lung membrane provides better lung protection than conventional treatment for severe postpneumonectomy noncardiogenic acute respiratory distress syndrome. J Thorac Cardiovasc Surg 2008;6:1362–71.

92. Mallick A, Elliot S, McKinlay J, et al. Extracorporeal carbon dioxide removal using the Novalung in a patient with intracranial bleeding. Anaesthesia 2007; 62:72–4.

93. McKinlay J, Chapman G, Elliot S, et al. Pre-emptive Novalung-assisted carbon dioxide removal in a patient with chest, head and abdominal injury. Anaesthesia 2008;63:767–70.

94. Hammell C, Forrest M, Barrett P. Clinical experience with a pumpless extracorporeal lung assist device. Anaesthesia 2008;63:1241–4.

95. Elliot SC, Paramasivam K, Oram J, et al. Pumpless extracorporeal carbon dioxide removal for life-threatening asthma. Crit Care Med 2007;35:945–8.

96. Hughes C, Weavind L, Banerjee A, et al. Intraoperative risk factors for acute respiratory distress syndrome in critically ill patients. Anesth Analg 2010;111: 464–7.

97. Gollege G, Goldstraw P. Renal impairment after thoracotomy: incidence, risk factors and significance. Ann Thorac Surg 1994;58:524–8.

98. Kuitunen A, Venato A, Suojaranta-Ylinen R, et al. Acute renal failure after cardiac surgery: evaluation of the RIFLE classification. Ann Thorac Surg 2006;81:542–6.

99. Reimer C, McRae K, Seitz D, et al. Perioperative acute kidney injury in pneumonectomy: a retrospective cohort study. Can J Anaesth 2010;57(S1):A802743.

100. Ishikawa S, Greisdale DEG, Lohser J. Acute kidney injury after lung resection surgery: incidence and perioperative risk factors. Anesth Analg 2012;114: 1256–62.

101. Blank RS, Huffmayer JL, Jaeger JM, et al. Anesthesia for esophageal surgery [Chapter 30]. In: Slinger P, editor. Principles and practice of anesthesia for thoracic surgery. New York: Springer; 2011.

102. Chappell D, Jacob M, Hofmann-Kiefer K, et al. A rational approach to perioperative fluid management. Anesthesiology 2008;109(4):723–40.

103. Cense HA, Lagarde SM, de Jong K, et al. Association of no epidural analgesia with post-operative morbidity and mortality after transthoracic esophageal cancer resection. J Am Coll Surg 2006;202:395–400.

104. Al-Rawi OY, Pennefather S, Page RD, et al. The effect of thoracic epidural bupivacaine and an intravenous adrenalin infusion on gastric tube blood flow during esophagectomy. Anesth Analg 2008;106:884–7.

105. Holte K, Sharrock NE, Kehlet H. Pathophysiology and clinical implications of perioperative fluid excess. Br J Anaesth 2002;89(4):622–32.

106. Theodorou D, Drimousis PG, Larentzakis A, et al. The effects of vasopressors on perfusion of gastric graft after esophagectomy. J Gastrointest Surg 2008;12: 1497.

107. Klijn E, Niehof S, de Jong J, et al. The effect of perfusion pressure on gastric tissue blood flow in an experimental gastric tube model. Anesth Analg 2010; 110:541–6.

108. Hiltebrand LB, Koepfli E, Kimberger O, et al. Hypotension during fluid restricted abdominal surgery. Anesthesiology 2011;114:557–64.
109. Oohashi S, Endoh H. Does central venous pressure or pulmonary capillary wedge pressure reflect the status of circulating blood volume in patients after extended transthoracic esophagectomy? J Anesth 2005;19(1):21–5.
110. Kobayashi M, Ko M, Kimura T, et al. Perioperative monitoring of fluid responsiveness after esophageal surgery using stroke volume variation. Expert Rev Med Devices 2008;5:311–6.
111. Wei S, Tian J, Song X, et al. Association of perioperative fluid balance and adverse surgical outcomes in esophageal cancer and esophagogastric junction cancer. Ann Thorac Surg 2008;86(1):266–72.
112. Starling EH. On the absorption of fluids form the connective tissue spaces. J Physiol 1896;19:312–26.
113. Woodcock TE, Woodcock TM. Revised Starling equation and the glycocalyx model of transvascular fluid exchange. Br J Anaesth 2012;108:384–94.
114. Kregenow DA, Rubenfeld GD, Hudson LD, et al. Hypercapnic acidosis and mortality in acute lung injury. Crit Care Med 2006;34:1–7.
115. Curley G, Laffey JG, Kavanagh BP. Bench-to-bedside: carbon dioxide. Crit Care 2010;14:220.
116. Faller S, Ryter SW, Choi AM, et al. Inhaled hydrogen sulfide protects against ventilator-induced lung injury. Anesthesiology 2010;113:104–15.
117. Waerhaug K, Kuzkov VV, Kuklin VN, et al. Inhaled aerosolised recombinant human activated protein C ameliorates endotoxin-induced lung injury in anesthetised sheep. Crit Care 2009;13:R51.
118. Matthay M. ß-Adrenergic agonist therapy as a potential treatment for acute lung injury. Am J Respir Crit Care Med 2006;173:254–5.
119. Perkins GD, McAuley DF, Thickett DR, et al. The ß-agonist lung injury trial. Am J Respir Crit Care Med 2006;173:281–7.
120. Bernard GR. Acute respiratory distress syndrome: a historical perspective. Am J Respir Crit Care Med 2005;172:798–806.

Advances in Therapy for Acute Lung Injury

Vera von Dossow-Hanfstingl, MD

KEYWORDS

- Acute lung injury • Lung protective ventilation • Ventilator-induced lung injury
- Extracorporeal support • ECMO • iLA

KEY POINTS

- Despite recent advances in the therapy for acute lung injury and adult respiratory distress syndrome, the mortality remains high.
- The iatrogenic risk of ventilator-induced lung injury might contribute to this high mortality because, even in patients ventilated with low tidal volumes less than 6 mL/kg, the lungs are hyperinflated.
- Extracorporeal membrane oxygenation and interventional lung assist allow ultraprotective ventilation strategies. However, these assists have different technical aspects and different indications.

INTRODUCTION

The incidence for acute lung injury (ALI) and adult respiratory distress syndrome (ARDS) is much higher than previously published.[1–5] Rubenfeld and colleagues[1] reported 78.9 cases per 100 000 people per year for ALI and 58.7 cases per 100 000 people per year for ARDS. The in-hospital mortality for patients with ALI ranges between 38.5% (34.9%–42.2%) and 41.1% (36.7%–45.4%) for those with ARDS.[5] Despite major advances in thoracic surgery, intraoperative anesthetic management, and perioperative critical care over the past 20 years, ALI and ARDS are responsible for most respiratory-related deaths after thoracic surgery.[6,7] Previous published studies that used the American-European consensus conference definition of ALI/ARDS[6] reported an overall prevalence rate of 2.2% to 4.2% in patients who underwent thoracic surgery.[6,7] The mortality rate from ALI/ARDS in these patients ranged from 52% to 65%.[6–9]

It became obvious that a multimodal therapeutic approach is necessary. Randomized trials confirmed an oxygenation benefit for several therapeutic approaches: lung protective ventilation, positive end-expiratory pressure (PEEP), prone position,

Department of Anesthesiology, Ludwig Maximilian University, Marchioninistrasse 15, Munich 81377, Germany
E-mail address: vera.dossow@med.uni-muenchen.de

Anesthesiology Clin 30 (2012) 629–639
http://dx.doi.org/10.1016/j.anclin.2012.08.008   **anesthesiology.theclinics.com**
1932-2275/12/$ – see front matter

restrictive fluid administration, inhalational pulmonary vasodilators, and extracorporeal lung support.[10–16] All of these approaches can be included in a multimodal algorithm.[16] However, lung protective ventilation with a tidal volume of 6 mL/kg predicted body weight and a plateau pressure of 30 cm H_2O or less remains the only proven therapy to decrease mortality in ARDS.[17] Although most of the studies failed to demonstrate an outcome benefit for extracorporeal lung support, Peek and collegues,[18] for the first time, found a decreased mortality in patients with severe ARDS treated with extracorporeal membrane oxygenation (ECMO). Since the 2009 H1N1 virus pandemic, there is increasing enthusiasm for ECMO as a first-line treatment strategy for ARDS.[18–21] Recently, a pumpless extracorporeal lung support system, the *interventional lung assist* (iLA; Novalung GmbH, Talheim, Germany) was developed, which provides effective carbon dioxide elimination.[22] However, the outcome benefit still remains to be determined in randomized studies.

This article focuses on recent advances in lung protective strategy, including prevention of ventilator-associated injury and the role of extracorporeal lung support.

Ventilator-Induced Lung Injury

The application of high inspiratory pressures and high tidal volumes are known to contribute to ventilator-induced lung injury (VILI).[23–25] The main forces responsible for VILI are the regional overdistention caused by volutrauma and barotrauma as well as recruitment and under-recruitment of collapsed alveoli (atelectasis). Furthermore, physical stress by mechanical ventilation induces the release of inflammatory mediators directly from the lung into the circulation. The complexity of these alterations is described by the term *biotrauma*. In addition, ventilation strategies that aim to maximize the recruitment of dependent regions through the application of high PEEP put nondependent regions at risk of injury from overdistension.[26,27] The open lung strategy can be performed either by stepwise increases in PEEP or by recruitment maneuver to prevent tidal recruitment/derecruitment.[27–29] Nevertheless, in 3 randomized trials, high PEEP levels failed to be associated with improved mortality.[30–32] One meta-analysis revealed an increased survival in patients with severe ARDS (<200 mm Hg) and higher PEEP levels (34.1 vs 39.1, $P<.049$).[33] This finding was supported by the study of Villar and colleagues.[13]

Limitation of tidal volume and inspiratory pressure (Pinsp) may not be sufficient to avoid hyperinflation, and PEEP is likely to increase hyperinflation in some patients and might have a failed outcome benefit for most of the studies.[34] Thus, the need of a protective ventilation strategy according to an individual patient's lung mechanics became obvious.[29] The clinical relevance was underlined by Gattinoni and colleagues[26] with the concept of stress and strain, a mechanical phenomenon that refers to small areas of a body.[35] *Stress* is defined as the internal distribution of the counterforce per unit of area that balances and reacts to an external load. The associated deformation of the structure is called *strain*, which is defined as the change in size referred to the initial status.[35] Gattinoni and colleagues[26] pointed out that the clinical equivalent of stress is transpulmonary pressure (airway pressure minus pleural pressure) and the clinical equivalent of strain is the ratio of volume change to the functional residual capacity presenting the resting lung volume.[26,27] For a given plateau pressure or tidal volume/ideal body weight, stress and strain may vary largely because of the variability of chest wall elastance and the resting lung volume.[26]

Chiumello and colleagues[25] measured stress and strain in all of their patients with ALI/ARDS. They noted that, in a small collective of patients, strain values were higher than 2 even with low tidal volume less than 6 mL/kg. They concluded that, for these patients, safe mechanical ventilation does not exist and that extracorporeal support might be considered.[25,26] Recently, Terragni and collegues[34] demonstrated that even low tidal volume of 6 mL/kg ideal body weight may be potentially injurious. Moreover, Grasso and colleagues[27] used the stress index and found that hyperinflation in all patients with ARDS during ARDS network strategy and PEEP was decreased. Talmor and colleagues[28] used transpulmonary pressure measurements to increase PEEP compared with the ARDS network strategy. Oxygenation was significantly improved with transpulmonary pressure measurement, and there was a strong trend toward increased survival and shorter mechanical ventilation.

In summary, introducing the measurement of stress and strain into the clinical practice might be helpful to clarify the safe limits of mechanical ventilation for each individual patient. The concept of an individualized ventilation might have an impact for a more precise indication of extracorporeal support in context with lung protective ventilation strategies. However, as Plataki and colleagues[29] pointed out in their review, further clinical research on the impact of biophysical determinants of lung injury on patient outcomes is needed.

EXTRACORPOREAL LUNG SUPPORT

In patients with ARDS with severe hypoxemia, the implementation of lung protective ventilation strategies is frequently limited by a dilemma: The reduced oxygenation usually requires high end-expiratory pressure, which limits carbon dioxide elimination with the risk of severe hypercapnia and further contributes to VILI.[36] However, the effects of hypercapnia have not yet been conclusively clarified. Hypercapnia results in pulmonary and cardiac vasoconstriction, peripheral arterial and cerebral vasodilatation, delivery from catecholamines, reduction of renal perfusion, and triggers respiratory drive.[36] These adverse pathophysiological consequences could result in organ damage, such as myocardial insufficiency, renal failure, or restriction of liver/intestine circulation caused by systemic hypercapnia.[36] Therefore, it became obvious to avoid secondary organ damage. In patients with severe ARDS and life-threatening hypoxemia, a pump-driven veno-venous ECMO is indicated. Recently, a pumpless extracorporeal lung support system was developed using an arteriovenous bypass with an integrated gas exchange membrane. This system provides effective carbon dioxide elimination but only moderate improvement in oxygenation.[37]

INDICATIONS FOR ECMO

The most common indication for ECMO in respiratory failure includes ARDS with severe hypoxemia (Pao_2/F_iO_2 <100 mm Hg), primary graft failure after lung transplantation, and severe lung contusion after trauma, which are all refractory to conventional mechanical ventilation.[38–40] Among thoracic surgery, respiratory complications (ALI, ARDS, bronchopleural fistula) remain the major cause of morbidity and mortality of lung surgery.[40]

According to the Extracorporeal Life Support Organization, ECMO should be initiated in hypoxic respiratory failure when the risk of mortality is 50% or greater, the Pao_2/F_iO_2 is less than 150 mm Hg (Murray Score: 2–3, F_iO_2 >90%), or the Pao_2/F_iO_2 is less than 80 mm Hg (Murrey Score 3–4, F_iO_2 >90%).[41] In Australia, the New South Wales Department of Health recommended immediate veno-venous ECMO for refractory hypoxemia (Pao_2/F_iO_2 <60) or hypercarbia ($Paco_2$ >100 mm Hg).[42] Deja and colleagues[16] included fast-entry criteria for ECMO (Pao_2/F_iO_2 50 mm Hg and PIP >35 cm H_2O over 2 hours) in their ARDS-treatment algorithm.

However, the institution of ECMO is appropriate if the organ failure is thought to be reversible with therapy and rest on ECMO. If lung function does not recover due to a progressive lung disease, ECMO might be instituted as bridging for transplant.[43]

TECHNICAL ASPECTS OF ECMO

An ECMO circuit is designed to pump and oxygenate blood and remove carbon dioxide. The ECMO pump works to push blood through the oxygenator and back to patients.[44,45] It also works to augment venous outflow to the circuit. Two different pumps are used in the ECMO circuit: centrifugal pumps and roller pump.[44,45] The main advantage of a centrifugal pump is that there is no excessive negative pressures on the blood, less cavitation, and less hemolysis.[45] However, increases in systemic vascular resistance or kinking of the ECMO circuit can cause dramatic decrease of flow.[45]

Membrane Oxygenator

The most commonly used gas exchange membrane is the hollow fiber oxygenation.[45,46] Its tight hollow-fiber membrane made of polymethylpentene eliminates plasma leaks. It effectively prevents the formation of microbubbles.[45,46] A coating reduces the risk of clotting. A lower pressure gradient across the membrane decreases the risk for hemolysis. Membrane function is monitored by the premembrane and postmembrane pressure differences and the gas exchange function.[44]

ECMO CANNULATION

It is important to insert the largest possible cannula (21–23 F) to maintain adequate flow (60–120 mL/kg/min) because gravity and not the pump primarily determine venous outflow.[36] This outflow would be from 25% to 75% of the cardiac output, providing sufficient oxygenation and decarboxylation.[36]

ECMO should be inserted in a *veno-venous* configuration in case of respiratory failure with severe hypoxia (no major cardiac dysfunction) or can be used as a *veno-arterial* (VA) configuration (providing both respiratory and cardiac support).[46] The use of VA ECMO in case of adequate cardiac function may cause severe hypoxia in the upper part of the body (brain and heart) in the setting of a severe pulmonary shunt.[45]

Peripheral cannulation should be strictly percutaneous by the Seldinger technique[36,45,46]: It reduces bleeding complication and allows simple decannulation after weaning. Mostly, the femoral vein is used as outflow tract, and oxygenated blood via the ECMO circuit is returned to the right atrium via the right internal jugular vein (inflow).[46] Blood that returns via the superior vena cava remains deoxygenated. A bicaval dual-lumen catheter is now available (Avalon Elite, Avalon laboratories LLC, Rancho, Dominguez, California) and can be safely used to provide adequate veno-venous ECMO support in patients with ARDS.[47,48] This dual-lumen cannula has the advantage of single-site cannulation and avoids the femoral vascular access.[48] Furthermore, blood recirculation flow is very small. The double-lumen cannula can be successfully placed with transthoracic echocardiographic guidance.[49]

VENTILATOR SETTINGS DURING VENO-VENOUS ECMO

Hypoxia is treated by increasing the ECMO flow rate and the F_iO_2 of the ECMO circuit and not by altering the F_iO_2 and PEEP on the ventilator. Attempts should be made to wean the F_iO_2 on the ventilator (keeping arterial oxygen saturation >85%) and to maintain a lung protective strategy with adequate PEEP (>10 cm H_2O to prevent alveolar collapse), low plateau pressures (<25 cm H_2O), low tidal volumes, and low respiratory rates to prevent VILI.[33] $Paco_2$ control should be via the ECMO fresh gas flow of the oxygenator and not by altering the respiratory rate on the ventilator.[36,45,46]

WEANING ECMO (ACCORDING TO DEJA AND COLLEAGUES AND VON DOSSOW-HANFSTINGL AND COLLEAGUES)
Monitoring for Anticoagulation

Patients treated with ECMO do require low-level heparinization to prevent clotting of the cannula, tubing, and particularly the oxygenator **Box 1**. An activated partial thromboplastin time of 50 to 60 seconds and 0.2 to 0.3 IU/mL for heparinemia (anti-Xa activity) as well as a platelet count greater than 80 × 10 9/L is reasonable.[36,45,46] In case of heparin-induced thrombocytopenia, argatroban seems to be an adequate alternative for anticoagulation during ECMO.[50] Regular measurement of the clotting profile, platelet count, and hemoglobin should be performed as least twice per day. Hemolysis is another well-recognized complication of ECMO, with an incidence of 5% and 8% and should be regularly monitored.[51] This monitoring is done by regular (daily) checking of the plasma-free hemoglobin.[36]

COMPLICATIONS ASSOCIATED WITH ECMO

The most common *patient-related complications* associated with ECMO are life-threatening thrombosis and excessive bleeding caused by the need of systemic heparin therapy.[37,47,52] Lidegran and collegues[53] found intracranial lesions (infarction, hemorrhage) within the first 7 days after ECMO initiation. Ischemia of the lower limb occurs with VA-ECMO using cannulation of the femoral artery. *Mechanical complications* with the ECMO circuit include thrombus formation in the oxygenator, shaking of the cannula caused by hypovolemia, air embolism, and oxygenator and pump failure.[44]

ILA
Indication for iLA

The iLA can be applied to give the injured or diseased lung a chance to heal (bridge to recovery) or it might be used as a bridge to transplant in an end-stage lung disease.[36,54–57] There are numerous published case reports and retrospective studies of patients with ALI and ARDS successfully treated with iLA and the ultraprotective lung ventilation strategy.[55–62] Experimental animal studies revealed contrasting results.[63,64] Although Dembinski and collegues[63] failed to demonstrate a benefit with the

---

Box 1
Weaning of ECMO

Weaning of ECMO

F_iO_2 less than 0.4 to 0.6

PaO_2 greater than 80 mm Hg

Target ventilator settings

BIPAP: PEEP ± 12 cm H_2O; PIP less than 30 cm H_2O; Vt: 4 to 6 mL/kg

RR spontaneous approximately 5 breaths per minute

Procedure

- Reducing blood flow 0.5 l/min every 12 hours to minimal blood flow 0.5 to 1.0 l/min
- $PaCO_2$ less than 60 mm Hg, reducing gas flow and F_iO_2 over membrane
- ECMO trial off: gas flow 0.5 to 1 l/min over 15 minutes; criteria fulfilled: discontinue ECMO

Abbreviations: BIPAP, Biphasic Positive Airway pressure; PEEP, positive end-expiratory pressure; PIP, peak inspiratory pressure; Vt, tidal volume.

ultraprotective ventilation strategy with iLA (6 mL/kg vs 3 mL/kg, PEEP 5 cm H_2O), Iglesias and colleagues[64] showed, in a postpneumonectomy-ARDS model, improved lung protection with 2.3 mL/kg, PEEP 15 cm H_2O, reduced lung cytokine release, and survival at the end of the study. The different levels of PEEP in the previously mentioned studies might account for the contrasting results. It is recommended to keep the PEEP between 15 and 20 cm H_2O to prevent derecruitment.[16,65,66] Muellenbach and colleagues[67] retrospectively analyzed 22 patients with ARDS with iLA and ultraprotective ventilation strategy (3 mL/kg and high PEEP). Seventy-two percent of the patients in this study were discharged from the intensive care unit. However, apart from these small studies, the outcome benefit is still lacking.

Technical Aspects

Pumpless extracorporeal lung assist, iLA, is an arteriovenous shunt with carbon dioxide elimination as the primary function owing to the arterial inflow blood. The principle is simple diffusion alongside a semipermeable membrane. Blood flows over an exterior surface (1.5 m^2) of the device fibers and the ventilating gas (oxygen sweep) flows into these fibers.[36] It is driven by the partial pressure gradient of carbon dioxide and oxygen, which is connected to an oxygen supply of 10 to 12 L/min. The iLA is a low-pressure–gradient device to operate without a pump. Adequate mean arterial blood pressure is mandatory (60–80 mm Hg).[58–60] The heparin-coated cannulas are inserted by the Seldinger technique into the femoral vessels. Flow rates range between 1.5 and 2.0 l/min (ie, approximately 20% of cardiac output).[36] Because the cannulas and the lung-assist device are heparin coated, only low-dose thromboembolic prophylaxis is necessary.[68] Although the iLA device effectively eliminates CO_2, oxygenation is limited.[37]

WEANING CRITERIA ILA (ACCORDING TO DEJA AND COLLEAGUES AND VON DOSSOW-HANFSTINGL AND COLLEAGUES)
Complications

Ischemia and compartment syndrome of the lower limb are associated with large cannulas (>15 F) that were initially used **Box 2**.[22,69] It is recommended to measure the vascular diameter of the femoral vessels by ultrasound to define the appropriate site of cannulas.[69]

Box 2
Weaning of iLA

Ramsay sedation score 0/-1

F_iO_2 less than 0.4

$Paco_2$ less than 60 mm Hg

Target ventilator settings

BIPAP: PEEP $\pm$ 12 cm H_2O; PIP less than 30 cm H_2O; Vt: 4 to 6 mL/kg; RR 14 $\pm$ 2 breaths per minute

RR spontaneous approximately 5 breaths per minute

Procedure

1. Reducing oxygen flow iLA 1 l/min in steps

2. Weaning iLA oxygen flow less than 2 l/min: iLA 6 hours without gas flow

3. iLA trial off: criteria fulfilled: discontinue iLA

OTHER THERAPEUTIC RECOMMENDATIONS
Analgosedation

Daily interruption of analgosedation was associated with improved outcome (ie, shorter mechanical ventilation and shorter stay in the intensive care unit).[70] This finding is important in patients requiring extracorporeal lung support with respect to early detection of new neurologic deficits (infarction, hemorrhage).[36] Daily monitoring of analgosedation improves outcome.[71] Therefore, daily assessment of the level of sedation and analgesia is strongly recommended in all critical care patients, especially those on extracorporeal lung support.

Spontaneous Breathing

Spontaneous breathing activity improved lung function and damage in different experimental models of ALI/ARDS compared with controlled mechanical ventilation.[72–74] In clinical trials, the combination of unsupported spontaneous breathing with mandatory cycles improves lung function, reduces the need for analgosedation, and allows weaning, but there is no effect on mortality.[73]

In contrast, the multicenter randomized clinical trial of Papazian and collegues[75] found that the use of neuromuscular blocking agents in the first 48 hours of severe ARDS was associated with a decreased mortality. Even if there is strong evidence to avoid spontaneous breathing in patients with severe ARDS for the first 48 hours, it may be useful in patients with less severe ARDS or ALI. In addition, patients with expected prolonged ventilatory support, early tracheotomy to facilitate patients' comfort might be performed.[36,76]

PERSPECTIVES

Important aspects of lung protective ventilation and prevention of VILI has been studied in multiple experimental and clinical studies. It became obvious that there is a need for individual adjustment of ventilator settings. In addition, the role of extracorporeal lung support in the context of an algorithm approach on patients' outcomes remains to be determined in further studies.

REFERENCES

1. Rubenfeld GD, Caldwell E, Peabody E, et al. Incidence and outcomes of acute lung injury. N Engl J Med 2005;353:1685–93.
2. Luhr OR, Antonsen K, Karsson M, et al. Incidence and mortality after acute respiratory failure and acute respiratory distress syndrome in Sweden, Denmark, and Iceland. Am J Respir Crit Care Med 1999;159:1849–61.
3. Lewandowski K, Metz J, Deutschmann C, et al. Incidence, severity and mortality of acute respiratory failure in Berlin, Germany. Am J Respir Crit Care Med 1999; 151:1121–5.
4. Kanazawa M. Acute lung injury: clinical concept and experimental approaches to pathogenesis. Keio J Med 1996;45:131–9.
5. Luce JM. Acute lung injury and the acute respiratory distress syndrome. Crit Care Med 1998;26:369–76.
6. Bernard GR, Artigas A, Brigham KL, et al. The American-European Consensus Conference on ARDS. Definitions, mechanism, relevant outcomes, and clinical trial coordination. Am J Respir Crit Care Med 1994;149:818–24.
7. Kutlu CA, Williams EA, Evans TW, et al. Acute lung injury and acute respiratory distress syndrome after pulmonary resection. Ann Thorac Surg 2000;69:376–80.

8. Ruffini E, Parola A, Papalia E, et al. Frequency and mortality of acute lung injury and acute respiratory distress syndrome after pulmonary resection for bronchogenic carcinoma. Eur J Cardiothorac Surg 2001;20:30–7.

9. Dulu A, Pastores S, Park B, et al. Prevalence and mortality of acute lung injury and ARDS after lung resection. Chest 2006;130:73–8.

10. Amato MB, Barbas K, Hopper L, et al. Effect of a protective-ventilation strategy on mortality in the acute respiratory distress syndrome. N Engl J Med 1998;338:347–54.

11. Gattinoni L, Tognoni G, Pesenti A, et al. Effect of prone positioning on the survival of patients with acute respiratory failure. N Engl J Med 2001;345:568–73.

12. Wiedemann HP, Wheeler AP, Bernard GR, et al. Comparison of two fluid-management strategies in acute lung injury. N Engl J Med 2006;354:2564–75.

13. Villar J, Kacmarek RM, Pérez-Méndez L, et al. A high positive end-expiratory pressure, low tidal volume ventilatory strategy improves outcome in persistent acute respiratory distress syndrome: a randomized, controlled trial. Crit Care Med 2006;34:1311–8.

14. Weissmann N, Gerigk B, Kocer O, et al. Hypoxia-induced pulmonary hypertension: different impact of iloprost, sildenafil, and nitric oxide. Respir Med 2007; 101:2125–32.

15. Lewandowski K, Rossaint R, Pappert D, et al. High survival rate in 122 ARDS patients managed according to clinical algorithm including extracorporeal membrane oxygenation. Intensive Care Med 1997;23:819–35.

16. Deja M, Hommel M, Weber-Carstens S, et al. Evidence-based therapy of severe acute respiratory distress syndrome: an algorithm-guided approach. J Int Med Res 2008;3:211–21.

17. Acute Respiratory Distress Syndrome Network. Ventilation with lower tidal volumes as compared with traditional tidal volumes for acute lung injury and the acute respiratory distress syndrome. N Engl J Med 2000;351:327–36.

18. Peek GJ, Mugford M, Tiruvoipati R, et al. Efficacy and economic assessment of conventional ventilatory support versus extracorporeal membrane oxygenation for severe adult respiratory failure (CESAR): a multicentre randomized controlled trial. Lancet 2009;374:1351–63.

19. Noah MA, Peek GJ, Finney SJ, et al. Referral to an extracorporeal membrane oxygenation center and mortality among patients with severe 2009 influenza (H1N1). JAMA 2011;306:1659–68.

20. Cianchi G, Bonizzoli M, Pasquini A, et al. Ventilatory and ECMO treatment of H1N1-induced severe respiratory failure: results of an Italian referral ECMO center. BMC Pulm Med 2011;11:2.

21. Forrest P, Ratchford J, Burns B, et al. Retrieval of critically ill adults using extracorporeal membrane oxygenation: an Australian experience. Intensive Care Med 2011;37:824–30.

22. Bein T, Weber F, Philipp A, et al. A new pumpless extracorporeal interventional lung assist in critical hypoxemia/hypercapnia. Crit Care Med 2006;34:1372–7.

23. Ngiam N, Kavanagh BP. Ventilator-induced lung injury: the role of gene activation. Curr Opin Crit Care 2012;18:16–22.

24. Plötz FB, Slutzky AS, van Vught AJ, et al. Ventilator-induced lung injury and multiple system organ failure: a critical review of facts and hypothesis. Intensive Care Med 2004;30:1865–72.

25. Chiumello D, Carlesso E, Cadringher P, et al. Lung stress and strain in ALI/ARDS. Am J Respir Crit Care Med 2008;178:346–55.

26. Gattinoni L, Carlesso E, Cadringher P, et al. Physical and biological triggers of ventilator-induced lung injury and its prevention. Eur Respir J Suppl 2003;47:15s–25s.

27. Grasso S, Stripoli T, De Michele M, et al. ARDSnet ventilatory protocol and alveolar hyperinflation: role of positive end-expiratory pressure. Am J Respir Crit Care Med 2007;176:761–7.
28. Talmor D, Sarge T, O'Donell CR, et al. Mechanical ventilation guided by esophageal pressure in acute lung injury. N Engl J Med 2008;359:2095–104.
29. Plataki M, Hubmayr RD. The physical basis on ventilator-induced lung injury. Expert Rev Respir Med 2010;4:373–85.
30. Brower RG, Lanken PN, MacIntyre N, et al. Higher versus lower positive end expiratory pressures in patients with the acute respiratory distress syndrome. N Engl J Med 2004;351:327–36.
31. Meade MO, Cook DJ, Guyatt GH, et al. Ventilation strategy using low tidal volumes, recruitment maneuvers, and high positive end-expiratory pressure for acute lung injury and acute respiratory distress syndrome: a randomized controlled trial. JAMA 2008;299:637–45.
32. Mercat A, Richard JC, Vielle B, et al. Positive end-expiratory pressure setting in adults with acute lung injury and acute respiratory distress syndrome: a randomized controlled trial. JAMA 2008;299:646–55.
33. Briel M, Meade M, Mercat A, et al. Higher versus lower positive end-expiratory pressure in patients with acute lung injury and acute respiratory distress syndrome: a systematic review and meta-analysis. JAMA 2010;303:865–73.
34. Terragni PP, Del Sorbo L, Mascia L, et al. Tidal volume lower than 6 ml/kg enhances lung protection: role of extracorporeal carbon dioxide removal. Anesthesiology 2009;111:826–35.
35. Wilson TA. Solid mechanics. In: American Physiological Society, editor. Handbook of physiology: a critical, comprehensive presentation of physiological knowledge and concepts. Baltimore (MD): Waverly Press; 1986. p. 35–9.
36. von Dossow-Hanfstingl V, Deja M, Zwissler B, et al. Postoperative management: extracorporeal ventilatory therapy (Ch. 43). In: Slinger P, editor. Thoracic anesthesia. Heidelberg (NY): Springer Verlag; 2012. p. 635–48.
37. Meyer A, Strueber M, Fischer S. Advances in extracorporeal ventilation. Anesthesiol Clin 2008;26:381–91.
38. Madershahian N, Wittwer T, Strauch J, et al. Application of ECMO in multitrauma patients with ARDS as rescue therapy. J Card Surg 2007;22:180–4.
39. Kshettry VR, Kroshus TJ, Hertz MI, et al. Early and late airway complications after lung transplantation: incidence and management. Ann Thorac Surg 1997;63:1576–83.
40. Khan NU, Al-Aloul M, Khasati N, et al. Extracorporeal membrane oxygenator as a bridge to successful surgical repair of bronchopleural fistula following bilateral sequential lung transplantation: a case report and review of the literature. J Cardiothorac Surg 2007;2:28.
41. ELSO guidelines. Available at: http://www.elso.med.umich.edu.Guidelines.html. Accessed September 15, 2011.
42. NSW indications for ECMO referral. Available at: http://amwac.health.nsw.gov.au/policies/pd/2010/pdf/PD2010_028pdf. Accessed March, 2010.
43. Marasco SF, Lukas G, Mc Donald M, et al. Review of ECMO (extra corporeal membrane oxygenation) support in critically ill adult patient. Heart Lung Cric 2008;17(Suppl 4):S41–7.
44. Allen S, Holena D, Mc Cunn M, et al. A review of fundamental principles and evidence base in the use of extracorporeal membrane oxygenation (ECMO) in critically adult patients. J Intensive Care Med 2011;26:13.
45. Freckner B, Palmér P, Lindén V. Extracorporeal respiratory support and minimally invasive ventilation in severe ARDS. Minerva Anestesiol 2002;68:381–6.

46. Combes A, Bacchetta M, Brodie D, et al. Extracorporeal membrane oxygenation for respiratory failure in adults. Curr Opin Crit Care 2012;18:99–104.

47. Diaz-Guzmann E, Lynch J, Hoopes CW, et al. Venovenous extracorporeal membrane oxygenation in acute respiratory failure: do we need a new configuration? J Thorac Cardiavasc Surg 2012;143:993–4.

48. Wang D, Zhou X, Liu X, et al. Wang-Zwische double –lumen cannula – toward a percutaneous and ambulatory paracorporeal artificial lung. ASAIO J 2008;54: 1722–5.

49. Bermudez CA, Rocha RV, Sappington PL, et al. Initial experience with single cannulation for veno-venous extracorporeal oxygenation in adults. Ann Thorac Surg 2010;90:991–5.

50. Beiderlinden T, Treschan T, Goerlinger K, et al. Argatroban in extracorporeal membrane oxygenation. Artif Organs 2007;31:154–74.

51. Oliver WC. Anticoagulation and coagulation management for ECMO. Semin Cardiothorac Vasc Anesth 2009;13:154.

52. Thiara AP, Hoel TN, Kristiansen F, et al. Evaluation of oxygenators and centrifugal pumps for long-term pediatric extracorporeal membrane oxygenation. Perfusion 2007;22:323–6.

53. Lidegran MK, Mosskin M, Ringertz HG, et al. Cranial CT for diagnosis of intracranial complications in adult and pediatric patients during ECMO: clinical benefits in diagnosis and treatment. Acad Radiol 2007;14:62–71.

54. Conrad SA, Zwischenberger JB, Grier LR, et al. Total extracorporeal arteriovenous carbon dioxide removal in acute respiratory failure: a phase I clinical study. Intensive Care Med 2001;27:340–51.

55. Von Mach MA, Kaes J, Omogbehin B, et al. An update on interventional lung assist devices and their role in acute respiratory distress syndrome. Lung 2006;184:169–75.

56. Dschietzig T, Laule M, Melzer C, et al. Long-term treatment of severe respiratory failure with an extracorporeal lung assist- a case report. Intensivmed 2005;42: 365–70.

57. Brederlau J, Anetseder M, Wagner R, et al. Pumpless extracorporeal lung assist in severe blunt chest trauma. J Cardiothorac Vasc Anesth 2004;18(6):777–9.

58. Fischer S, Hoeper MM, Tomaszek S, et al. Bridge to lung transplantation with the extracorporeal membrane ventilator Novalung in the veno-venous mode: the initial Hannover experience. ASAIO J 2007;53(2):168–70.

59. Fischer S, Hoeper MM, Bein T, et al. Interventional lung assist: a new concept of protective ventilation in bridge to lung transplantation. ASAIO J 2008;54:3–10.

60. Mattheis G. New technologies for respiratory assist. Perfusion 2003;18(4): 245–51.

61. Iglesias M, Martinez E, Badia JR, et al. Extrapulmonary ventilation for unresponsive severe acute respiratory distress syndrome after pulmonary resection. Ann Thorac Surg 2008;85:237–44.

62. Taylor K, Holtby H. Emergency interventional lung assist device for pulmonary hypertension. Anesth Analg 2009;109:382–5.

63. Dembinski R, Hochhausen N, Terbeck S, et al. Pumpless extracorporeal lung assist for protective mechanical ventilation in experimental injury. Crit Care Med 2007;35:2359–66.

64. Iglesias M, Jungebluth P, Petit C, et al. Extracorporeal lung membrane provides better lung protection than conventional treatment for severe postpneumonectomy noncardiogenic acute respiratory distress syndrome. J Thorac Cardiovasc Surg 2008;135:1362–71.

65. Jungebluth P, Iglesias M, Go T, et al. Optimal positive end-expiratory pressure during pumpless extracorporeal lung membrane support. Artif Organs 2008; 32:885–90.

66. Caironi P, Cressoni M, Chiumello D, et al. Lung opening and closing during ventilation in acute respiratory distress syndrome. Am J Respir Crit Care Med 2010; 181:578–86.

67. Muellenbach RM, Kredel M, Wunder C, et al. Arteriovenous extracorporeal lung assist as integral part of a multimodal concept: a retrospective analysis of 22 patients with ARDS refractory to standard care. Eur J Anaesthesiol 2008;25: 897–904.

68. Moerer O, Quintel M. Protective and ultra-protective ventilation: using pumpless interventional lung assist. Minerva Anestesiol 2011;77:537–44.

69. Zimmermann M, Bein T, Arlt A, et al. Pumpless extracorporeal interventional lung assist in patients with acute respiratory distress syndrome: a prospective pilot study. Crit Care Med 2009;13:R10.

70. Kress JP, Pohlmann AS, O'Connor MF. Daily interruption of sedative infusions in critically ill patients undergoing mechanical ventilation. N Engl J Med 2000;342: 1471–7.

71. Kastrup M, von Dossow V, Seeling M, et al. Key performance indicators in intensive care medicine. A retrospective matched cohort study. J Int Med Res 2009; 37:1267–84.

72. Carvalho NC, Güldner A, Bead A, et al. Effects of different levels of spontaneous breathing activity during biphasic positive airway pressure ventilation on lung function and inflammation in experimental lung injury. Am J Respir Crit Care Med 2011;183:A6233.

73. Gama de Abreu M, Cuevas M, Spieth PM, et al. Regional lung aeration and ventilation during pressure support and biphasic positive airway pressure ventilation in experimental lung injury. Crit Care 2010;14:R34.

74. Putensen C, Zech S, Wrigge H, et al. Long-term effects of spontaneous breathing during ventilatory support in patients with acute lung injury. Am J Respir Crit Care Med 2001;164:43–9.

75. Papazian L, Forel JM, Gacouin A, et al. Neuromuscular blockers in early respiratory distress syndrome. N Engl J Med 2010;363:1107–16.

76. Trouillet JL, Luyt CE, Guiguet M, et al. Early percutaneous tracheostomy versus prolonged intubation of mechanically ventilated patients after cardiac surgery: a randomized trial. Ann Intern Med 2011;154:373–83.

Fluid Management in Thoracic Surgery

Cait P. Searl, BSc, MA, MBChB, MRCP, FRCA[a],*, Albert Perrino, MD[b]

KEYWORDS

- Thoracic surgery • Fluid management • Acute kidney injury • Acute lung injury

KEY POINTS

- Fluid management in thoracic surgery remains controversial with level 1 evidence for benefit or harm from the commonly practised fluid restriction lacking.
- Acute lung injury following thoracic surgery is multifactorial in causation and not simply due to excess fluid.
- Individualized goal-directed fluid management may provide opportunities for reducing morbidity and mortality in thoracic surgery.

The role of perioperative fluid management in perioperative complications of thoracic surgery has long been the subject of debate, largely concentrated on the pulmonary complications of thoracic surgery. Since Zeldin and colleagues[1] postulated in 1984 a cause-and-effect relationship between overzealous fluid administration during surgery and the syndrome of postpneumonectomy pulmonary edema, it has been fashionable to blame the anesthesiologist for drowning the patient when acute lung injury (ALI) occurs following thoracic surgery. They advised that, "the most important thing we can do in terms of recognition of this problem is to watch our anesthesiologists as they start loading the patients up with fluids." The effects of fluids on other organ systems have played a lesser role in the arguments about fluid therapy until recently as the effects on renal and cardiac function have been increasing recognized as important considerations to patient outcome following thoracic surgery.

Despite increasingly ill patients with higher rates of comorbidity receiving operations, in-hospital mortalities of less than 2% following lobectomy and less than 6% for pneumonectomy have remained unchanged for decades.[2] This rate suggests that anesthesiologists are getting some things right but at least some of this improvement is down to our surgical colleagues. Improvements in surgical technique and technology, such as thoracoscopic approaches, are advances that should be recognized. For example, qualified cardiothoracic surgeons who have either purely or

[a] Newcastle upon Tyne Hospitals NHS Foundation Trust, NE7 7DN, UK; [b] Yale University School of Medicine, New Haven, CT 06510, USA
* Corresponding author.
E-mail address: Cait.Searl@nuth.nhs.uk

Anesthesiology Clin 30 (2012) 641–655
http://dx.doi.org/10.1016/j.anclin.2012.08.009
1932-2275/12/$ – see front matter © 2012 Elsevier Inc. All rights reserved.

mainly thoracic surgical practices achieve better results than nonspecialized surgeons.[3] This is consistent with other evidence[4,5] showing that hospitals with high volumes of any complex procedure have better short-term and long-term results. The main complications have shifted from cardiac and surgical complications toward infectious complications, multiorgan dysfunction and, ALI/adult respiratory distress syndrome (ARDS)[6] and hence the focus on these to further improve outcomes.

To create future outcome improvements, the practices common today should be reexamined in light of the current literature base. Such evidence-based practice is designed to apply the best available evidence gained from the scientific method to clinical decision making, in the form of evidence-based guidelines at the organizational or institutional level or evidence-based decision making by the individual health care provider. In the United States, evidence is divided into level I (evidence obtained from at least 1 properly designed randomized controlled trial) through to level III (opinion of respected authorities), as shown in **Table 1**. The UK National Health Service uses a similar system categorizing evidence from A to D. This article examines the use of evidence-based fluid management to improve outcomes following thoracic anesthesia.

THE STARTING POINT: FLUID BALANCE IN THE PERIOPERATIVE PERIOD

Surgery elicits a stress response of combined endocrine and inflammatory origin with several of the hormones involved exerting major influences on the distribution of body fluids. In general terms, the endocrine response leads to conservation of sodium and water and to the excretion of potassium, the principal mediators being antidiuretic hormone (ADH), aldosterone, and the renin-angiotensin II system. Increased ADH leads to increased water reabsorption at the kidney with consequent decreases in diuresis and plasma sodium levels after surgery, whereas increase in aldosterone and renin increases conservation of sodium and excretion of potassium.[7,8] Weight gain and edema formation is therefore a frequent complication of major surgical procedures with incidences as high as 40%. Negative fluid balances (mean -244 mL) were recorded in a study in the setting of lung respective surgery[9] using a restrictive fluid

Table 1 Ranking the quality of evidence			
United States	Preventative Task Force	National Health Service	United Kingdom
Level I	Evidence from at least 1 randomized controlled trial	Consistent randomized controlled trial, cohort study	Level A
Level II-1	Evidence from well-designed controlled trial, no randomization	Case-control study; outcomes research; consistent retrospective cohort studies; extrapolation from level A studies	Level B
Level II-2	Evidence from well-designed cohort or case-control analytical studies	Case-series studies or extrapolation from level B studies	Level C
Level II-3	Evidence from multiple time series with or without interventions	—	—
Level III	Expert opinion	Expert opinion	Level D

regimen on day 1. On day 2, postoperative modest positive fluid balances (averaging +968 mL), patient weight gain, and changes in transthoracic bioimpedance confirmed that significant fluid retention was occurring during the postoperative period.

The problem of fluid retention leading to total excess body water and associated weight gain has been exacerbated by a tradition of routine infusions of large volumes of crystalloids during surgery. This fluid strategy was intended to maintain an adequate circulating volume to ensure organ perfusion and oxygen delivery to the tissues, based on the premise that the patient would be hypovolemic from the combination of prolonged preoperative fasting and third-space losses during surgery.[10] Fluid loading has also been triggered in response to anesthesia-induced hypotension (both general and neuroaxial).

All 3 reasons for fluid loading warrant reexamination. Prolonged preoperative fasting has become a practice that should be relegated to the past. Fasting for 6 hours for solid food and only 2 hours for oral fluids, including carbohydrate-laden fluids, is not only safe but improves outcomes.[11] Even in the presence of prolonged fasting, there is no good evidence to support the administration of large fluid load. There is no evidence of changes in blood volume related to fasting in healthy individuals.[12] The concept of third-space losses has also been largely discredited. This hypothesis[10] claimed that, during surgery, fluid becomes sequestered in traumatized tissues and the gastrointestinal tract, areas called the third space. Trials measuring changes in extracellular volume have consistently failed to show a need for volume expansion.[13] In addition, anesthesia-related hypotension is known to respond poorly to volume loading and is best managed by the administration of vasoconstrictors.[12,14,15]

Although fluid restriction has become the norm in thoracic surgery, elsewhere in surgical practice the volume of administered intraoperative fluids remains highly variable. Bundgaard-Neilsen and colleagues[16] recently reviewed studies comparing restrictive with liberal fluid regimens and their effects on postoperative outcome. Of the 7 randomized trials that were identified, none of which were of lung resections, 6 involved major abdominal surgery and 1 involved knee arthroplasty. They highlighted the lack of definition of liberal or restrictive, with fluid input varying from 2750 to 5388 mL in the liberal groups and 998 to 2740 mL in the restrictive groups. The difficulty of interpreting these studies is in the lack of a common definition of restrictive and liberal and the variation in design, types of fluid administered, indications for administering additional fluid, and outcome variables studied. These studies also excluded a crucial group of patients: those considered at high–risk. Nevertheless, there is a suggestion of better outcomes when fluid is restricted. Three of the studies showed improved outcome with restrictive regimens, whereas 2 showed benefit in selected outcomes and 2 showed no difference. The studies showing no difference used only crystalloid, whereas the 5 showing benefit had included colloid boluses in addition to crystalloid fluids. Improvements noted included faster returns of gastrointestinal function, beneficial effect in pulmonary function, and postoperative hypoxemia. Although overall benefit is not clearly proven, the evidence suggests that restrictive fluid regimens seem to do no harm. This conclusion is not established and is not the conclusive endorsement espoused by restrictive fluid regimen advocates. A continuing concern with restrictive regimens of fluid management is the potential for inadequate preload of the heart leading to a lowered cardiac output and hence poor organ perfusion. For the anesthesiologist, achieving the balance between excessive and inadequate fluid administration is important because both extremes can lead to harm (**Fig. 1**). For lung resection surgeries, fluid management is of even greater importance because of the high comorbidity of the patients and the potential for ALI.

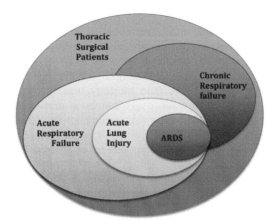

Fig. 1. Following thoracic surgery, 2 clinical patterns of ALI (sometimes overlapping) can be distinguished that develop within 48 to 72 hours after surgery, and a more delayed form developing in the presence of postoperative complications such as aspiration or infection. It is the former that perioperative fluid management seeks to prevent.

STRATEGIES OF FLUID MANAGEMENT: AVOIDING ALI

The diagnosis of ALI/ARDS relies on specific criteria (**Box 1**)[17] but this includes a wide spectrum of injury and causes. Following thoracic surgery, 2 clinical patterns of ALI can be distinguished (sometimes overlapping) that develop within 48 to 72 hours after surgery, and a more delayed form developing in the presence of postoperative complications such as aspiration or infection.[6] It is the former that perioperative fluid management seeks to prevent. In this group of patients (**Fig. 2**), an acute on chronic pattern of respiratory failure may occur with ALI and ARDS developing de novo following surgery or on a background of already chronic respiratory failure in a variety of lung diseases, most commonly chronic obstructive pulmonary disease. The incidence of ALI continues to be reported as between 2% and 4% but with a reduction over the last 2 decades in resulting mortality from universal to around 40%. This decrease can be attributed to improved management of the injury once it has occurred.

ALI and ARDS are the catastrophic responses of the lung to an injury that can be a direct insult to the lung (eg, surgical handling or ventilator induced) or caused by

---

Box 1
ARDS and ALI definitions

American Consensus Conference Diagnostic Criteria for ARDS and ALI

- Acute onset
- Bilateral infiltrates on chest radiograph consistent with pulmonary edema
- Hypoxemia:
  - ALI: Pao_2/forced inspiratory oxygen (Fio_2) ratio <300
  - ARDS: Pao_2/Fio_2 ratio <200
- Absence of heart failure
  - No clinical evidence of left atrial hypertension
  - If measured, pulmonary occlusion pressure <18 mm Hg

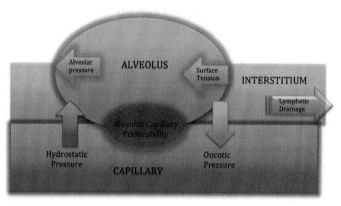

Fig. 2. Determinants of development of alveolar edema.

indirect damage to the alveolar epithelium. There is an initiation of an inflammatory cascade within the alveolar-capillary endothelium and epithelium. A wide range of inflammatory cells, cytokines, and chemokines has been implicated in the process. The resulting damage to the alveolar-capillary membrane results in edema and alveolar flooding, leading eventually to hyaline membrane formation and fibrosis.[18,19]

In the healthy lung, the prevention of alveolar flooding can, simplistically, be regarded (see **Fig. 3**) as primarily the result of 3 factors:

- Capillary hydrostatic pressure
- Oncotic pressure (colloid osmolar pressure)
- Alveolar-capillary permeability

Perturbations in these domains can result in transit of fluid from the vasculature into the alveolar space. An increase in capillary hydrostatic pressure and/or a decrease in oncotic pressure causes an imbalance in the equilibrium between intravascular and extravascular water. The presence of inflammatory mediators increases alveolar-capillary permeability, which, in combination with the imbalance of the other 2 factors, allows more fluid than normal to cross into the alveolae. This process in turn disrupts the surfactant barrier that normally maintains surface tension within the alveolus and exacerbates atelectasis with alveolar collapse.

If, rather than considering how ALI might be treated once present, consideration were given to how its occurrence might be prevented, each of these factors should be considered.

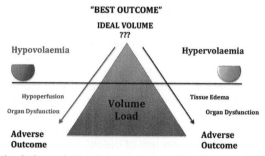

Fig. 3. Achieving the balance between excessive and inadequate fluid administration is important because both extremes can lead to harm.

Reduce Capillary Hydrostatic Pressure: Fluid Restriction

Zeldin and colleagues'[1] conclusions that tackling postthoracotomy pulmonary edema starts by reducing hydrostatic pressure through fluid restriction do not seem unreasonable if the evidence from treating established ARDS is considered. Reducing capillary hydrostatic pressure by targeting fluid replacement therapy to pulmonary artery (PA) occlusion pressure (wedge pressure)[20] and central venous pressure (CVP)[21] may be associated with an improved outcome in already established ALI. In contrast, a persistently positive fluid balance[22] and increased extravascular water[23] are associated with worse outcomes, which is consistent with experimental evidence from as long ago as 1942[24] showing that pulmonary edema following lung resection could be induced by plasma infusion, suggesting that Zeldin and colleagues'[1] supposition was correct. However, Zeldin and colleagues[1] drew their conclusions from a case series of 10 patients, only 4 of whom had adequate fluid data from which to draw any conclusion (level 3 evidence, at best). It has been shown in larger studies, including a cohort analysis of risk factors by Licker and colleagues,[25] that increased fluid administration is associated with the development of ALI. This evidence is better but does not show a causative relationship or that fluid restriction is the correct response. To date, randomized controlled trials have not addressed this issue. Further, despite recognition that postpneumonectomy pulmonary edema is a form of ALI and therefore has a multifactorial causation, restriction of intravenous fluids has continued without consideration of the lack of benefit, or even potential other harm, that might be associated with this approach. That the opposite (ie, overadministration of fluid) is harmful does not confer benefit to restricting fluids.

Increase Oncotic Pressure by Colloid Infusion

If the evidence for manipulating capillary hydrostatic pressure through the restriction of fluid infusion remains unproven, how about evidence for manipulating the oncotic pressure? If the simplistic model of fluid being drawn back in the intravascular space through a higher colloidal osmotic pressure is to be accepted, is there any evidence to support this and, if so, which colloid should be used?

Colloid solutions used in clinical practice are divided into the semisynthetic colloids containing macromolecules such as polysaccharides or polypeptides derived from either plants or animal (gelatins, dextrans, hydroxyethyl starches [HESs]) and the naturally occurring human plasma derivatives (human albumin solutions, plasma protein fraction, fresh frozen plasma, and immunoglobulin solutions).[26] The role of different types of colloids in fluid resuscitation and management is as controversial in anesthetic and critical care as the debate between use of crystalloid and colloid. The relative merits of the 2 classes center around the increase in edema associated with crystalloid therapy and the known adverse effects (eg, hemostatic impairment, anaphylaxis, renal impairment) of some synthetic colloid solutions.

The case for the use of colloid rather than crystalloid solutions was undermined by the publication in 1988 of a systematic review[27] of randomized controlled trials of resuscitation with colloids compared with crystalloids. The results suggested that the use of colloids was associated with an increased absolute risk of mortality of 4% (4 extra deaths in 100 patients treated). However, these were studies using both colloids and crystalloid solutions that were not directly comparable and not reflective of solutions currently in use. Studies[28,29] in other surgical disciplines and settings of ALI/ARDS have not suggested benefit from the use of colloid. When the effects on pulmonary edema formation were compared between crystalloid and colloid fluids, there was no difference in septic or nonseptic patients with or at risk of ALI/ARDS. Provided that fluid overloading is prevented, the type of fluid used for volume loading in mechanically venti- lated patients does not affect pulmonary edema formation in patients with ALI following cardiac and major vascular surgery. The more recent Cochrane Systematic Review[30,31] did reflect more modern practice, although it did not suggest a mortality increase, failed to show benefit in absolute outcome, concluding that there is no evidence from random- ized controlled trials that fluid resuscitation with colloids reduces death compared with resuscitation with crystalloids following surgery. The colloids studied included albumin, plasma protein fraction, HES, modified gelatin, and dextran. The investigators also concluded that, because they are more expensive than crystalloids, it is hard to see how their continued use can be justified outside the context of randomized controlled trials. These studies were focused on nonthoracic surgeries and many featured an inten- sive care unit (ICU) population admitted for sepsis. This finding further limits the useful- ness of these findings to the thoracic anesthesiologist.

That the use of colloid rather than crystalloid does not have absolute benefit in terms of mortality does not exclude the possibility of colloid being beneficial in the presence of pulmonary injury. In surgical patients, Verheij and colleagues[29] compared volume loading with saline, gelatin 4%, HES 6%, and albumin 5%. Compared with the other fluid types, HES ameliorated increased pulmonary permeability.[29] This result is consis- tent with an earlier comparison study between gelatin and HES that showed decreased microvascular permeability and better pulmonary function in the patients treated with HES.[30] In addition, this effect was confirmed in a study showing that HES resuscitation in patients with early ARDS not only significantly improved their hemodynamics and cardiac output without worsening pulmonary edema and pulmonary mechanics but also attenuated membrane permeability.[32] The same investigators and others have fol- lowed through to investigate the role of HES in potentially attenuating lung injury. In animal models,[33,34] HES reduced high-tidal-volume mechanical ventilator–induced lung injury and neutrophil infiltration and pulmonary edema compared with infusions of crystalloid. This basic research provides new avenues to explore the role of HES in patients having thoracic surgery but confirmation of efficacy is needed in ALI attenuation in clinical practice and confirmation of lack of harm to other organ systems, including the kidneys, before colloids can be recommended as a treatment of pulmonary injury.[26,27,30]

Prevent Increases in Alveolar-Capillary Permeability

These suggested effects of HES on membrane permeability suggest the third approach to preventing and tackling lung injury during thoracic surgery: how to prevent an increase in alveolar-capillary permeability. ALI is commonly seen in the dependent, ventilated lung rather than in the operated lung. In a series of patients with ALI/ARDS following lobectomy, 8/9 patients had increased density in the nonoperated lung on chest radiography.[35] This finding suggests that ventilator-induced lung injury and other factors unrelated to surgical resection play a role in lung injury and are potential targets of therapy. Mechanical ventilation, and in particular one-lung ventilation (OLV), is well recognized as a source of lung injury operating in part at the alveolar-capillary level. High-tidal-volume ventilation is thought to cause disruption of the alveolar-capillary barrier with overdistension, tensile strain, and shear stress.[36] It is also well recognized that ventilation produces an inflammatory reaction.[37] This has led to the current prac- tice of lung-protective ventilation based on evidence from the management of ALI and ARDS following ARDS Network studies.[38] This strategy involves achieving lung venti- lation tidal volume 6 to 8 mL/kg ideal body weight or less, preferably using the pressure- limiting benefits of pressure-controlled ventilation. Extrapolating from the evidence for ventilating patients with ALI/ARDS with pressure-controlled ventilation, this is in a group of patients who, by definition, have poor lung function. The next question is whether this can be extrapolated to OLV.

Although the scientific evidence suggests that traditional ventilator settings are dangerous even for healthy lungs, no level 1 study criteria has shown demonstrable clinical benefits to using low-pressure, low-volume ventilation in OLV settings. The role of anesthetic[39] and other agents that are administered to patients should also be considered, along with their effects on the inflammatory response and contribution to disruption of the alveolar-capillary membrane integrity.

In summary, the evidence suggests that the cause and perioperative management of ALI are more complex than simple fluid management. A multimodal approach, focused on ventilation settings, surgical approach, and fluid therapy, targeting the inflammatory mechanisms at the root of ALI, offers the best hope to reduce the incidence of this tragic complication.

FLUID MANAGEMENT AND THE KIDNEYS

The dangers of acute renal injury (acute kidney injury [AKI]) after thoracic surgery have largely been underappreciated. The adoption of standardized diagnostic criteria for AKI along with the understanding that even those patients with low-grade renal impairment face worsened outcomes has led to a reexamination of the role of thoracic surgery fluid management with respect to AKI. The development of the Acute Kidney Injury Network (AKIN) and renal risk, injury, failure, loss, end-stage disease (RIFLE) classifications systems for AKI has provided a means by which to rank the severity of renal injury in the perioperative period.[40,41] By examining the relative changes in serum creatinine and glomerular filtration rate the RIFLE criteria rank AKI (from mildest to most severe) as risk, injury, failure, loss, and end-stage renal disease. The more recent AKIN criteria comprise 3 stages that correspond with the risk, injury, and failure stages of RIFLE. The widespread adoption of these classification systems (**Table 2**)[41] has aided in understanding both the incidence and impact of perioperative AKI.

Of particular importance to cardiothoracic anesthesiologists are data showing worsened outcomes in patients developing perioperative AKI, even in its mildest forms, compared with those patients who do not develop AKI. In a retrospective study of long-term outcomes following thoracic surgeries, AKI was associated with an adjusted

Table 2		
Classification/staging system for acute kidney injury		
Stage	**Serum Creatinine Criteria**	**Urine Output Criteria**
1	Increase in serum creatinine of more than or equal to 0.3 mg/dL ($\geq$26.4 μmol/L) or increase to more than or equal to 15.0%–200% (1.5-fold to 2-fold) from baseline	Less than 0.5 mL/kg per hour for more than 6 h
2	Increase in serum creatinine to more than 200%–300% (>2-fold to 3-fold) from baseline	Less than 0.5 mL/kg per hour for more than 12 h
3	Increase in serum creatinine to more than 300% (>3-fold) from baseline (or serum creatinine of $\geq$4.0 mg/dL [$\geq$354 μmol/L] with an acute increase of at least 0.5 mg/dL [44 μmol/L])	Less than 0.3 mL/kg per hour for 24 h or anuria for 12 h

hazard ratio of 1.60 (1.18–2.17) for long-term survival compared with an absence of AKI.[42] Perhaps most concerning is that even those patients who completely recovered from their AKI showed worse outcomes than those patients without perioperative AKI. Thus, perioperative care plans targeted to avoid any degree of renal injury are warranted.

The reported incidence of perioperative AKI in lung resection surgery varies widely from institution and patient group. A retrospective analysis of 401 patients admitted to the University of Florida ICU following thoracic surgery showed a 33% incidence of AKI.[42] A 1129-patient trial from Vancouver, Canada, using the AKIN classification system found a 14% incidence of AKI following pneumonectomy and a 6% incidence in lesser resections.[43] Patients with AKI had increased complication rates and prolonged lengths of stay. Swiss investigators using the RIFLE classification found a 7% incidence of AKI following lung resection surgery with higher ASA (American Society of Anesthesiologists) score and poor pulmonary function as markers of greatest risk.[44] As with the previous studies, AKI led to increased rates of ICU admissions, death, and cardiothoracic complications.

The cause of perioperative AKI remains unclear and the hazards of either excessive or inadequate fluid therapy should be considered. General anesthetics exert an inhibitory effect on renal hemodynamics and function, as reflected by a depression of glomerular filtration rate, urinary volume, and sodium excretion.[45] Because the kidneys are responsible for the excretion of most administered fluids, renal functional demands are increased in a state of fluid overload. Excretion of fluid excess in the range of 1.5 to 2 L may take 2 days even in healthy volunteers, and possibly more in postsurgical patients.[46] Ishikawa and colleagues[43] found that patients having thoracic surgery who developed AKI received more intraoperative crystalloid than those without AKI, but this association was likely caused by the length of surgery and other factors particular to this group. At this time, the role of fluid excess in postoperative renal morbidity remains undetermined.

Total intraoperative volume of infused crystalloid was not independently associated with AKI in a large retrospective observational study of patients undergoing lung resection surgery. However, thoracic surgery with restrictive fluid therapy may lead to an environment of renal hypoperfusion secondary to inadequate fluids and hemodynamics. Because data are lacking to determine the incidence and impact of renal hypoperfusion on perioperative kidney injury, it is prudent to carefully monitor hemodynamics and urine flow rates and promptly treat unstable hemodynamics to minimize the risks for prolonged renal hypoperfusion.

There is limited and contradictory evidence on the use of synthetic colloids and provocation of acute renal failure in the perioperative period. A retrospective study suggested an association between administration of HES and AKI after lung resection surgery.[43] As noted by the investigators, this association should be treated with caution because only a small number of patients had received HES. A retrospective study of patients who had cardiac surgery similarly found that HESs may be associated with a modest impairment of renal function.[47] These studies are in contrast with randomized trials and a US Food and Drug Administration registration trial in the perioperative period of HES that did not find evidence for renal injury in thoracic or other surgeries.[48–50]

Recent literature provides new guidance for the anesthesiologist on how to appropriately prescribe colloids in the perioperative setting.[51] One issue relates to the volume of HES administered. Studies using lower volumes of HES (approximately 1000 mL in the first 48 hours) showed HES not to be associated with AKI or the need for renal replacement therapy.[52,53] In contrast, studies showing increased renal injury with HES typically used higher dosages, up to 70 mL/kg.[54,55] Second, HES solutions are hyperoncotic and provide little free water. Avoidance of a hyperoncotic state, which will predictably result in an osmotic necrosis-based kidney injury, is essential.[52,56,57] HES use therefore seems most appropriate when used as a part of a multimodal volume resuscitation strategy and not as the sole fluid agent, as was the case in many large HES trials that found HES harmful.[54,55]

FLUID MANAGEMENT AND THE HEART

Although cardiac complications account for a large percentage of perioperative morbidity, the effect of fluid restriction on these complications is unknown. Intraoperative interventions have significant effects that may have implications for postoperative sequelae. During OLV in a healthy subject, there is a progressive, if modest, increase in pulmonary arterial pressure without changes in the systemic pressures. Although these changes are of no significance in well individuals, OLV in patients with significant parenchymal lung disease and baseline pulmonary hypertension produces more pronounced and potentially significant effects. With lung resection, pulmonary arterial ligation causes an initial increase in PA pressure and pulmonary vascular resistance (PVR) and hence an acute increase in right ventricular afterload. Right ventricular ejection fraction tends to continue to decrease over the first few days after surgery. This decrease has been presumed to be consequent on raised afterload and occurs despite normalization of PA pressure and PVR.[58] Development of postoperative heart failure is assumed to be a consequence of right heart disease and secondary to the increase in right ventricular afterload.[59] Although pressure overload is presumed to be the cause, the role of volume overload should not be forgotten as a consequence of overzealous fluid administration.

INDIVIDUALIZED, GOAL-DIRECTED FLUID MANAGEMENT

Although the evidence seems to suggest that a restrictive fluid regimen is at least not generally harmful, this general approach to treating patients does not fit the heterogeneity of a typical clinical practice. Anesthesiologists traditionally relied on easily measurable parameters, typically a combination of heart rate and blood pressure, to indicate fluid status. Hypotension combined with tachycardia triggered fluid boluses because hypovolemia was assumed to be present. However, these indicators are neither specific nor sensitive markers of fluid status and hence a strategy based solely on these can often result in overzealous fluid loading with overall detrimental effects. CVP measurements do not give an accurate assessment of blood volume or predict the response to a fluid challenge either by the absolute value or the rate of change of CVP.[60] In the 1980s, Shoemaker and colleagues[61] used the PA catheter (PAC) to measure tissue oxygen delivery in high-risk surgical patients with the intention of achieving supranormal oxygen delivery with to improve outcomes. Although the initial results were encouraging, the PAC can cause an increase in morbidity and mortality and its pressure-based measurements have many of the same limitations as does CVP. Large outcome studies based on PA-based pressure measurements have not shown benefit.[62]

With the advent of less invasive methods such as esophageal Doppler and pulse contour of monitoring flow-based hemodynamic parameters[63] interest has revived in goal-directed therapy. The intention of goal-directed therapy in the present context is to prevent tissue oxygen debt by maintaining tissue perfusion, and thus avoid perioperative and postoperative complications. The nonthoracic surgical literature provides increasing support to this approach,[64] suggesting the importance of individualized goal-directed fluid therapy and hemodynamic management. The common approach is fluid therapy individualized to patients based on objective feedback on their fluid responsiveness. However, the validity of these parameters is not clear in surgery requiring thoracotomy or in lung resection. In thoracic patients, the questions remain as to which method to use to determine hemodynamic status and which target to achieve.

A recent small study (27 patients in total)[65] suggested that using a volume strategy orientated to stroke volume variation as measured using the PiCCO (Pulse Contour Cardiac Output) system did not result in pulmonary fluid overload or deleterious reduction of pulmonary function during thoracic surgery requiring lateral thoracotomy and OLV. However, there was no comparison group, limiting this study to showing that stroke volume variation–guided fluid management in thoracic surgery may be useful but requires further investigation. Similarly the Flo Trac/Vigileo system, which uses an analysis of the peripheral arterial pulse to calculate cardiac output via comparison with algorithms, may also be useful and less invasive than other forms of cardiac output monitoring. This method does not require calibration but this may also be a limiting factor. In a direct comparison study with continuous cardiac output monitoring via thermodilution-calibrated pulmonary arterial measurement there was no clinical equivalence.[66] Nevertheless the arterial pulse waveform analysis does allow tracking of changes in cardiac output and has potential as a trend monitor.

In the intraoperative setting, the use of the esophageal Doppler monitor seems to be the most promising minimally invasive technique for measuring dynamic cardiovascular performance because it is supported by the most evidence. Positive outcome studies in colorectal surgery have resulted in the use of esophageal Doppler being recommended for use in the United Kingdom (National Institute for Health and Clinical Excellence [NICE] Guidelines on Intravenous Fluid Therapy for Adult Surgical Patients [GIFTASUP]),[67,68] the United States (Medicare and Medicaid), and Europe (Enhanced Recovery After Surgery [ERAS]).[69] Esophageal Doppler monitoring uses Doppler ultrasound technology to analyze the blood flow in the descending aorta. The probe is placed in the esophagus and aligned with the blood flow to produce a flow velocity profile for each heart beat, producing a waveform that is used in conjunction with a nomogram of biometric data to derive a value for stroke volume. This Doppler monitoring allows noninvasive beat-to-beat measurements and therefore continuous cardiac output monitoring. Concerns about the effects OLV might have on measurements have been dispelled because a pilot study of esophageal Doppler in thoracic surgical patients showed its ability to detect and guide hemodynamic management in these patients.[70] Esophageal Doppler has also been used to guide intraoperative fluid management successfully while comparing different colloid regimens in thoracic surgery,[48] again showing the potential this method has for optimizing fluid management and hemodynamic status.

SUMMARY

The debate on the appropriate fluid therapy for lung resection surgeries has been argued from concerns about excess intraoperative fluid administration and its impact on ALI to concerns about inadequate tissue perfusion and AKI with restricted fluid protocols. Better understanding of the pathophysiology of ALI and the hazards inherent to both extremes in volume status has led efforts toward goal-directed, individualized therapies designed to achieve optimal hemodynamic status. Such strategies offer opportunities for improved outcomes, although, unlike in abdominal and orthopedic surgery, data are lacking for thoracic surgery. The role for colloids both as a volume expander and potential protective agent against ALI is similarly receiving revived interest. Here again, clinical investigations are required to show and define the beneficial or harmful effects of colloids. The evidence for the impact of fluid therapy as a means to improve outcome is encouraging and supports the undertaking of properly designed perioperative fluid trials in thoracic surgeries. Such work offers hope that optimal fluid strategies can be defined and reduce the adverse events that have affected patients having lung resection. Until such studies are completed, the debate about proper fluid management in these cases will continue.

REFERENCES

1. Zeldin RA, Normandin D, Landtwing D, et al. Post-pneumonectomy pulmonary oedema. J Thorac Cardiovasc Surg 1984;87:359–65.
2. Boffa DJ, Allen MS, Grab JD, et al. Data from the Society of Thoracic Surgeons General Thoracic Surgery database: the surgical management of primary lung tumours. J Thorac Cardiovasc Surg 2008;135:247–54.
3. Goodney PP, Lucas FL, Stukel TA, et al. Surgeon specialty and operative mortality with lung resection. Ann Surg 2005;241:179–84.
4. Urbach DR, Baxter NN. Does it matter what a hospital is high volume for? Specificity of hospital volume-outcome associations for surgical procedures: analysis of administrative data. BMJ 2004;328:737–40.
5. Lien YC, Huang MT, Lin HC. Association between surgeon and hospital volume and in-hospital fatalities after lung cancer resections: the experience of an Asian country. Ann Thorac Surg 2007;83:1837–43.
6. Licker M, Fauconnet P, Villiger Y, et al. Acute lung injury and outcomes after thoracic surgery. Curr Opin Anaesthesiol 2009;22:61–7.
7. Desborough JP. The stress response to trauma and surgery. Br J Anaesth 2000; 85:109–17.
8. Wilmore DW. Metabolic responses to severe surgical illness: an overview. World J Surg 2000;24:705–11.
9. Cagini L, Capozzi R, Tassi V, et al. Fluid and electrolyte balance after major thoracic surgery by bioimpedance and endocrine evaluation. Eur J Cardiothorac Surg 2011;40:e71–6.
10. Shires T, Williams J, Brown F. Acute change in extracellular fluids associated with major surgical procedures. Ann Surg 1961;154:803–10.
11. Brady M, Kinn S, Stuart P. Preoperative fasting for adults to prevent perioperative complications. Cochrane Database Syst Rev 2003;(4):CD004423.
12. Jacob M, Chappell D, Conzen P, et al. Blood volume is normal after pre-operative overnight fasting. Acta Anaesthesiol Scand 2008;52:522–9.
13. Brandstrup B, Svensen C, Engquist A. Haemorrhage and operation and operation cause a contraction of the extracellular space needing replacement – evidence and implications. A systematic review. Surgery 2006;139:419–32.
14. Tatara T, Tashiro C. Quantitative analysis of fluid balance during abdominal surgery. Anesth Analg 2007;104:347–54.
15. Tuman KJ, McCarthy RJ, March RJ, et al. Effects of phenylephrine or volume loading on right ventricular function in patients undergoing myocardial revascularisation. J Cardiothoracic Vascular Anesthesia 1995;9:2–8.
16. Bundgaard-Neilsen M, Secher NH, Kehlet H. Liberal' vs. 'restrictive' perioperative fluid therapy – a critical analysis of the evidence. Acta Anaesthesiol Scand 2009; 53:843–51.
17. Bernard GR, Artigas A, Brigham KL, et al. The American-European consensus conference on ARD: definitions, mechanisms, relevant outcomes and clinical trial co-ordination. Intensive Care Medicine 1994;20:225–32.

18. Ware LB, Matthay MA. The acute respiratory distress syndrome. N Engl J Med 2000;342:1334–49.

19. Luce JM. Acute lung injury and the acute respiratory distress syndrome. Crit Care Med 1998;26:369–76.

20. Humphrey H, Hall J, Sznajder I, et al. Improved survival in ARDS patients associated with a reduction in pulmonary capillary wedge pressure. Chest 1990;97:1176–80.

21. National Heart Lung and Blood Institute Acute Respiratory Distress Syndrome Clinical Trials Network. Comparison of two fluid-management strategies in acute lung injury. N Engl J Med 2006;354:1564–75.

22. Rosenberg AL, Deschert RE, Park PK, et al. Review of a large clinical series. Association of cumulative fluid balance on outcome in acute lung injury. A retrospective review of the ARDS Net Tidal Volume Study Cohort. J Intensive Care Med 2009;24:35–46.

23. Davey-Quinn A, Gedney J, Whiteley S, et al. Extravascular lung water and acute respiratory distress syndrome: oxygenation and outcome. Anaesth Intensive Care 1999;27:357–62.

24. Gibbon JH, Gibbon MH. Experimental pulmonary edema following lobectomy and plasma infusion. J Thorac Surg 1942;12:694–704.

25. Licker M, De Perrot M, Spiliopoulos A, et al. Risk factors for acute lung injury after thoracic surgery for lung cancer. Anesth Analg 2003;97:1558–65.

26. Grocott MP, Mythen MG, Gan TJ. Perioperative fluid management and clinical outcomes in adults. Anesth Analg 2005;100:1093–106.

27. Schierhout G, Roberts I. Fluid resuscitation with colloid or crystalloid solutions in critically ill patients: a systematic review of randomized trials. Br J Med 1988;316:961–4.

28. Van der Heijden M, Verheij J, Amerongen GP, et al. Crystalloid or colloid fluid loading and pulmonary permeability, oedema and injury in septic and nonseptic patients. Crit Care Med 2009;37:1275–81.

29. Verheij J, van Lingen A, Raijmakers PG, et al. Effect of fluid loading with saline or colloids on pulmonary permeability, oedema and lung injury score after cardiac or major vascular surgery. Br J Anaesth 2006;96:21–30.

30. Perel P, Roberts I. Colloids versus crystalloids for fluid resuscitation in critically ill patients. Cochrane Database of Systematic Reviews 2012;(6):CD000567.

31. Rittoo D, Gosling P, Burnley S, et al. Randomised study comparing the effects of hydroxyethyl starch solution with Gelofusine on pulmonary function in patients undergoing abdominal aortic aneurysm surgery. Br J Anesth 2004;92:61–6.

32. Huang CC, Kao KC, Hsu KH, et al. Effects of hydroxyethyl starch resuscitation on extravascular lung water and pulmonary permeability in sepsis-related acute respiratory distress syndrome. Crit Care Med 2009;37:1948–55.

33. Li LF, Huang C, Liu YY, et al. Hydroxyethyl starch reduces high stretch ventilation-augmented lung injury via vascular endothelial growth factor. Transl Res 2011;157:293–305.

34. Balkamou X, Xanthos T, Strompoulis K, et al. Hydroxyethyl starch 6% (130/0.4) ameliorates acute lung injury in Swine haemorrhagic shock. Anesthesiology 2010;113:1092–8.

35. Padley SP, Jordan SJ, Goldstraw P, et al. Asymmetric ARDS following pulmonary resection: CT findings – initial observations. Radiology 2002;223:468–73.

36. Frank JA, Matthay MA. Science review: mechanisms of ventilator induced injury. Crit Care 2003;7:233–41.

37. Ranieri VM, Suter PM, Tortorella C, et al. Effects of mechanical ventilation on inflammatory mediator in patients with acute respiratory distress syndrome: a randomised controlled trial. JAMA 1999;282:54–61.

38. The Acute Respiratory Distress Syndrome Network. Ventilation with lower tidal volumes as compared with traditional tidal volumes for acute lung injury and the acute respiratory distress syndrome. N Engl J Med 2000;342:1301–8.

39. Schilling T, Kozian A, Kretzschmar M, et al. Effects of propofol and desflurane anaesthesia on the alveolar inflammatory response to one-lung ventilation. Br J Anaesth 2007;99:368–75.

40. Bellomo R, Ronco C, Kellum JA, et al. Acute renal failure – definition, outcome measures, animal models, fluid therapy and information technology needs: the Second International Consensus Conference of the Acute Dialysis Quality Initiative (ADQI) group. Crit Care 2004;8:R204.

41. Mehta RL, Kellum JA, Dhah SV, et al. Acute Kidney Injury Network: report of an initiative to improve outcomes in acute kidney injury. Crit Care 2007;11:R31.

42. Hobson CE, Yavas S, Segal M, et al. Acute kidney injury is associated with increased long term mortality after cardiothoracic surgery. Circulation 2009;119: 2444–53.

43. Ishikawa S, Griesdale DE, Lohser J. Acute kidney injury after lung resection surgery: incidence and perioperative risk factors. Anesth Analg 2012;114:1256–62.

44. Licker M, Cartier V, Robert J, et al. Risk factors of acute kidney injury according to RIFLE criteria after lung cancer surgery. Ann Thorac Surg 2011;91:844–51.

45. Cousins MJ, Skowronski G, Plummer SL. Anaesthesia and the kidneys. Anaesth Intensive Care 1983;11:292–5.

46. Holte K, Sharrock NE, Kehlet H. Pathophysiology & clinical implications of perioperative fluid excess. Br J Anaesth 2002;89:622–32.

47. Winkelmayer WC, Glynn RJ, Levin R, et al. Hydroxyethyl starch and change in renal function in patients undergoing coronary artery bypass graft surgery. Kidney Int 2003;64:1046–9.

48. Abdallah MS, Assad OM. Randomised study comparing the effect of hydroxyethyl starch HES130/0.4, HES 200/0.5 and modified fluid gelatin for perioperative volume replacement in thoracic surgery: guided by transoesophageal Doppler. EJCTA 2010;4:76–84.

49. Godet G, Lehot JJ, Janvier G, et al. Safety of HES 130/0.4 (Voluvens) in patients with preoperative renal dysfunction undergoing abdominal aortic surgery: a prospective, randomized, controlled, parallel-group multicentre trial. European Journal of Anesthesiology 2009;25:986–94.

50. Mahmood A, Gosling P, Vohra RK. Randomized clinical trial comparing the effects on renal function of hydroxyethyl starch or gelatin during aortic aneurysm surgery. Br J Surg 2007;94:427–33.

51. Kaplan LJ. To dose or not to dose: that is the (starch) question…. Crit Care 2010; 14:148.

52. Boussekey N, Darmon R, Langois J, et al. Resuscitation with low volume hydroxyethyl starch 130 kDa/0.4 is not associated with acute kidney injury. Crit Care 2010;14:R40.

53. Sakr Y, Payen D, Reinhart K, et al. Effects of hydroxyethyl starch administration on renal function in critically ill patients. Br J Anaesthesia 2007;98(2):216–24.

54. Brunkhorst F, Engel C, Bloos F, et al. German Competence Network Sepsis (SepNet): intensive insulin therapy and pentastarch resuscitation in severe sepsis. N Engl J Med 2008;358:125–39.

55. Schortgen F, Lacherade JC, Bruneel F, et al. Effects of hydroxyethylstarch and gelatin on renal function in severe sepsis: a multicentre randomised study. Lancet 2001;357:911–6.

56. Schortgen F, Girou E, Deye N, et al, CRYCO Study Group. The risk associated with hyperoncotic colloids in patients with shock. Intensive Care Med 2008;34:2157–68.
57. Wiedermann CJ, Dunzendorfer S, Gaioni LU, et al. Hyperoncotic colloids and acute kidney injury: a meta-analysis of randomized trials. Crit Care 2010;14:R191.
58. Heerdt PM, Malhotra J. The right ventricular response to lung resection. In: Slinger P, editor. Progress in thoracic anesthesia. Lippincott Williams & Williams; 2004.
59. De Decker K, Jorens PG, Van Schil P. Cardiac complications after noncardiac thoracic surgery: an evidence-based current review. Ann Thorac Surg 2003;75: 1340–8.
60. Marik PE, Baram M, Vahid B. Does central venous pressure predict fluid responsiveness? A systemic review of the literature and the tale of seven mares. Chest 2008;134:172–8.
61. Shoemaker WC, Appel PL, Kram HB, et al. Prospective trial of supranormal values of survivors as therapeutic goals in high-risk surgical patients. Chest 1988;94:1176–86.
62. Sandham JD, Hull RD, Brant RF, et al. Trial of the use of pulmonary-artery catheters in high-risk surgical patients. N Engl J Med 2003;348:5–14.
63. Matthews L, Singh KR. Cardiac output monitoring. Ann Card Anaesth 2008;11: 56–68.
64. Bungaard-Neilsen M, Ruhnau B, Secher NH, et al. Flow-related techniques for pre-operative goal-directed fluid optimisation. Br J Anaesth 2007;98:38–44.
65. Haas S, Eichhorn V, Hasbach T, et al. Goal-directed fluid therapy using stroke volume variation does not result in pulmonary fluid overload in thoracic surgery requiring one lung ventilation. Critical Care Research & Practice 2012. Article ID 687018.
66. Hamm JB, Nguven BV, Ross G, et al. Assessment of a cardiac output device using arterial pulse waveform analysis, Vigileo, in cardiac surgery compared to pulmonary arterial thermodilution. Anesth Intensive Care 2010;38:295–301.
67. National Institute for Health and Clinical Excellence (NICE) guidance. Available at: http://guidance.nice.org.uk/MTG3. Accessed July 3, 2012.
68. Powell-Tuck J, Gosling P, Lobo DN, et al. 'British Consensus Guidelines on Intravenous Fluid Therapy for Adult Surgical Patients (GIFTASUP)'. Available at: http://www.bapen.org.uk/pdfs/bapen_pubs/giftasup.pdf. Accessed July 3, 2012.
69. Lassen K, Soop M, Nygren J, et al. Consensus review of optimal perioperative care in colorectal surgery: enhanced Recovery After Surgery (ERAS) Group recommendations. Arch Surg 2009;144:961–9.
70. Diaper J, Ellenberger C, Villiger Y, et al. Transoesophageal Doppler monitoring for fluid and hemodynamic treatment during lung surgery. J Clin Monit Comput 2008; 22:367–74.

Transesophageal Echocardiography in Noncardiac Thoracic Surgery

Breandan Sullivan, MD*, Ferenc Puskas, MD, PhD,
Ana Fernandez-Bustamante, MD, PhD

KEYWORDS

- Noncardiac thoracic surgery • Transesophageal echocardiography
- Lung resection surgery • Thoracic aortic surgery

KEY POINTS

- Transesophageal echocardiography (TEE) is a minimally invasive monitor that has multiple applications in the operating room and in the intensive care unit.
- Although there is a lack of evidence in TEE improving outcomes outside of cardiac surgery, TEE is rapidly becoming a more common monitor in the operating room for critically ill patients undergoing high-risk surgery.
- For patients undergoing noncardiac thoracic surgery, TEE offers multiple additional benefits such as: rapid and reliable monitoring of right heart function; monitoring of lesions that can predict adverse outcomes (aortic atheromas); and assistance in placing extracorporeal membrane oxygenation cannulas.

▶ Clip 1. Midesophageal right ventricular (LV) inflow outflow view. Clip 2. Transgastric LV short axis view. Clip 3. Transgastric LV short axis. Clip 4. Reperfusion of the left lung during a double lung transplant for idiopathic pulmonary fibrosis. Video clips accompany this article at http://www.anesthesiology.theclinics.com/

INTRODUCTION

In the last decade, transesophageal echocardiography (TEE) has become essential in cardiac surgery, and has expanded its role in other areas of surgical care (Videos 1–4, available in online version of this article). TEE aids in diagnosis in hemodynamically unstable patients and in guiding fluid resuscitation in trauma patients. Additionally, they can help narrow differential diagnosis in critically ill patients. Outside of cardiac

Department of Anesthesiology and Critical Care Medicine, University of Colorado School of Medicine, Mail Stop B113, 12401 East 17th Avenue, Room 727, Aurora, CO 80045, USA
* Corresponding author.
E-mail address: breandan.sullivan@ucdenver.edu

Anesthesiology Clin 30 (2012) 657–669
http://dx.doi.org/10.1016/j.anclin.2012.08.007   **anesthesiology.theclinics.com**

surgery, TEE has been used in postcardiac arrest in the operating room and in the intensive care unit (ICU) and diagnoses the etiology of the arrest with extremely high accuracy.[1] TEE is also used routinely to assess for clot or tumor extension in the inferior vena cava during nephrectomy for renal cell carcinoma.[2] It is commonly used to assess for the presence of intracardiac shunt in patients with refractory hypoxemia as well as patients with a likelihood of left-sided cardiac thrombus. However, outside of cardiac surgery, TEE is not routinely used to guide resuscitation or as a monitor for continuous cardiac monitoring in noncardiac surgery. Despite the expanded role of TEE in the operating room and the ICU, there are no randomized trials that the authors could identify that have tested TEE as a routine monitor in noncardiac thoracic surgery; however in high-risk surgeries with medically complicated patients, TEE adds an additional level of monitoring with which few can disagree. This article presents multiple applications of TEE that can assist both the anesthesiologist and the surgeon through major noncardiac thoracic surgery. It highlights how TEE can be used as an adjuvant to lung resection surgery; TEE as a monitor during lung transplantation; TEE to assess patients for extracorporeal membrane oxygenation (ECMO); TEE for thoracic aortic surgery; and TEE in the assessment of patients with acute pulmonary hypertension undergoing noncardiac thoracic surgery.

CURRENT MONITORING PRACTICES IN THORACIC SURGERY

Continuous cardiac output monitors are showing a great emergence in the operating room. There are numerous trials trying to assess the outcomes of managing patients with a goal-directed strategy. Unfortunately, pulmonary artery catheters (PACs) remain the most common continuous cardiac output monitor that anesthesiologists rely on, and there is no uniformly accepted practice of managing the data generated from these catheters. PACs are placed in patients with low ejection fractions undergoing major surgery or patients in whom fluid status and cardiac function are difficult to interpret. In a landmark trial published in 2003 in the *New England Journal of Medicine,* PACs were compared with the standard of care in high-risk elderly surgery patients.[3] In a subgroup of thoracic surgery patients, the mortality rate was increased in the patients who were managed with PACs, although in all groups there was no increased mortality. The authors concluded that there was no benefit to the management of high-risk elderly patients with the addition of PACs.

Many clinicians believe that PACs will allow them to guide therapy in an appropriate patient population. In addition to the tremendous variability of interpretation of data generated by PAC measurements, numerous other studies exist that show no benefit in patients being managed with these invasive monitors compared with patients managed without PACs. In 2005, the ESCAPE trial (Evaluation of Heart Failure and Pulmonary Artery Catheterization Effectiveness trial) randomized 433 patients with symptomatic heart failure to clinical decision making with or without a PAC and revealed no difference in the amount of patient days alive or days out of hospital during the first 6 months.[4] Similar studies showing a lack of benefit can be found in the critical care literature as well.[5–7] However, many clinicians still rely on PACs to manage patients who are not improving despite aggressive interventions.

If PACs were not beneficial in the management of heart failure patients and in the management of high-risk thoracic surgery patients, then how would a TEE be beneficial? The degree of correlation between hemodynamic variables taken from TEE and PAC is relatively unresolved, largely owing to a scarcity of data providing their direct, real-time comparison. Su and colleagues[8] used both TEE and PAC to simultaneously measure cardiac output every 15 minutes in patients undergoing routine coronary artery bypass graft (CABG). The results of that study indicate that there is good agreement between cardiac output measurements obtained from TEE compared with the continuous cardiac output obtained from PAC. Alternatively, Ali and colleagues[9] showed poor correlation between estimated pulmonary artery wedge pressures by TEE and those generated by PAC. This study was limited by being retrospective in nature and therefore did not offer the exact timing between numbers generated by TEE versus PAC to produce an accurate correlation. These studies also do not address the benefit that a TEE can provide in assessment of overall left ventricular (LV) systolic function, right ventricular (RV) systolic function, the presence of pericardial or pleural effusions, valvular dysfunction, and clot in transit.

Despite the widespread use of TEE during cardiac surgery, the PAC remains the most common tool for continuous cardiac monitoring postoperatively, and probably the most common tool to evaluate high-risk thoracic surgery patients in the operating room. Crucial decisions are often made by clinicians on the basis of PAC-generated numbers, many of which have significant impact on patients' overall care (eg, choice of vasoactive drugs, decision to administer fluid vs blood, decision to extubate). In survey questionnaires, Jain and colleagues[10,11] demonstrated that there is significant heterogeneity among intensivists in selecting an intervention based on PAC data and that the addition of echocardiography information may influence which intervention is chosen.

The use of PACs is becoming increasingly controversial, as their use carries significant risk of complication, and numerous studies have failed to show a positive outcome benefits.[5] As such, the routine use of the PAC is being phased out of use in the management of critically ill patients (as evidenced by a 65% and 63% reduction in the use of PAC among medical ICU (MICU) and surgical ICU (SICU) patients, respectively, between the years 1993 and 2004).[12] However, anesthesiologists seem to differ from intensivists in this regard. A survey performed by Jacka and colleagues[13] among 345 cardiac anesthesiologists in 2002, revealed that the PAC was used and preferred more than twice as frequently as TEE during cardiac surgery.

The most recent American Society of Anesthesiologists (ASA) practice guidelines for perioperative TEE are broadly applicable and are not very prescriptive. A slightly modified list of the recommendations follows.[14]

The authors believe that for noncardiac thoracic surgery TEE offers an increased level of monitoring and is superior to the PAC.

Noncardiac Surgery

A TEE may be used when the surgery or the patient's cardiovascular comorbidities may result in severe hemodynamic, pulmonary, or neurologic compromise.

If equipment and the expertise to use the equipment are readily available, a TEE should be used when life-threatening circulatory instability persists and is unresponsive to conventional interventions.

Intraoperative Right Heart Evaluation During Thoracic Surgery

TEE is the only monitor that can provide simultaneous biventricular monitoring. The authors are advocating focused attention to the right ventricle during thoracic surgery; however any time a TEE is placed intraoperatively, a standard 20-view examination should be performed.[15] Unexpected hypotension during thoracic surgery can be the manifestation of right heart dysfunction. Acute right heart dysfunction can result from hypoxia and hypercarbia during 1 lung ventilation or during clamping of a branch of the pulmonary artery during pneumonectomy or lung transplantation. Direct monitoring of pulmonary pressure is not useful, because it tells an incomplete story. Only the visualization of the right ventricle with TEE allows a direct assessment of RV function, and only the visualization of the problem can aid the anesthesiologist to assess what treatment is needed. Assessing the right heart function has 3 key elements: free wall motion, tricuspid annular plane systolic excursion (TAPSE), and interventricular septal function.

Free wall motion
Free wall motion requires the contraction on circumferential and longitudinal RV fibers. This can best be assessed in the midespophageal RV inflow–outflow view (omniplane 40–60°) (**Fig. 1**).

Tricuspid annular plane systolic excursion
The efficacy of longitudinal contraction can be best assessed in the midesophageal 4-chamber view. In this view, the right and left ventricles are visualized; the right and left atria are seen as well. In patients with RV failure, the intra-atrial septum can be seen bowing into the left atrium. However, special attention should be devoted to the tricuspid annulus. By measuring the length the lateral aspect of the tricuspid annulus moves in 1 cardiac cycle, one can quickly assess the systolic function of the right ventricle. This is an accurate and validated measurement that can be done quickly and is easily repeated (**Fig. 2**).

Intraventricular septal function
This is best assessed in the deep transgastric LV short axis view also known as the midpapillary short axis view. The TEE probe should be advanced into the stomach and retroflexed. The shape of the septum is important to note, especially if the septum appears to be flattened, making the left ventricle into a D shape. This is a sign of either pressure or volume overload of the right ventricle. In peak systole, if the shape of the left ventricle resembles a D, this is evidence of pressure overload; if the D shape is more pronounced in end diastole, this is evidence of volume overload (**Fig. 3**).[16–18]

The simplicity of this focused right heart evaluation allows a single anesthesiologist to perform multiple examinations quickly and have both visual cues as well as objective numbers to quickly quantitative right heart function. This abbreviated examination is meant to provide a practical approach to monitoring a patient who needs frequent

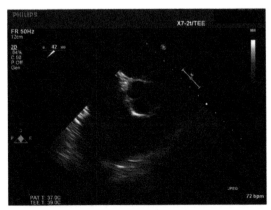

Fig. 1. Midesophageal right ventricular inflow outflow view. This is a good view for assessing the free wall of the right ventricle. This view shows the free wall of the right ventricle with good systolic motion and overall good RV function.

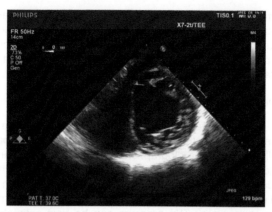

Fig. 2. Transgastric LV short axis view. In this view the left ventricle forms a more pronounced D in the diastole, indicating that the right ventricle is experiencing acute volume overload. If the D shape is more pronounced in the systole, that is more indicative of acute pressure overload.

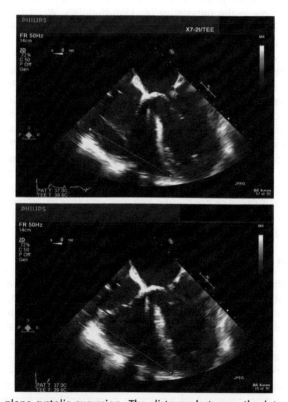

Fig. 3. Tricuspid plane systolic excursion. The distance between the lateral aspect of the tricuspid annulus in the 4-chamber view is measured in systole and diastole. This measurement can be done quickly and easily and provides the echocardiographer with an objective measurement of RV function.

evaluation and intervention on hemodynamic and ventilator management. The anesthesiologist taking care of the patient undergoing noncardiac thoracic surgery does not have the luxury of the pure echo cardiographer capable of acquiring repeated 3-dimensional clips and making complex calculations and estimations without the responsibility of taking care of the patient.

TEE FOR ACUTE PULMONARY HYPERTENSION

TEE is a useful diagnostic technique for acute pulmonary hypertension (PHTN) secondary to pulmonary emboli (PE) if a recent TEE examination can be used as a reference. Occasionally, the echo cardiographer can pick up clot-in-transit, evidence of tricuspid or pulmonic valve endocarditis with mobile thrombus, or mobile thrombus on an indwelling catheter or transvenous pacemaker. In addition to the detailed examination described previously to examine RV function, the following examination should be included. Pulmonary artery (PA) pressure can be best estimated with spectral Doppler in the upper esophageal (UE) aortic arch short-axis (SA) view at approximately 90°. By turning the probe slightly to the left and retroflexing the alignment with the pulmonary artery, blood flow is best. Pulse wave Doppler (PWD) across the pulmonic valve (PV) may show a rapid early PA systolic flow acceleration and midsystolic slowing. Suggestive signs of a sudden increase in PA or right ventricle pressure are RV dilatation, decrease in RV contractility, increase in tricuspid regurgitation, or development of reversed systolic flow in the hepatic veins. Unfortunately, all of these changes are usually subtle, or interpretation is challenging due to the effect of different flow angle alignments, and therefore of limited diagnostic value without (or sometimes even with) a recent previous TEE examination. Despite the challenge, TEE may still provide valuable information for differential diagnosis in emergency situations where a central or massive PE is considered,[19,20] or to follow up after initiation of PHTN therapeutic measures (ie, inhaled nitric oxide).[21] Some authors have reported the combination of TEE with intravenous contrast (contrast-enhanced, or CE-TEE) to enhance the visualization of PE.[22] Finally, in a patient in whom there is a reasonable suspicion of a pulmonary embolism, the evidence of a McConnell sign provides a test with 77% sensitivity and 94% specificity to detect an acute PE in the setting of right heart dysfunction. The echo finding is described in midesophageal 4-chamber view at zero degrees. The echo cardiographer should closely examine the RV free wall. Patients with an acute PE will have akinesis of his or her middle free wall with preserved motion of his or her apex of their right ventricle. Although this finding was originally described in transthoracic echocardiography, it can also be used with a TEE.[23]

LUNG RESECTION SURGERY AND PNEUMONECTOMY

The majority of thoracic noncardiac surgery involves resection of cancer in patients with nonmetastatic disease. Unless there is a special indication, there is rarely a role for TEE in patients undergoing video-assisted thorascopic surgery/thoracotomy for a wedge resection or lobectomy. However, if the cancer is extensive, and if the decision is made to progress to a pneumonectomy, a TEE may help the anesthesiologist in hemodynamic management.

Pneumonectomy is a high-risk procedure that carries a perioperative mortality rate of 5% to 15%. Common perioperative complications of pneumonectomy include atrial arrhythmias, post-thoracotomy pain syndrome, persistent bronchopleural fistula, and postoperative respiratory failure requiring mechanical ventilation. The presence of postoperative pulmonary edema greatly increases the patient's risk of death. The pulmonary edema can be multifactorial: cardiac overload, barotrauma, large volume resuscitation with an impaired left ventricle, disruption of lymphatic drainage, and inflammation from surgery causing a capillary leak. Continuous cardiac monitoring during these cases may help guide anesthesiologists in their management decisions. Vigilant monitoring of left and right heart function during these cases, as well as a protective lung ventilation strategy, may decrease the risk of postoperative pulmonary edema and mortality. TEE views that would be especially beneficial for continuous monitoring would be first the standard 20-view examination as described by Shanewise and colleagues,[15] followed by a focused evaluation of the right ventricle as described previously.[24]

LUNG TRANSPLANTATION

TEE serves multiple roles in the management of patients undergoing lung transplantation. TEE improves the decision-making ability of the anesthesiologist to decide whether to initiate cardiopulmonary bypass. There is some suggestion from the literature that cardiopulmonary bypass leads to worse perioperative mortality and in some series worse 1- year mortality.[25] The decision to initiate cardiopulmonary bypass is usually based on a combination of factors: acid–base status, oxygenation, ventilation, change in pulmonary artery pressures, and change in systemic arterial blood pressure. Hemodynamic, oxygenation, and ventilation derangements can result in right heart failure. Once the patient develops right heart failure, it is extremely important to treat aggressively with inotropic support and possibly inhaled pulmonary artery vasodilators, and to maintain an adequate mean arterial blood pressure to ensure right heart perfusion. However, even in the setting of a dramatic change in pulmonary artery pressures, sometimes the right ventricle is able to maintain its contractility and avoid hemodynamic collapse (**Fig. 4**). TEE can greatly assist the anesthesiologist in managing RV function during lung transplantation. TEE also allows the anesthesiologist to assess pulmonary artery anastomosis, assess flow in all 4 pulmonary veins, evaluate for intra-cardiac air (**Fig. 5**) or thrombus, and assist in assessment of sudden unexplained shock.[26] Patients with severe emphysema can rapidly develop hemodynamic collapse from auto-positive end-expiratory pressure and pulmonary tamponade.[27]

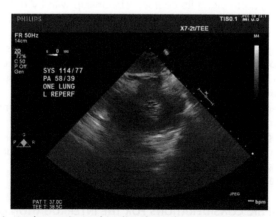

Fig. 4. Transgastric LV short axis. In this clip, the pulmonary artery pressures have acutely doubled, and the values of the systemic blood pressure and pulmonary artery pressure are listed on the echo clip. Clearly the left ventricle is functioning well, and there is no sign of septal wall dysfunction in the setting of the acute rise in the pulmonary artery pressure that the PAC is recording.

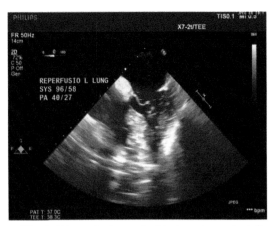

Fig. 5. Reperfusion of the left lung during a double lung transplant for idiopathic pulmonary fibrosis. In this 4- chamber view, there is air seen from the pulmonary veins moving across the tricuspid valve into the left ventricle.

TEE FOR THORACIC AORTIC SURGERY

TEE allows an evaluation of nearly the entire thoracic aorta, with some limitations of the distal ascending and proximal arch portions due to airway interposition. Epiaortic echocardiography is extremely useful to obtain accurate measurements of local lesions in cases where access is available. The 6 views recommended by the Society of Cardiovascular Anesthesiologists and American Society of Echocardiography (SCA/ASE) are[28]:

1. The Midesophageal (ME) ascending aorta Short Axis (SAX) view, for a cross-section measurement of the diameter and wall thickness of the ascending aorta. It also allows the visualization of the superior vena cava (SVC) and main and right pulmonary arteries.
2. The ME ascending aorta Long Axis (LAX) view, for evaluating the relative diameter of the ascending aorta along its course, relationship with LV outflow tract (LVOT) diameter, ascending aorta contour, wall thickness, and blood flow pattern. It occasionally allows visualization of the right coronary artery (RCA).
3. The Upper Esophageal (UE) aortic arch SAX view allows the cross-section interrogation of portions of the aortic arch and branch vessels in terms of diameter, wall thickness, and location of atherosclerotic plaques, but also the visualization of the pulmonary artery and innominate vein.
4. The UE aortic arch LAX view is useful to define the aortic arch dimension, contour and outlet of branch vessels, and blood flow pattern.
5. The descending aorta SAX view allows interrogation of the cross-sectional diameter, wall thickness and structure and flow patterns, and left pleural effusions.
6. The descending aorta LAX view complements the series of SAX views, providing a longitudinal evaluation of the descending aorta.

ECHOCARDIOGRAPHIC CONSIDERATIONS FOR THE INTERROGATION OF THE THORACIC AORTA DURING THORACIC SURGERY
Atherosclerosis

TEE has a critical role in the diagnosis of atherosclerotic plaques and their morphology located in the thoracic aorta.[29] These plaques can be responsible for systemic embolisms, contributing to episodes of stroke or acute renal insufficiency.[30–32] Atherosclerotic lesions of the ascending aorta and aortic arch are associated with postoperative stroke after cardiac surgery.[32,33] Strokes secondary to retrograde embolisms have been also suggested in patients with atherosclerosis of the descending aorta. Complex plaques ($\geq$4 mm thickness, ulcerated or mobile) have an embolic high-risk source of stroke after Harloff and colleagues[30] showed retrograde flow arising from these complex plaques by 3-dimensional magnetic resonance imaging (MRI). Less clear is the predictive value for future vascular events (ischemic stroke) of the presence of atherosclerotic lesions in the aortic arch of proximal descending aorta in the general stroke-free population.[34] Performing TEE and/or epiaortic evaluation of the thoracic aorta is nonetheless valuable and complementary to preoperative magnetic resonance angiography (MRA) before any aortic thrombectomy,[29,35] thoracic endovascular aneurysm repair (TEVAR),[36] placement of an intra-aortic balloon pump (IABP),[31] or aortic instrumentation (cannulation or cross-clamping).[37,38]

Atherosclerosis of the thoracic aorta can also reflect the spread and severity of the atherosclerotic disease in other locations. In a recent study combining TEE aortic assessment and coronary angiography, the presence of complex atherosclerosis plaque in the descending aorta showed the strongest association with the incidence of coronary artery disease (CAD) (defined by presence of $\geq$70% stenosis in $\geq$1 coronary vessel), even stronger than hypertension or diabetes mellitus.[39]

Aneurysm and Dissection

TEE can complement angiographic techniques in the diagnosis of the location, extension and morphology of aortic aneurysms and dissection, and the presence of atherosclerosis, and/or clots. The latter can modify the surgical intervention in terms of deciding location of aortic instrumentation[40] and precise thoracic endovascular aneurysm repair (TEVAR) procedures.[36] The presence of aortic insufficiency by TEE aortic valve assessment can guide decisions of aortic valve-sparing versus valve replacement surgery in ascending aneurysms.[41,42]

Trauma

TEE has been mostly replaced by computed tomography (CT)/MRA for the diagnosis of blunt trauma of the thoracic aorta, although it may be helpful in certain occasions.[43,44]

INITIATION OF ECMO

ECMO is most frequently used as mechanical support for primary cardiac dysfunction but is also used for the treatment acute respiratory failure when oxygenation and carbon dioxide removal are no longer sufficient (eg, 2009 H1N1 epidemic) as a bridge to recovery.[45] There are also considerable efforts being made in the development of simpler ECMO circuits for chronic use, so-called artificial lungs, as hundreds of patients die every year due to the lack of organs while being on the lung transplant list. ECMO or artificial lung circuits when placed for oxygenation can be very different, but they have a common feature that they require either percutaneous venoarterial (V-A) or venovenous (V-V) cannula placement.[46] V-A systems are also capable of providing circulatory support, while V-V systems are purely for respiratory support. For both A-V and V-V ECMO, the venous cannula or 1 of the venous cannulas is positioned centrally in the right atrium (RA). TEE is used in guiding and confirming correct cannula placement. The primary TEE view used is the bicaval view, which is obtained by turning the TEE probe to the right at the mid-\esophageal position and by opening the omniplane to 100° to 120°. The venous cannula (first the guidewire), when placed from the femoral vein, should be seen coming into the RA from the inferior vena cava (IVC). The IVC can be confused with the coronary sinus if the probe is over-rotated to the right. To confirm that the IVC is visualized, the TEE probe should be pushed down toward the stomach, and the IVC should be visualized as it traverses the liver. The ECMO cannula should be seen coming through the IVC, through the liver, into the RA. If a V-V ECMO is used, one of the cannula is placed into RA via the internal jugular vein. The same bicaval view is used to visualize the SVC-RA junction. Larger portions of the proximal SVC can be seen by slightly pulling the TEE probe up while maintaining the bicaval view. In 2009, a dual-lumen bicaval (AvalonElite, Avalon Laboratories, LLC, Rancho Dominguez, California) cannula was approved and introduced to clinical practice. It is a percutaneous, single-site (internal jugular), V-V device that has a proximal and distal drainage port, and an infusion port between the 2 drainage ports. When correctly positioned with TEE guidance, the proximal drainage port sits in the SVC at the SVC-RA junction, while the cannula tip points toward the IVC for distal drainage. The inflow jet from the infusion port should be directed toward the tricuspid valve. Again, the bicaval view can be used to guide cannulation (first guidewire than cannula placement) and confirm correct cannula position. Recently a case of pericardial tamponade from RV injury was described during Avalon cannula placement, emphasizing the importance of direct and continuous TEE visualization during cannulation until the institution of ECMO.[47]

SUMMARY

TEE is a minimally invasive monitor that has multiple applications in the operating room and in the ICU. Although there is a lack of evidence of TEE improving outcomes outside of cardiac surgery, TEE is rapidly becoming a more common monitor in the operating room for critically ill patients undergoing high-risk surgery. For patients undergoing noncardiac thoracic surgery TEE offers multiple additional benefits such as: rapid and reliable monitoring of right heart function, monitoring of lesions that can predict adverse outcomes (aortic atheromas), and assistance in placing ECMO cannulas.

SUPPLEMENTARY DATA

Supplementary data related to this article can be found online at doi:http://dx.doi.org/10.1016/j.anclin.2012.08.007.

REFERENCES

1. Memstsoudis S, Rosenberg P, Loffler M. The usefulness of transesophageal echocardiography during intraoperative arrest in noncardiac surgery. Anesth Analg 2006;102:1653–7.
2. Oikawa T, Shimazui T, Joharuka A, et al. Intraoperative transesophageal echocardiography for inferior vena caval tumor throbus in renal cell carcinoma. Int J Urol 2004;11:189–92.
3. Sandham JD, Hull RD, Brant RF, et al. A randomized, controlled trial of the use of pulmonary artery catheters in high-risk surgical patients. N Engl J Med 2003;348:5–14.
4. Binanay C, Califf RM, Hasselblad V, et al. Evaluation study of congestive heart failure and pulmonary artery effectiveness: the ESCAPE trial. JAMA 2005;294:1625–33.

5. Richard C, Warszawski J, Anguel N, et al. Early use of the pulmonary artery catheter and outcomes in patients with shock and acute respiratory distress syndrome: a randomized controlled clinical trial. JAMA 2003;290:2713–20.

6. Rhodes A, Cusack RJ, Newman PJ, et al. A randomized, controlled trial of the pulmonary artery catheter in critically ill patients. Intensive Care Med 2002;28:256–64.

7. Ranucci M. Which cardiac surgical patients can benefit from placement of a pulmonary artery catheter? Crit Care 2006;10(Suppl 3); S6 pages 1–8.

8. Su N, Huang CJ, Tsai P, et al. Cardiac output measurement during cardiac surgery: esophageal Doppler versus pulmonary artery catheter. Acta Anaesthesiol Scand 2002;40:127–33.

9. Ali M, Royse AG, Connelly K, et al. The accuracy of transesophageal echocardiography in estimating pulmonary capillary wedge pressure in anaesthetized patients. Anaesthesia 2012;67:122–31.

10. Jain M, Upadhyay D, Balagani R, et al. Cardiologists use pulmonary artery catheter information to make homogenous treatment decisions. J Intensive Care Med 2007;22(5):251–6.

11. Jain M, Canham M, Upadhyay D, et al. Variability in interventions with pulmonary artery catheter data. Intensive Care Med 2003;29(11):2059–62.

12. Greenberg SB, Murphy GS, Vender JS. Current use of the pulmonary artery catheter. Curr Opin Crit Care 2009;15(3):249–53.

13. Jacka MJ, Cohen MM, To T, et al. The use of and preferences for the transesophageal echocardiogram and pulmonary artery catheter among cardiovascular anesthesiologists. Anesth Analg 2002;94(5):1065–71.

14. American Society of Anesthesiologists and Society of Cardiovascular Anesthesiologists Task Force on Transesophageal Echocardiography. Practice guidelines for perioperative transesophageal echocardiography. An updated report by the American Society of Anesthesiologists and the Society of Cardiovascular Anesthesiologists Task Force on Transesophageal Echocardiography. Anesthesiology 2010;112(5):1084–96.

15. Shanewise JS, Cheung AT, Aronson S, et al. ASE/SCA guidelines for performing a comprehensive intraoperative multiplane transesophageal echocardiography examination: recommendations of the American Society of Echocardiography Council for Intraoperative Echocardiography and the Society of Cardiovascular Anesthesiologists Task Force for Certification in Perioperative Transesophageal Echocardiography. Anesth Analg 1999;89(4):870–84.

16. Otto CM. Echocardiographic evaluation of the left and right ventricular systolic function. Philadelphia: W.B. Saunders Company; 2000.

17. Jardin F, Dubourg O, Bourdarias JP. Echocardiographic pattern of acute cor pulmonale. Chest 1997;111(1):209–17.

18. Little WC, Reeves RC, Arciniegas J, et al. Mechanism of abnormal interventricular septal motion during delayed left ventricular activation. Circulation 1982;65(7):1486–91.

19. Lengyel M. Should transesophageal echocardiography become a routine test in patients with suspected pulmonary thromboembolism? Echocardiography 1998;15(8 Pt 1):779–86.

20. Pruszczyk P, Torbicki A, Pacho R, et al. Noninvasive diagnosis of suspected severe pulmonary embolism: transesophageal echocardiography vs spiral CT. Chest 1997;112(3):722–8.

21. Riedel B. The pathophysiology and management of perioperative pulmonary hypertension with specific emphasis on the period following cardiac surgery. Int Anesthesiol Clin 1999;37(2):55–79.

22. Izrailtyan I, Clark J, Swaminathan M, et al. Case report: optimizing intraoperative detection of pulmonary embolism using contrast-enhanced echocardiography. Can J Anaesth 2006;53(7):711–5.

23. McConnell MV, Solomon SD, Rayan ME, et al. Regional right ventricular dysfunction detected by echocardiography in acute pulmonary embolishm. Am J Cardiol 1996;78:469–73.

24. Slinger P. Update on anesthetic management for pneumonectomy. Curr Opin Anaesthesiol 2009;22(1):31–7.

25. Nagendran M, Maruthappu M, Sugand K. Should double lung transplant be performed with or without cardiopulmonary bypass. Interact Cardiovasc Thorac Surg 2011;12:799–805.

26. Gonzalez-Fernandez C, González-Castro A, Rodriguez-Borregan JC, et al. Pulmonary venous obstruction after lung transplantation. Diagnostic advantages of transesophageal echocardiography. Clin Transplant 2009;23:975–80.

27. Miranda A, Zink R, McSweeney M. Anesthesia for lung transplantation. Semin Cardiothorac Vasc Anesth 2005;9(3):205–12.

28. Savage RM. Comprehensive textbook of perioperative transesophageal echocardiography. 2nd edition. Philadelphia: Wolters Kluwer/Lippincott Williams & Wilkins Health; 2011.

29. Krishnamoorthy V, Bhatt K, Nicolau R, et al. Transesophageal echocardiography-guided aortic thrombectomy in a patient with a mobile thoracic aortic thrombus. Semin Cardiothorac Vasc Anesth 2011;15(4):176–8.

30. Harloff A, Simon J, Brendecke S, et al. Complex plaques in the proximal descending aorta: an underestimated embolic source of stroke. Stroke 2010; 41(6):1145–50.

31. Nowak-Machen M, Rawn JD, Shekar PS, et al. Descending aortic calcification increases renal dysfunction and in-hospital mortality in cardiac surgery patients with intra-aortic balloon pump counterpulsation placed perioperatively: a case control study. Crit Care 2012;16(1):R17.

32. Bergman P, van der Linden J. Atherosclerosis of the ascending aorta as a major determinant of the outcome of cardiac surgery. Nat Clin Pract Cardiovasc Med 2005;2(5):246–51 [quiz: 269].

33. Sugioka K, Matsumura Y, Hozumi T, et al. Relation of aortic arch complex plaques to risk of cerebral infarction in patients with aortic stenosis. Am J Cardiol 2011; 108(7):1002–7.

34. Russo C, Jin Z, Rundek T, et al. Atherosclerotic disease of the proximal aorta and the risk of vascular events in a population-based cohort: the Aortic Plaques and Risk of Ischemic Stroke (APRIS) study. Stroke 2009;40(7):2313–8.

35. Namura O, Sogawa M, Asami F, et al. Floating thrombus originating from an almost normal thoracic aorta. Gen Thorac Cardiovasc Surg 2011;59(9):612–5.

36. Rousseau H, Chabbert V, Maracher MA, et al. The importance of imaging assessment before endovascular repair of thoracic aorta. Eur J Vasc Endovasc Surg 2009;38(4):408–21.

37. Royse AG, Royse CF. Epiaortic ultrasound assessment of the aorta in cardiac surgery. Best Pract Res Clin Anaesthesiol 2009;23(3):335–41.

38. Yamaguchi A, Adachi H, Tanaka M, et al. Efficacy of intraoperative epiaortic ultrasound scanning for preventing stroke after coronary artery bypass surgery. Ann Thorac Cardiovasc Surg 2009;15(2):98–104.

39. Gu X, He Y, Li Z, et al. Relation between the incidence, location, and extent of thoracic aortic atherosclerosis detected by transesophageal echocardiography and the extent of coronary artery disease by angiography. Am J Cardiol 2011;107(2):175–8.

40. Attaran S, Safar M, Saleh HZ, et al. Cannulating a dissecting aorta using ultrasound-epiaortic and transesophageal guidance. Heart Surg Forum 2011; 14(6):E373–5.

41. Bossone E, Evangelista A, Isselbacher E, et al. Prognostic role of transesophageal echocardiography in acute type A aortic dissection. Am Heart J 2007; 153(6):1013–20.

42. Gologorsky E, Karras R, Gologorsky A, et al. Transesophageal echocardiography after contrast-enhanced CT angiography in the diagnosis of type A aortic dissection. J Card Surg 2011;26(5):495–500.

43. Benjamin ER, Tillou A, Hiatt JR, et al. Blunt thoracic aortic injury. Am Surg 2008; 74(10):1033–7.

44. Demetriades D, Velmahos GC, Scalea TM, et al. Diagnosis and treatment of blunt thoracic aortic injuries: changing perspectives. J Trauma 2008;64(6):1415–8 [discussion: 1418–9].

45. Combes A, Pellegrino V. Extracorporeal membrane oxygenation for 2009 influenza A (H1N1)-associated acute respiratory distress. Seminars in respiratory and critical care medicine 2011;32(2):188–94.

46. Sadahiro T, Oda S, Nakamura M, et al. Trend in and perspectives on extacorporeal membrane oxygenation for severe adult respiratory failure. Gen Thorac Cardiovasc Surg 2012;60:192–201.

47. Hirose H, Yamane K, Marhefka G, et al. Right ventricular rupture caused by malposition of the Avalon cannula for venovenous extracorporeal memebrane oxygenation. J Cardiothorac Surg 2012;7:36.

How to Choose the Double-Lumen Tube Size and Side: The Eternal Debate

Alessia Pedoto, MD

KEYWORDS

- Small DLT • Big DLTs • Right-sided DLTs • Left-sided DLTs • Airway damage
- Lung isolation • Margin of safety

KEY POINTS

- Big double-lumen tubes (DLTs) are usually placed for most cases of lung isolation, leaving the small tubes for patients with short stature.
- Some controversy has been generated about the practice of using small-size DLTs for any individual independent of height, weight, and gender. Airway trauma and rupture have been proposed to be associated with this practice.
- Left-sided DLTs are commonly used for isolating the lung because of their alleged higher margin of safety.
- Proponents of the routine use of right-sided DLTs for left-sided procedures advocate this practice to increase the level of comfort of the anesthesiologist and to learn how to manage potential problems during one-lung ventilation.

INTRODUCTION

Double-lumen tubes (DLTs) are the most commonly used devices to provide lung isolation.[1–3] DLTs are bifurcated tubes with a tracheal and a bronchial lumen, disposable, and made of polyvinyl chloride (PVC). Different sizes (28F, 32F, 37F, 39F, and 41F catheter), sides (left vs right), and manufacturers (Rusch [Teleflex Medical, Seattle, WA, USA], Mallinckrodt [Mallinckrodt Inc, St Louis, MO, USA], Sheridan [Hudson RCI, Highcombe, UK], and Portex [Smiths Medical, Dublin, OH, USA]) are available. Left-sided DLTs are used more often than right-sided.

Although disposable DLTs have been used for many years, there is still controversy regarding performance, efficiency, and outcome among thoracic and nonthoracic anesthesiologists. Strong opinions exist on the best size to use and when a right-sided DLT is indicated.

This article provides a review of the current data from the literature and opinions from experts on this topic.

Department of Anesthesiology and Critical Care Medicine, Memorial Sloan-Kettering Cancer Center, Room M 301, 1275 York Avenue, New York, NY 10065, USA
E-mail address: pedotoa@mskcc.org

Anesthesiology Clin 30 (2012) 671–681
http://dx.doi.org/10.1016/j.anclin.2012.08.001
1932-2275/12/$ – see front matter © 2012 Elsevier Inc. All rights reserved.

anesthesiology.theclinics.com

THE CONUNDRUM OF THE SIZE

Little evidence is available in the literature on how to choose the size of a DLT. Recommendations are mainly based on old teachings, which ultimately dictate clinical practice. Most thoracic and nonthoracic anesthesiologists chose the DLT size based on patient height and gender, or on their personal experience. Measuring the tracheal or bronchial diameter has been suggested as a more precise way to determine the size of the DLT.[4–8] Tracheal diameter should be measured at the level of the clavicles on the posterior–anterior chest radiograph.[4] The bronchial diameter should be measured on the computed tomography scan within 1 to 2 mm of carina,[5,7] because the left mainstem is not clearly visible on the chest radiograph in 50% to 70% of cases. Independent of the imaging used, the measurement obtained is amplified as a result of the radiograph technique; therefore, the final value should be corrected. Several mathematical formulas have been proposed to accomplish this goal.[4,6,7] Although measuring radiograph films has a theoretical scientific background, it may not be practical. Moreover, this approach may work for most white patients, but it does not seem to be as effective in the Asian population, especially if female.[9]

The main concern of using an inappropriate size DLT is the potential of causing airway trauma and rupture. This can occur as a direct consequence of either a too big or too small DLT or indirectly, by delivering inappropriate minute ventilation during one-lung ventilation and causing auto positive end-expiratory pressure. Experts in the field remain divided between using small versus big DLTs. The supporters of using a small DLT (35F or 37F catheter) advocate the use of this size based on the assumption that it is easy to place, fits all patients, and does not seem to be associated with an increased incidence of airway damage.[10] In case of difficult airway or for small patients, a small device may be easier to use. The proponents of a bigger size (39F and 41F catheter) argue that if the DLT is too small, it will cause airway injury because of (1) the need to use high pressures in the bronchial cuff to achieve lung isolation; (2) a higher incidence of dislodgment, causing either failure to isolate the lung or ventilator-induced lung injury; (3) the inability to suction secretions; and (4) an increased resistance during mechanical ventilation, which could lead to auto positive end-expiratory pressure.[11] Airway edema and trauma, and hoarseness and sore throat have been reported with the use of DLTs and big single-lumen endotracheal tubes.[12,13]

Most of the data on airway rupture and the use of DLTs come from isolated case reports.[14–21] This is a rare but potentially catastrophic event, with a less than 1% incidence. It usually occurs in the membranous part of the trachea or the left mainstem bronchus. Presentation signs and symptoms include mediastinal and subcutaneous emphysema and tension pneumothorax, difficulty ventilating, and respiratory insufficiency.[11] Mediastinitis and sepsis may be later complications. The cause still remains multifactorial. Fitzmaurice and Brodsky[11] reviewed 33 case reports in 1999, and found that overinflation of the bronchial cuff was the main culprit for airway rupture in most of the cases. Airway trauma was more common with Robertshaw, Carlens, and White DLTs. For these devices, the use of a big size was mainly implicated. Airway rupture was uncommon with PVC DLTs. However, when it occurred, it seemed to be associated more with the use of small DLTs. In the latter group, most of the patients had either comorbidities that placed them at risk of airway trauma (eg, spontaneous pneumothorax[19]), or had traumatic insertions with multiple blind attempts,[14,15,18] or with the stylet left in place.[16,21] Mallinckrodt DLTs were used in most of the cases of traumatic PVC DLT injury.

Airway trauma has been reported during intubation and extubation. **Table 1** summarizes potential causes. Several factors can be implicated, other than the device

Table 1
Summary of potential causes for airway trauma

DLT	Operator	Patient	Trachea
Inappropriate size	Inexperience	Women	Tracheomalacia
Bronchial cuff overinflation	Multiple attempts	Short stature	Steroid/chest radiotherapy
Stylet not removed	Blind technique	Obesity	Endoluminal tumors
Malposition	Forceful placement	Chronic obstructive pulmonary disease	
Memory bend		Age >50	
Use of an exchange catheter		Coughing/moving	

Data from Kim HK, et al. Left mainstem bronchial rupture during one-lung ventilation with Robertshaw double lumen endobronchial tube: a case report. Korean J Anesthesiol 2010;59(Suppl):S21–5; and Kim J, Lim T, Bahk JH. Tracheal laceration during intubation of a double-lumen tube and intraoperative fiberoptic bronchoscopic evaluation through an LMA in the lateral position: a case report. Korean J Anesthesiol 2011;60(4):285–9.

itself. Operator experience is a very important component. Other factors contributing to airway rupture include forceful insertion; multiple attempts, especially if blind and with the stylet in place; and the use of a tube exchanger. This complication seems to be more common in women, obese patients, short stature, presence of chronic obstructive pulmonary disease, age older than 50 years, and with patient movement or coughing during placement.[11,22,23] Tracheomalacia, immunosuppression, tracheal tumors, and the use of steroid or chest radiotherapy are also risk factors for tracheal rupture.

Other causes of airway trauma include pressure in the bronchial cuff, memory bend and stylet, and technique of insertion. Regarding pressure in the bronchial cuff, the higher the pressure in the cuff, the worse the damage. It seems counterintuitive to think that the more air in the bronchial cuff, the higher the pressure generated and the chance of causing damage. Cuff overinflation has been associated with airway damage in several studies.[11] Roscoe and colleagues[24] looked at the pressures generated by 1-mL increments of air in the bronchial cuff of different size DLTs and blockers in an in vitro model. A maximum volume of 6 mL for the DLTs and 10 mL for the blockers was used. Static and dynamic compliance curves were measured. Small-size DLTs required more volume in the cuff to have an underwater seal, generating higher pressures than bigger size tubes. However, the highest pressures needed to achieve a seal to 25 mm Hg pressure ranged from 12 to 24 mm Hg. This was lower than the accepted threshold for mucosal ischemia of 30 mm Hg.

Regarding memory bend and stylet, all DLTs have a premade memory bend for the bronchial side that is evident after the stylet is removed. The memory bend has been implicated in causing damage during intubation[25] or extubation.[26] If the DLT is not turned in a timely fashion after passing the vocal cords, its tip may lodge on the tracheal rings and if forced cause injury. A similar mechanism has been proposed during extubation, when the tip of the tube can injure the vocal cords. This can occur with any size adult DLT, because the deflection of the bronchial tip is approximately 3 cm in most DLTs (**Fig. 1**).[25]

Technique of insertion is another cause of airway trauma. Blind insertion of the DLT can cause airway trauma or rupture, especially if forceful. A common practice is to

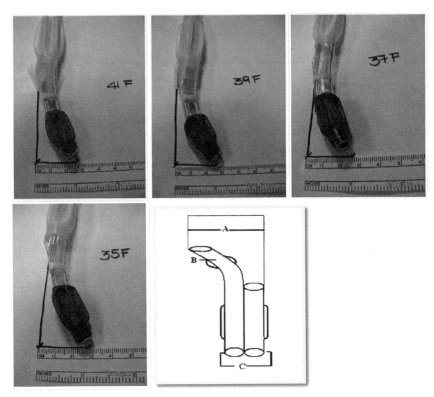

Fig. 1. Memory bend of a left-sided DLT (Sheridan), after removing the stylet. (*Adapted from* Lohser J, Brodsky JB. Tracheal perforation from double-lumen tubes: size may be important. Anesth Analg 2005;101(4):1243–4. [author reply: 1244–5]; with permission.)

insert the DLT by direct laryngoscopy, and after the blue cuff has passed vocal cords the stylet is removed, the tube turned depending on the side used (counterclockwise for left DLTs and clockwise for right DLTs), and pushed until it meets resistance. Inexperienced operators, leaving the stylet in place, weakened tracheal tissue, or endotracheal or endobronchial tumors can all contribute to airway damage. The use of fiberoptic bronchoscopy has decreased this potential complication, allowing confirmation of the final position after blind insertion or assisting in positioning the device under direct vision, especially in cases of endobronchial lesions. New DLTs with a built-in camera in the distal tracheal lumen are being developed to facilitate positioning during insertion and during the case.

Sore throat, hoarseness, and vocal cord and bronchial injuries have been demonstrated by Knoll and colleagues[12] to be more frequent (44% of cases) with the use of DLTs compared with endotracheal tubes and bronchial blockers. None of the patients in the study had either bronchial or vocal cord rupture. The DLT size used in this study was chosen according to Brodsky's criteria,[8] ranging from 37F to 41F. All the data were combined for the DLT group; therefore, it was not possible to discern if there was any relationship between size and severity of the damage. Amar and colleagues[10] did a prospective observational study as a result of a change in clinical practice in their institution. A small DLT (35F) was used in every patient independent of height and gender, and was compared with a bigger size (37F and 39F). There was no difference in the incidence of desaturation, tube malposition, and lung isolation failure between the groups. Despite the presence of more females in the 35F DLT group, no differences were found between genders when data were analyzed by height. No patient had major airway complications at the end of the case or in the postoperative period. Therefore, they concluded that the use of a small DLT was feasible independent of patient size and gender.

Pros and Cons of the Size Chosen

There are specific case scenarios where a big DLT is indicated, such as lung transplantation; lung volume reduction surgery (especially in case of severe emphysema or with copious secretions); or for thoracoabdominal aneurysm repair. Big DLTs may have the advantage of allowing better suctioning of secretions, faster lung collapse, and cause less work of breathing when patients resume spontaneous ventilation at the end of the case. Small DLTs may work better for Asian females; difficult airways with cervical or carinal compression or stenosis; when an awake fiber optic (FOB) intubation is needed; or in the presence of a fresh tracheostomy (<7 days) or laryngoplasty or vocal cord medialization. In case of carinal distortion with left mainstem compression, the placement of a big size DLT may be difficult.

Conclusion

The choice of which DLT size to use still remains a personal one, based on experience and comfort level. Ultimately, the size should be customized to the patient characteristics and pathology. Careful insertion of the DLT, paired with the use of the FOB as an aid for placement and positioning, removal of the stylet after the bronchial cuff passes the vocal cords, and avoiding overinflation of the bronchial cuff are all useful pointers to decrease potentially catastrophic events.

LEFT VERSUS RIGHT: WHICH SIDE TO USE?

Left-sided DLTs are commonly used for thoracic procedures because of their reliability and alleged safety margin. This may be especially true for nonthoracic anesthesiologists with limited bronchoscopic experience. The margin of safety has been defined by Benumof and colleagues[27] as "the length of tracheobronchial tree over which the DLT may be moved or positioned without obstructing a conducting airway." Because of the length of the left mainstem bronchus (4.4–4.9 cm), left-sided DLTs are thought to have a larger margin of safety for positioning and quality of lung isolation. When the margin of safety was studied for three brands of DLT (Mallinckrodt, Sheridan, and Rusch), it was found that left-sided tubes had a safety margin of 16 to 19 mm, whereas right-sided tubes varied between 1 and 4 mm (Rusch) and 8 mm (Mallinckrodt).[27] These values were size dependent (**Fig. 2**). They concluded that left-sided DLTs were more reliable and easier to manage compared with right-sided tubes. Routine use of right-sided DLT is still frowned up on by most anesthesiologists and surgeons. Because of the variable takeoff of the right upper lobe (**Fig. 3**), right-sided DLT may be difficult to position properly and may dislodge during the case, especially with surgical manipulation of the carina. Ideally, a well-positioned right-sided DLT should allow ventilation of all three lobes of the right lung and complete isolation of the left lung. The right mainstem bronchus has a straighter angle compared with the trachea and a wider lumen (see **Fig. 3**) explaining the ease of placement, which is comparable with a right mainstem intubation. Correct positioning may be more challenging because of the anatomy of the right mainstem bronchus, especially if the right upper lobe takeoff is very close to the carina or above it (<2.3 cm distance). The presence of a porcine bronchus, which takes off above the carina, represents the only absolute contraindication for a right-sided DLT placement.

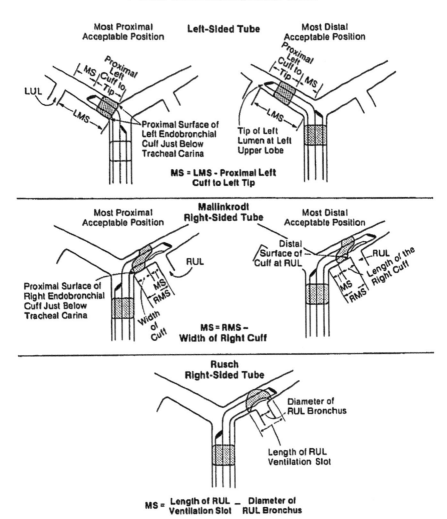

The Margin of Safety (MS) in Positioning Double-Lumen Endotracheal Tubes

Left-Sided Tube

Most Proximal Acceptable Position — Most Distal Acceptable Position

LUL

Proximal Surface of Left Endobronchial Cuff Just Below Tracheal Carina

Tip of Left Lumen at Left Upper Lobe

MS = LMS - Proximal Left Cuff to Left Tip

Mallinkrodt Right-Sided Tube

Most Proximal Acceptable Position — Most Distal Acceptable Position

RUL

Proximal Surface of Right Endobronchial Cuff Just Below Tracheal Carina

Distal Surface of Cuff at RUL

Length of the Right Cuff

MS = RMS - Width of Right Cuff

Rusch Right-Sided Tube

Diameter of RUL Bronchus

Length of RUL Ventilation Slot

$$MS = \frac{Length\ of\ RUL}{Ventilation\ Slot} - \frac{Diameter\ of}{RUL\ Bronchus}$$

Fig. 2. Margin of safety for left and right DLT placement and the most proximal and most distal acceptable position for the DLT. (*Top*) Left-sided DLTs. (*Middle*) Mallinckrodt right-sided DLT. (*Lower*) Rusch right-sided DLT. LMS, length of the left mainstem bronchus; MS, margin of safety in positioning the DLT; RMS, length of the right mainstem bronchus; RUL, right upper lobe. (*From* Benumof JL, Partridge BL, Salvatierra C, et al. Margin of safety in positioning modern double-lumen endotracheal tubes. Anesthesiology 1987;67(5):729–38; with permission.)

Several brands of right-sided DLTs are commercially available, with different bronchial cuff configurations and length (**Fig. 4**). Mallinckrodt has the more forgiving shape to accommodate the DLT in the proper position because of the shape of the bronchial cuff in relation to the side orifice for the right upper lobe. Broncho-Cath tubes by Mallinckrodt have been modified to increase their safety margin, by widening the opening of the right upper lobe orifice.[28] The Cliny (Create Medic, Yokohama, Japan) has

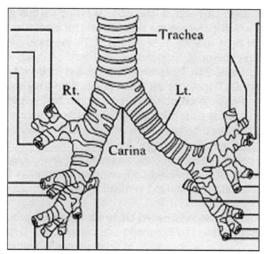

Fig. 3. Tracheobronchial tree anatomy.

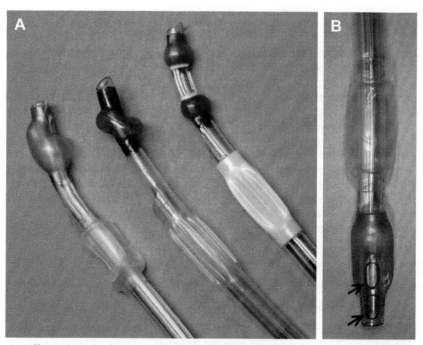

Fig. 4. Different brands of commercially available right-sided DLTs. From left to right, manufacturers are Portex, Mallinckrodt, and Sheridan (*A*), and Cliny (*B*). ([*A*] *From* Ehrenfeld JM, Walsh JL, Sandberg WS. Right- and left-sided Mallinckrodt double-lumen tubes have identical clinical performance. Anesth Analg 2008;106(6):1847–52; with permission; and [*B*] *From* Hagihira S, Takashina M, Mashimo T. Application of a newly designed right-sided, double-lumen endobronchial tube in patients with a very short right mainstem bronchus. Anesthesiology 2008;109(3): 565–8; with permission.)

created a new right-sided DLT with a long oblique bronchial cuff and two orifices for the right upper lobe, which increases the success rate for placement and positioning in patients with a short right mainstem bronchus.[29] To increase the success rate for proper positioning, the fiberoptic bronchoscope should be used.

Indications for right-sided DLT placement are listed in **Box 1**. For these cases, blockers or left-sided DLT may not be suitable because they would be positioned on the surgical site. Possible bronchial injury, trauma to the tumor with bleeding, and difficulty in the surgical dissection or repair may represent potential problems. In case of extrinsic bronchial compression or distortion, it may be difficult to place a left-sided DLT or a blocker. Furthermore, the device chosen may need to be periodically withdrawn to check the site of surgical repair. In case of left bronchial sleeve resection, the presence of a left-sided DLT requires withdrawal from the airway to allow suturing the anastomosis, making ventilation of the right lung difficult after the airway is opened.

Some centers routinely use right-sided DLTs for left-sided procedures with good results. This was demonstrated by Erhenfeld and colleagues.[1] This group conducted a retrospective review on the performance of right- versus left-sided DLTs when used for contralateral thoracic procedures. No difference in hypoxia, hypercapnia, or high airway pressures was found. The same group also demonstrated that there was no difference in incidence of these complications when frequent and infrequent DLT users were compared.[30] However, when these events occurred, they were more severe and prolonged among the infrequent users.

How to Avoid Placing a Right-Sided DLT if Absolutely Indicated

Several options have been proposed to avoid the use of a right-sided DLT when there is an absolute indication. Right mainstem intubations with a single-lumen tube, placing a left-sided DLT very close to the carina, or careful placement of a blocker have been suggested. However, they all have some downsides that may contraindicate their use. Right mainstem intubation has been suggested as an alternative to the use of a right-sided DLT. As shown in **Fig. 5**, the length and size of the cuff of a regular endotracheal tube may not be appropriate for ventilating the right lung and to properly isolate the left. Specifically, the total length of the endotracheal tube may not be sufficient to reach the mainstem bronchus; the cuff may be too big to fit completely in the right mainstem, with possible herniation above the carina or occlusion of the take-off of the right upper lobe; and finally the tip of the endotracheal tube beyond the cuff is longer, causing lobar ventilation. Indications for mainstem intubation include pediatric airway (below the limits of commercially available DLT size); critical airway in patients

---

Box 1
Indications for right-sided DLT placement

Left bronchial disease or damage

    Left endobronchial tumors

    Penetrating or blunt trauma to left mainstem bronchus

    Prior left mainstem reconstruction (transplantation or sleeve resection)

    Kinking of the left bronchus after left upper lobectomy

Left bronchial compression

    Thoracic aortic aneurysm

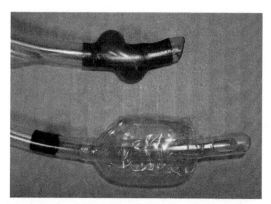

Fig. 5. Comparison between the cuff of a Rusch 7.0 I.D. single-lumen endotracheal tube and a right double-lumen tube (Mallinkrodt Broncho-Cath 39F). The cuff starts are aligned. The single-lumen endotracheal tube extends far beyond the distal end of the right-sided DLT cuff.

already intubated (where changing the DLT would be problematic, such as unstable neck or difficult airway); and in case of distorted or damaged trachea.

In the case of careful insertion of a left-sided DLT in the left mainstem, the DLT is placed in the contraindicated area. Careful positioning away from the lesion with the aid of a fiberoptic bronchoscope can be done. However, the DLT is positioned in the proximity of the lesion and potentially can cause damage or be damaged during surgery. The left-sided DLT may need to be withdrawn in case of bronchial resection or repair, potentially causing the inability to ventilate the contralateral side. It also needs to be readvanced in case lung isolation is still required (ie, sleeve resection, lung transplantation), with the potential of injuring the anastomosis.

The use of a blocker may not be a safe practice because it needs to be placed in the operative side. Placement may be difficult because of airway pathology or distortion, with potential injury of the bronchus, tumor, or existing anastomosis. Moreover, the blocker may periodically require being withdrawn to check for the surgical repair and prevent being stapled in the specimen. In case of extrinsic compression, blockers may be difficult to insert and do not seal properly.

Conclusion

The routine use of a right-sided DLT for left-sided procedures is a standard of practice in some institutions. It requires (1) a patient with the appropriate right bronchial anatomy, (2) experience with the use of the fiberoptic bronchoscope and a bronchoscopic knowledge of the airway anatomy, (3) a familiarity with the technique, and (4) an open-minded surgeon. Elective use of this device has the advantage of helping the anesthesiologist to build the confidence and skills to use and troubleshoot right-sided tubes when absolutely indicated. It also helps to demonstrate to surgical colleagues that the device works. Key points for successful right-sided DLT placement are as follows:

1. The choice an appropriate size and brand
2. Identification of the carina with the bronchoscope through the tracheal lumen
3. Identification of the bronchial cuff in the right mainstem bronchus
4. Matching of the opening of the bronchial side of the DLT and the right upper lobe take-off
5. Secure "taping job" after the right-sided DLT is properly positioned to avoid dislodgment

6. Holding the head and the tube in place during positioning in the lateral decubitus, avoiding flexion and extension
7. Reconfirm positioning with the fiberoptic scope once in the lateral decubitus, and resecure the tape if needed to avoid dislodgment after surgery has started

Despite all the evidence that right- and left-sided DLTs have similar performance, left-sided DLTs are still the most commonly used devices for lung isolation. Ultimately, successful use of a right-sided DLT remains in convincing skeptical surgeons and anesthesiologists that it functions satisfactorily.

REFERENCES

1. Ehrenfeld JM, Walsh JL, Sandberg WS. Right- and left-sided Mallinckrodt double-lumen tubes have identical clinical performance. Anesth Analg 2008;106(6): 1847–52.
2. Campos JH. Progress in lung separation. Thorac Surg Clin 2005;15(1):71–83.
3. Brodsky JB, Lemmens HJ. Left double-lumen tubes: clinical experience with 1,170 patients. J Cardiothorac Vasc Anesth 2003;17(3):289–98.
4. Brodsky JB, Lemmens HJ. Tracheal width and left double-lumen tube size: a formula to estimate left-bronchial width. J Clin Anesth 2005;17(4):267–70.
5. Hannallah M, Benumof JL, Silverman PM, et al. Evaluation of an approach to choosing a left double-lumen tube size based on chest computed tomographic scan measurement of left mainstem bronchial diameter. J Cardiothorac Vasc Anesth 1997;11(2):168–71.
6. Jeon Y, Ryu HG, Bahk JH, et al. A new technique to determine the size of double-lumen endobronchial tubes by the two perpendicularly measured bronchial diameters. Anaesth Intensive Care 2005;33(1):59–63.
7. Hannallah MS, Benumof JL, Ruttimann UE. The relationship between left mainstem bronchial diameter and patient size. J Cardiothorac Vasc Anesth 1995; 9(2):119–21.
8. Brodsky JB, Macario A, Mark JB. Tracheal diameter predicts double-lumen tube size: a method for selecting left double-lumen tubes. Anesth Analg 1996;82(4): 861–4.
9. Chow MY, Liam BL, Lew TW, et al. Predicting the size of a double-lumen endobronchial tube based on tracheal diameter. Anesth Analg 1998;87(1):158–60.
10. Amar D, Desiderio DP, Heerdt PM, et al. Practice patterns in choice of left double-lumen tube size for thoracic surgery. Anesth Analg 2008;106(2):379–83, table of contents.
11. Fitzmaurice BG, Brodsky JB. Airway rupture from double-lumen tubes. J Cardiothorac Vasc Anesth 1999;13(3):322–9.
12. Knoll H, Ziegeler S, Schreiber JU, et al. Airway injuries after one-lung ventilation: a comparison between double-lumen tube and endobronchial blocker: a randomized, prospective, controlled trial. Anesthesiology 2006;105(3):471–7.
13. Stout DM, Bishop MJ, Dwersteg JF, et al. Correlation of endotracheal tube size with sore throat and hoarseness following general anesthesia. Anesthesiology 1987;67(3):419–21.
14. Yuceyar L, Kaynak K, Canturk E, et al. Bronchial rupture with a left-sided polyvinylchloride double-lumen tube. Acta Anaesthesiol Scand 2003;47(5):622–5.
15. Kim HK, Jun JH, Lee HS, et al. Left mainstem bronchial rupture during one-lung ventilation with Robertshaw double lumen endobronchial tube: a case report. Korean J Anesthesiol 2010;59(Suppl):S21–5.

16. Kim J, Lim T, Bahk JH. Tracheal laceration during intubation of a double-lumen tube and intraoperative fiberoptic bronchoscopic evaluation through an LMA in the lateral position: a case report. Korean J Anesthesiol 2011;60(4):285–9.
17. Venkataramanappa V, Boujoukos AJ, Sakai T. The diagnostic challenge of a tracheal tear with a double-lumen endobronchial tube: massive air leak developing from the mouth during mechanical ventilation. J Clin Anesth 2011;23(1): 66–70.
18. Hannallah M, Gomes M. Bronchial rupture associated with the use of a double-lumen tube in a small adult. Anesthesiology 1989;71(3):457–9.
19. Huang CC, Chou AH, Liu HP, et al. Tension pneumothorax complicated by double-lumen endotracheal tube intubation. Chang Gung Med J 2005;28(7): 503–7.
20. Gilbert TB, Goodsell CW, Krasna MJ. Bronchial rupture by a double-lumen endobronchial tube during staging thoracoscopy. Anesth Analg 1999;88(6):1252–3.
21. Zinga E, Dangoisse M, Lechat JP. Tracheal perforation following double-lumen intubation: a case report. Acta Anaesthesiol Belg 2010;61(2):71–4.
22. Chen EH, Logman ZM, Glass PS, et al. A case of tracheal injury after emergent endotracheal intubation: a review of the literature and causalities. Anesth Analg 2001;93(5):1270–1, table of contents.
23. Liu H, Jahr JS, Sullivan E, et al. Tracheobronchial rupture after double-lumen endotracheal intubation. J Cardiothorac Vasc Anesth 2004;18(2):228–33.
24. Roscoe A, Kanellakos GW, McRae K, et al. Pressures exerted by endobronchial devices. Anesth Analg 2007;104(3):655–8.
25. Lohser J, Brodsky JB. Tracheal perforation from double-lumen tubes: size may be important. Anesth Analg 2005;101(4):1243–4 [author reply: 1244–5].
26. Benumof JL, Wu D. Tracheal tear caused by extubation of a double-lumen tube. Anesthesiology 2002;97(4):1007–8.
27. Benumof JL, Partridge BL, Salvatierra C, et al. Margin of safety in positioning modern double-lumen endotracheal tubes. Anesthesiology 1987;67(5):729–38.
28. Bussieres JS, Lacasse Y, Cote D, et al. Modified right-sided Broncho-Cath double lumen tube improves endobronchial positioning: a randomized study. Can J Anaesth 2007;54(4):276–82.
29. Hagihira S, Takashina M, Mashimo T. Application of a newly designed right-sided, double-lumen endobronchial tube in patients with a very short right mainstem bronchus. Anesthesiology 2008;109(3):565–8.
30. Jha S, Ehrenfeld J. Double lumen tubes: usage and performance by frequent and infrequent users. ISRN Anesthesiol 2011. http://dx.doi.org/10.5402/2011/586592.

Managing Hypoxemia During Minimally Invasive Thoracic Surgery

Jens Lohser, MD, MSc, FRCPC

KEYWORDS

- Hypoxemia • One-lung ventilation • Thoracoscopy

KEY POINTS

- An ever-increasing number of thoracic procedures are being performed through minimally invasive techniques.
- Although the incidence of hypoxemia during one-lung ventilation (OLV) has decreased over the years, it remains an issue in roughly 10% of cases.
- Algorithms for the management of OLV hypoxemia have to be adapted to the thoracoscopic approach, in particular the need for optimal surgical exposure.
- With appropriate planning and caution most of the treatment modalities for OLV hypoxemia can be applied to the thoracoscopy setting with some modifications.

INTRODUCTION

Minimally invasive approaches are gradually replacing most open surgical procedures. After being introduced into thoracic surgery as a diagnostic modality a century ago,[1] both video-assisted thoracoscopic surgery (VATS) and robot-assisted thoracoscopic surgery have since been described for every aspect of thoracic surgery: esophageal resections, mediastinal surgery, and all types of lung resections, including pneumonectomies.[2] The reported clinical benefits of VATS are perioperative decreases in blood loss, pain, inflammatory response, chest tube duration, and atrial fibrillation as well as improved postoperative pulmonary function and length of hospitalization.[3–5] Although operating room times tend to be increased for video-assisted procedures, the overall hospital costs are lower, which supports its widespread implementation.[3] Oncologic results seem to be equivalent to the open approach; however, few randomized studies have examined this aspect.[6,7]

Surgical exposure has traditionally been viewed as only a relative indication for lung isolation in thoracotomy procedures. In contrast, operative lung isolation or collapse is

Department of Anesthesiology, Pharmacology and Therapeutics, University of British Columbia, Vancouver General Hospital, JPP2 Room 2449, 899 West 12th Avenue, Vancouver, British Columbia, V5Z-1M9, Canada
E-mail address: jens.lohser@vch.ca

Anesthesiology Clin 30 (2012) 683–697
http://dx.doi.org/10.1016/j.anclin.2012.08.006   anesthesiology.theclinics.com
1932-2275/12/$ – see front matter © 2012 Elsevier Inc. All rights reserved.

essential to the successful performance of thoracoscopic procedures.[8] Hypoxemia used to be the primary concern associated with the provision of one-lung ventilation (OLV). However, its incidence has decreased significantly over the years, likely due to the increased use of fiberoptic bronchoscopy for confirmation of lung isolation and the use of anesthetic agents with less effect on hypoxic pulmonary vasoconstriction (HPV).[9] There has been some uncertainty in the literature on the true incidence of hypoxemia, in part because of its nonuniform definition and the large variability in reporting thresholds. Electronic medical records seem to indicate a higher rate of hypoxemia than that documented in manually recorded charts.[10] Clinically meaningful hypoxemia probably continues to occur in roughly 10% of patients during OLV.

THORACOSCOPY: WHAT IS DIFFERENT?

Whether surgery is performed through trocar sites or a full thoracotomy incision is immaterial to the redistribution of pulmonary blood flow by gravity and HPV. Similarly, the effect of lung isolation and OLV on the alteration of lung compliance and redistribution of ventilation is no different between open and closed approaches. The physiologic changes of OLV are beyond the scope of this article and have been reviewed in detail.[9,11]

The thoracic cavity remains partially closed during VATS procedures, because the incisions are essentially sealed by trocars and surgical instruments. This fact results in several pressure-related effects that distinguish thoracoscopic from open procedures. Although insertion of the trocars does breach the pleural interface, the presence of the instruments restricts the air inflow that is necessary for development of the surgical pneumothorax. Lung collapse is therefore delayed and often incomplete unless aided by applying suction to the open airway or facilitating air entry into the thorax by opening one of the trocars. The rate of lung collapse is maximal if OLV is preceded by complete denitrogenation.[12] Surgical suctioning reexpands the operative lung by creating negative intrathoracic pressure unless a vent is being used to decompress the hemithorax. Conversely, CO_2 insufflation, which is sometimes used to improve visualization, creates tamponade physiology at moderately low insufflation pressures of 5 to 15 mm Hg.[13] The main indication for the use of CO_2 insufflation is the inability to establish lung isolation (secondary to unfavorable airway anatomy or lack of appropriately sized device), which is why it is unusual outside of pediatric practice.

OLV management of the down-lung is unchanged from the thoracotomy settings and should focus on maintaining functional residual capacity (FRC) and open lung.[9] Because of the need for complete lung collapse for surgical exposure, techniques that involve partial or complete insufflation (continuous positive airway pressure [CPAP]) or ventilation (high-frequency jet ventilation [HFJV], two-lung ventilation [TLV]) of the operative lung are considered relatively contraindicated.

Surgical access to the lung is restricted, which complicates some of the interventions that have been described for the treatment of hypoxemia during thoracotomy procedures. Although mechanical restriction of the shunt fraction is still possible, it is significantly more difficult than in the open scenario. Lung retraction is feasible for the surgeons, whereas packing of the lung, which has been shown to improve shunt fraction,[14] is not. In the setting of refractory hypoxemia, the shunt fraction can be reduced by side-clamping the pulmonary artery (PA) or by distorting the PA anatomy with a sponge stick, both of which are feasible during thoracoscopy but more difficult than during open procedures.

What is not different between VATS and open procedures is the amount of intrathoracic trauma. External tissue trauma is reduced, resulting in improved postoperative lung function and earlier hospital discharge times. However, the intrathoracic surgical trauma is unchanged from the open approach, and there is "... no lessening in the complexity of the anesthetic process, [and] the degree of physiological trespass... ."[1] One needs to guard against the perception that procedures are just thoracoscopy, because there is no similarity between a VATS lobectomy and a VATS bullectomy in terms of the amount of tissue and vasculature that have to be resected and the potential for perioperative and immediate postoperative complications.

PREDICTORS FOR HYPOXEMIA DURING OLV

The physiologic changes associated with OLV for ventilation or perfusion during thoracoscopy are no different to those encountered during open thoracotomy. The predictors of hypoxemia for OLV are therefore unchanged from the open procedure (**Table 1**).

PREVENTATIVE MEASURES TO AVOID HYPOXEMIA

Because of the limited ability to use the operative lung for apneic oxygenation or ventilation, prevention of hypoxemia is crucial. Impaired HPV caused by hypocapnea, vasodilators, or excessive volatile anesthesia has to be avoided. Any shunt in the ventilated lung, because of derecruitment, is poorly tolerated. Appropriate and individualized ventilator settings focused on open-lung ventilation are essential (**Table 2**).[9]

The concept of open-lung ventilation originated in the intensive care literature and is an evolution of the management of patients with acute respiratory distress syndrome (ARDS). It consists of avoidance of cycling recruitment and derecruitment for lung injury prevention. In addition, open-lung ventilation maintains FRC and optimizes ventilation/perfusion (V/Q) matching and CO_2 elimination in the ventilated lung.[15,16] Although the shunt fraction primarily depends on the amount of perfusion through the collapsed operative lung, any additional shunt through the ventilated lung in excess of the physiologic 5% is poorly tolerated and usually preventable.

Derecruitment is a common reason for desaturation during OLV. The dependent ventilated lung is noncompliant because of extrinsic compression by abdominal and mediastinal contents and may be inadequately distended by low-tidal volume ventilation with insufficient positive end-expiratory pressure (PEEP). Application of a manual recruitment or vital capacity maneuver at a pressure of 30 to 40 cm H_2O has been shown to result in improved oxygenation during OLV.[15] Prolonged application of a vital capacity maneuver results in a reduced cardiac output, which routinely manifests as a transient dip in oxygen saturations, but may also result in significant hemodynamic instability.[17,18] When using a double-lumen tube (DLT), recruitment can be selectively applied to one lung at a time, which minimizes the intrathoracic pressure increase and associated hemodynamic effects.[19] Invasive arterial monitoring is beneficial for any

Table 1 Predictors of OLV hypoxemia	
Patient	**Procedure**

Preferential perfusion to operative lung
   ◦   Previous contralateral resection
	Preferential perfusion to operative lung
	   ◦ Right-sided surgery

Normal FEV$_1$	Supine position
Chronic vasodilator therapy	Vasodilator use
Poor oxygenation on TLV	Excessive volatile anesthesia (>>1 MAC)

Abbreviations: FEV$_1$, forced expiratory volume in first second of expiration; MAC, minimum alveolar concentration.

Table 2
OLV past and present

	Traditional OLV	Protective OLV	Comments
Emphasis	Oxygenation	Acute lung injury avoidance	
F_{IO_2}	1.0	0.5–0.8	Titrate as tolerated to stable Spo_2 >90%
Vt	10 mL/kg	4–6 mL/kg	Consider larger Vt if refractory hypoxia
P_{CO_2}	40 mm Hg	40–60 mm Hg	Cardiovascular instability possible at P_{CO_2} >70 mm Hg
PEEP	None	5–10 cm H_2O	
Ventilator mode	Volume control	Pressure regulated	Consider HFJV

Abbreviations: Vt, tidal volume.

recruitment maneuver in excess of 10 to 20 seconds. Recruitment maneuvers are successful in achieving improved oxygenation if atelectasis was present in the ventilated lung. This situation by definition indicates that ventilation, and in particular the amount of PEEP, was insufficient to prevent lung collapse. A positive recruitment maneuver should lead to an increase in the applied PEEP. A negative response may indicate adequate or excessive PEEP levels. Excessive PEEP may create or worsen air trapping in predisposed patients.[20] Dynamic air trapping may lead to hypotension because of pulmonary tamponade and can be detected by the presence of residual expiratory flow at the onset of inspiration (**Fig. 1**).[21]

Depressed cardiac output because of neuraxial anesthesia, excessive depth of anesthesia, or tamponade physiology from CO_2 insufflation impairs mixed venous oxygen concentrations, which is difficult to overcome in the setting of high shunt caused by OLV. Restoration of normal cardiac output with inotropic agents (eg, ephedrine) may be required.

TREATMENT OF HYPOXEMIA DURING THORACOSCOPY

The primary reason for desaturation is high shunt flow through the nonventilated lung. Resumption of TLV is therefore the most effective way to address the hypoxemia.

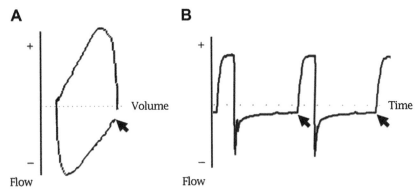

Fig. 1. Evidence of air trapping on spirometry. A flow-volume loop (A) and a flow-time trace (B) show that inspiration begins before complete exhalation of the previous breath (*blue arrow*), leading to gas trapping.

However, because TLV usually impairs exposure to the point that surgery has to be interrupted, other treatment modalities need to be considered unless hypoxemia is severe.

Hypoxemia during thoracoscopy should be addressed in stages (**Fig. 2**). First, any scenario should be temporized with increasing Fio_2 (fraction of inspired oxygen) and ensuring adequate hemodynamics. Immediate recruitment of the operative lung may be required, in cases of severe or symptomatic hypoxemia. With the situation temporized, the initial approach to hypoxemia during OLV is directed toward ensuring optimal ventilation of the nonoperative lung and appropriate circulatory parameters to support oxygen delivery. If hypoxemia persists, advanced interventions to manipulate pulmonary blood flow or use of the operative lung for oxygenation can be entertained.

Lower Fio_2 has become routine in light of concerns about oxygen toxicity and potential acute lung injury (ALI).[9] However, high Fio_2 is clearly required in the setting of hypoxemia, both to increase oxygen delivery and to act as a pulmonary vasodilator,[22] which may improve V/Q matching.

Whenever hypoxemia occurs, it is important to ensure right ventricular (RV) perfusion. HPV in response to OLV increases RV workload because of the increase in the pulmonary vascular resistance (PVR) in the operative lung.[23] Hypoxemia places further stress on the RV because of global pulmonary vascular constriction. Increasing RV systolic pressures cause gradual reductions in RV myocardial perfusion and can result in RV failure as a result of ischemia of the RV free wall. Systemic hypotension is poorly tolerated during periods of RV strain, because effective RV contraction depends on both the rigidity of the interventricular septum as support and the adequacy of the coronary perfusion pressure.[24] Systemic blood pressure support with inotropic agents

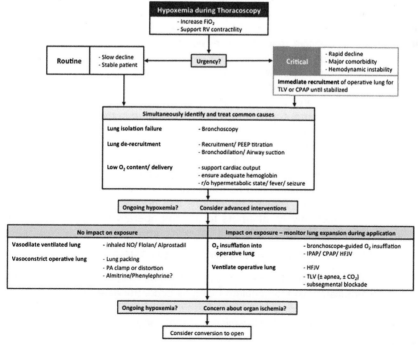

Fig. 2. OLV hypoxemia treatment pathway adapted to thoracoscopic surgery. See text for details. IPAP, intermittent positive airway pressure; NO, nitric oxide; PEEP, positive end-expiratory pressure; RV, right ventricular.

increases RV perfusion and contractility, and therefore the ability of the RV to cope with high afterload conditions.[24,25]

Rather than being a simple function of the degree of desaturation, the urgency of intervention is largely a judgment call based on the specific situation. A saturation of 88% to 90% may be inconsequential and well tolerated for a short wedge resection and in some cases may represent the baseline saturation in patients with advanced chronic obstructive pulmonary disease. On the other hand, a saturation of 90% to 94% may be insufficient in a patient with coronary artery disease and acute electrocardiographic changes or a patient with cerebrovascular disease and decreases in cerebral oximetry. Symptomatic hypoxemia or sudden severe hypoxemia should be stabilized with (at least transient) TLV.

IDENTIFY AND TREAT COMMON CAUSES

The first phase of hypoxemia assessment and treatment focuses on optimal ventilation of the nonoperative lung and appropriate circulatory parameters to support oxygen delivery. Loss of lung isolation, especially partial obstruction of the ventilated bronchus, results in hypoventilation and derecruitment. Lung isolation therefore needs to be confirmed as part of any assessment of OLV hypoxia. The need for fiberoptic bronchoscopy for confirmation depends on the clinical scenario and the index of suspicion for device malposition (ie, the side of surgery, the type of lung isolation device, and the initial adequacy of positioning of the device). In many cases, at least transient confirmation can be achieved by ensuring that ventilator parameters (pressures and volumes) are unchanged. Simultaneously, all ventilator settings should be reviewed to ensure that adequate alveolar ventilation is achieved. As discussed earlier, derecruitment has to be considered as one of the most likely reasons for any desaturation during OLV. Application of a manual recruitment or vital capacity maneuver at a pressure of 30 to 40 cm H_2O results in improved oxygenation in most patients.[15] A positive response to a recruitment maneuver should lead to an increase in the applied PEEP. Inadequate oxygen delivery caused by low cardiac output or low hemoglobin concentration must be ruled out. Transfusion is rarely necessary or justified for maintenance of oxygenation. However, cardiac output support is more commonly necessary. Anesthetic agents and neuraxial sympatholytics depress cardiac output, which may not be tolerated in the frail or hypovolemic patient. Avoidance of excessive anesthetic depth and correction of severe hypovolemia often suffices. Occasional support with inotropic agents (eg, ephedrine) may be necessary and helps to minimize fluid administration. Supranormal cardiac outputs are not indicated and may be detrimental for oxygenation.[26,27] If hypoxemia persists in the face of optimal perfusion and nondependent lung ventilation, advanced interventions may be required. These interventions can consist of manipulations of the shunt fraction, or alternatively, attempts to use the operative lung for oxygenation, the latter of which may interfere with surgical exposure.

ADVANCED INTERVENTIONS WITH NO IMPACT ON EXPOSURE

OLV results in a disruption of normal V/Q matching. Modulation of pulmonary blood flow, either vasodilation of the ventilated lung to accommodate more blood flow or vasoconstriction of the operative lung to further restrict the shunt fraction, can be attempted to more closely match baseline V/Q matching.

Vasodilators

The ventilated lung receives roughly 70% to 80% of the cardiac output during OLV as a result of gravity redistribution and HPV. The pulmonary vascular bed is capable of accepting large increases in blood flow because of its vast recruitable territory. During exercise, cardiac outputs of 30 Liters per minute (Lpm) can be accommodated without increases in pulmonary arterial blood pressure by decreasing PVR.[28] In theory, reducing PVR in the ventilated lung to accommodate more blood flow and thereby reduce the shunt flow across the nonventilated lung should improve oxygenation. In order to maintain HPV in the operative lung, these vasodilators need to be applied selectively to the ventilated lung, which can be achieved by using the inhalational route. Several inhalational pulmonary vascular dilators have been trialed, but only nitric oxide (NO), alprostadil (PGE1) and prostacyclin (PGI1, also known as epoprostenol or Flolan) have been evaluated in the OLV setting.[29] Oxygen itself is an effective pulmonary vascular dilator[22]; however, presumably it is already applied at maximal concentrations. Nitric oxide, an endothelium-derived relaxing factor, is a selective pulmonary vascular dilator. It has been shown to decrease PVR and pulmonary artery pressure (PAP) without affecting venous admixture in patients with normal and moderately increased mean PAP.[30] In studies of patients undergoing thoracic surgery with OLV, inhaled NO (iNO) of 20 ppm was unable to improve oxygenation unless combined with a vasoconstrictor.[31] This lack of oxygenation benefit was independent of F_{IO_2}.[32] In a piglet OLV study, an oxygenation benefit could be shown at concentrations of 4 ppm of iNO, but not higher concentrations.[33] Inhaled prostacyclin (PGI2) has been shown to be as effective as iNO in terms of pulmonary vasodilation in ARDS, cardiac surgery, an animal model of OLV, and lung transplantation.[34–36] As far as oxygenation is concerned, inhaled prostacyclin showed an 88% response rate for increases in P_{AO_2} (partial pressure of oxygen, alveolar)/F_{IO_2} ratio in a diverse population of intensive care unit patients during TLV,[37] but has not been evaluated for OLV. Alprostadil (PGE1) has a higher pulmonary clearance and therefore fewer systemic effects than prostacyclin. Inhaled PGE1 (10 ng/kg/min) has been shown to reduce PVR and improve oxygenation (with a decrease in shunt fraction from 25.9% to 17.4%) during first-graft implantation of double-lung transplants.[38] As a whole, the prostaglandins are significantly cheaper than NO, both in terms of drug cost and delivery system, and provide significant hospital savings.[39] In light of the variable efficacy and significant time required for setup of drug-delivery systems, inhaled agents cannot be relied on as a sudden rescue strategy; their use usually requires advance planning and preparation in the high-risk surgical candidate.

Vasoconstrictors

Even with maximal HPV about a quarter of the cardiac output continues to shunt through the nonventilated lung. This deoxygenated fraction mixes with the oxygenated blood from the ventilated lung and impairs arterial oxygen content. Additional decreases in pulmonary blood flow, and therefore the shunt fraction, can be achieved by pharmacologic means. Almitrine, a respiratory stimulant, which acts as a selective pulmonary vasoconstrictor when injected intravenously, has been shown to potentiate HPV and reduce shunt fraction. Moutafis and colleagues[40] showed that an intravenous infusion of 8 µg/kg/min of almitrine resulted in a P_{AO_2} of 325 mm Hg after 30 minutes of OLV (vs 178 mm Hg in a placebo group) without producing any adverse hemodynamic changes. When used in combination with 20 ppm of iNO an intravenous infusion of 16 µg/kg/min of almitrine resulted in a P_{AO_2} of 408 mm Hg after 30 minutes of OLV (vs 146 mm Hg in the control group).[31] Although almitrine is effective in improving oxygenation, high-dose infusions are associated with increases in PA pressures,[41] which is a potential safety concern, particularly because most of the published data are from small studies, which excluded patients with preexisting pulmonary hypertension. Almitrine remains a theoretical intervention in North America, where it is not commercially available. Other vasoconstrictors have been entertained; however, as none of them are pulmonary specific all result in concomitant systemic vasoconstriction. Phenylephrine infusions have been assessed in a small trial of patients with ARDS. An intravenous infusion of 50 to 200 μg/min did achieve a modest improvement in oxygenation, although only in 50% of patients, and predictably caused systemic vasoconstriction in all patients.[42]

Not having the benefit of larger studies that clearly establish a dose-response curve, as well as a safety profile, particularly in the patient with preexisting pulmonary hypertension and right heart dysfunction, it is difficult to recommend routine pharmacologic manipulation. Inhaled vasodilators may be entertained in high-risk patients, with alprostadil being the only agent that has been shown to improve oxygenation during OLV. There is no literature support for the use of vasoconstrictors other than almitrine for OLV hypoxemia and any such treatment would likely necessitate more invasive hemodynamic monitoring.

Beyond pharmacologic manipulation, PA flow can be mechanically manipulated. Clamping of the PA has been discussed as an intervention in cases of refractory hypoxemia during OLV. Specific surgical techniques for clamping the PA during VATS have been described.[43,44] Aside from physically clamping or side-clamping the artery, which requires hilar exposure, simple distortion of the anatomy can be effective in reducing pulmonary blood flow. Ishikawa and colleagues[14] have shown that packing the lung in the open scenario does improve oxygenation, likely by physically distorting the pulmonary arterial tree. Any reduction in the operative lung pulmonary blood flow comes at the potential cost of increased RV strain. In the study by Ishikawa and colleagues,[14] lung packing resulted in decreases in cardiac output and oxygen delivery.

ADVANCED INTERVENTIONS WITH POTENTIAL IMPACT ON EXPOSURE

Partial ventilation, or apneic oxygenation, of the operative lung is well known for thoracotomy procedures but is generally considered contraindicated in the thoracoscopy setting. Partial lung reinflation is required for these techniques in order for oxygen to be delivered past the conducting airway to the alveolar epithelium. However, this reinflation may interfere with surgical exposure. In order to avoid or minimize the impairment of the surgical exposure, reinflation can be limited to a subsegment of the lung that is remote to the surgical site or be minimally applied across the entire lung. Any reinflation must be monitored in real time on the thoracoscopy monitors. The amount of lung distention and the resulting impairment in surgical exposure are largely dependent on the underlying lung disease and the amount of elastic recoil in the lung tissue. After reinflation, oxygen can be delivered via CPAP circuit, fiberoptic bronchoscope, modified oxygen flush, or HFJV.

CPAP to the operative lung is a proven technique for improving oxygenation because it converts shunt lung to (partially) oxygenated lung, which participates in gas exchange.[45,46] CPAP is considered contraindicated in thoracoscopic procedures because it does require some lung recruitment from the fully atelectatic stage in order to deliver oxygen to the alveoli. In a trial of incremental CPAP titration during open thoracotomy, addition of CPAP resulted in predictable increases in oxygenation without interfering with the surgical field until CPAP pressures of 9 cm H_2O were reached.[47] Low CPAP pressures of 2 cm H_2O have been assessed during thoracoscopy and shown to result in minimal if any impairment of the operative field, with surgeons' satisfaction ranking 9 out of 10.[48] Beyond minimizing the inflation pressure, the amount of lung recruitment has to be limited in order not to impair the surgical field. Patients in whom lung collapse was difficult to achieve or required suction assistance, such as those with severe emphysematous disease, are not good candidates for intraoperative recruitment and CPAP. Similarly, surgeons may not be able to tolerate any degree of recruitment during procedures that require perfect hilar exposure (eg, lobectomies).

Various CPAP adaptations have been proposed to allow for oxygen insufflation without impairing surgical exposure. Russell[49] proposed intermittent positive airway pressurization (IPAP) with oxygen using oxygen tubing attached to a bacteriostatic filter on the nonventilated lumen of the DLT (**Fig. 3**). Occlusion of the filter end effectively closes the circuit and results in delivery of the set oxygen flow into the nonventilated lung, creating transient positive airway pressure and lung recruitment. Using 2 second inspirations at 2 Lpm oxygen flow 6 times per minute for up to 5 minutes, Russell was able to show a mean increase in Spo_2 of 7.2% in 10 patients during OLV. More importantly, he documented minimal lung motion and no impact on surgical exposure.[49]

Ku and colleagues[50] proposed subsegmental IPAP, specifically for the purposes of treating hypoxemia during thoracoscopy (**Fig. 4**). Using an oxygen source connected to the suction port of a fiberoptic bronchoscope, the investigators delivered IPAP (20 seconds at 5 Lpm) into a bronchopulmonary segment distant to the operative site (in their case, an apical bullectomy). This approach heavily relies on adequate knowledge of the subsegmental airway anatomy and clear communication with the surgical team. The amount of lung recruitment that occurs with the IPAP techniques depends on the amount of oxygen flow, the underlying lung disease, and the duration of the IPAP insufflation and therefore requires continuous observation on the surgical monitors. The specific oxygen flow rates and inspiratory times in **Figs. 3** and **4** are examples and need to be adapted to the clinical situation.

Simple oxygen insufflation into the bronchus for apneic oxygenation has been described[51] but does require residual alveolar recruitment. Application of oxygen at the time of complete lung collapse without recruitment does not result in improved oxygenation.[52]

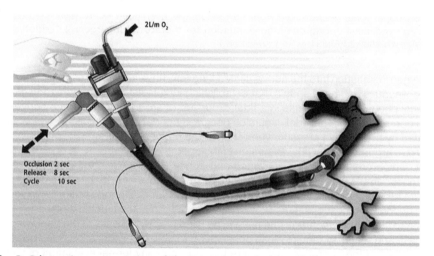

2L/m O₂

Occlusion 2 sec
Release   8 sec
Cycle   10 sec

Fig. 3. Schematic representation of the Intermittent Positive Airway Pressure technique. A bacteriostatic filter is attached to the 15-mm connector of the nonventilated DLT lumen. Tubing with an oxygen flow of 2 Lpm is connected to the sampling port of the filter. The open port of the filter is occluded for 2 seconds and open for 8 seconds. See text for details. (*Reproduced from* Russell WJ. Intermittent positive airway pressure to manage hypoxia during one-lung anaesthesia. Anaesth Intensive Care 2009;37(3):433; with permission.)

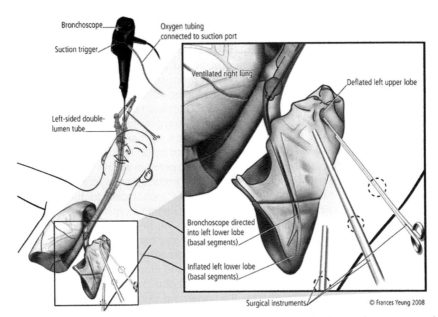

Fig. 4. Bronchoscope-directed segmental oxygen insufflation. The figure demonstrates the technique of insufflating oxygen directly into the left lower lobe basal segments using a fiberoptic bronchoscope during left-sided apical VATS bullectomy. An oxygen source with a flow of 5 Lpm is attached by standard tubing to the suction port of a 4-mm bronchoscope. The bronchoscope is then inserted into the left bronchial lumen of the DLT and guided into the basal segments of the left lower lobe bronchus. (*Insert*) When the suction trigger of the bronchoscope is activated, oxygen is insufflated into the segments of the lung remote from the site of surgery under direct visual observation by the thoracoscope. In this case, the basal segments of the left lower lobe were recruited and surgery could continue unimpeded on the left upper lobe. (*Reproduced from* Ku CM, Slinger P, Waddell TK. A novel method of treating hypoxemia during one-lung ventilation for thoracoscopic surgery. J Cardiothorac Vasc Anesth 2009;23(6):851; with permission.)

Oxygen insufflation into the nonventilated lung may have additional benefits. Pfitzner and colleagues[53,54] have shown that establishing lung isolation before creation of the surgical pneumothorax results in a tidal excursion of around 130 mL in the nonventilated operative lung. This tidal excursion occurs secondary to the cyclical midline shift initiated by the positive pressure ventilation of the nonoperative lung. These investigators have argued that the tidal excursion of the operative lung leads to nitrogen entrainment, which could delay lung collapse and impair HPV. Several investigators have described ambient pressure oxygen administration devices that create a closed system for the operative lung and have anecdotally reported good results for oxygenation during thoracoscopic surgeries in patients with advanced lung disease.[54,55] The caveat to these approaches is that have to be used prophylactically at the beginning of the case and that they require close observation to avoid pressurization (both positive or negative) of the operative lung. There has not been any formal evaluation of these techniques.

On rare occasions, lung isolation is not essential and ventilation of a lobe on the operative side may be possible using subsegmental blockade with a bronchial blocker. Diaphragm and lower chest-wall surgery is most likely to be amenable to this. More commonly, particularly for peripheral procedures such as wedge resections, TLV and intermittent apnea may be possible. CO_2 insufflation with TLV has been shown to be a suitable alternative to lung isolation in the setting of thoracoscopic sympathectomy,[56] prone esophagectomy[57] and pediatric VATS.[58] CO_2 insufflation at low pressures (1–2 mm Hg) has also been described as a means of improving exposure in the setting of pediatric OLV.[13,58] However, CO_2 insufflation pressures of 10 cm H_2O or more have been shown to be associated with cardiac indices below 2 Lpm/m^2 in adult patients.[13]

Another alternative to OLV is two-lung HFJV. HFJV via a single-lumen endotracheal tube has been shown to result in superior oxygenation and equivalent operative conditions for lung resection, esophagectomy, and minimally invasive coronary artery bypass graft (CABG).[59–61] HFJV has been used on the operative lung for thoracoscopic procedures without adverse effects on surgical exposure.[59,62] Two-lung HFJV does require a formal automated jet ventilator and a thorough understanding of its use.

In addition, HFJV has been described as a CPAP alternative for patients at high risk for perioperative desaturation during OLV.[63–65]

RISK OF HYPOXIA

OLV is associated with significant oxidative stress, irrespective of whether hypoxemia does occur. Even in the setting of normoxemia, OLV triggers an ischemia-reperfusion cascade and creates oxidative stress to both the lung and the heart[66,67] as well as histologic oxidative injury to the liver and the intestinal tract.[68] The amount of oxidative stress correlates with the duration of OLV and may therefore be increased in the face of prolonged operating times during VATS. Similarly, brain tissue oxygen saturations decrease during OLV even in normoxemic patients.[69,70] Reduced brain saturations have been associated with increased length of stay and major organ morbidity and mortality after CABG.[71] Intraoperative hypoxemia is likely to worsen the amount of oxidative stress and the severity of brain desaturations and therefore may adversely affect organ function and patient outcome. Although this is speculative, prolonged hypoxemia is likely to be harmful and should be treated.

Despite our best efforts, and because of the increasing number of patients presenting after previous contralateral resection, some patients may be difficult to oxygenate with the limited options that are available during thoracoscopic procedures. Furthermore, some of the partial ventilation techniques may worsen surgical exposure to the point that surgical progress is slowed and the risk of complications increased. Although a conversion may be undesirable, the morbidity of persistent hypoxemia outweighs that of a thoracotomy incision.

REFERENCES

1. Conacher ID. Anesthesia for thoracoscopic surgery. J Minim Access Surg 2007; 3(4):127–31.
2. Lee P, Mathur PN, Colt HG. Advances in thoracoscopy: 100 years since Jacobaeus. Respiration 2010;79(3):177–86.
3. Swanson SJ, Meyers BF, Gunnarsson CL, et al. Video-assisted thoracoscopic lobectomy is less costly and morbid than open lobectomy: a retrospective multi-institutional database analysis. Ann Thorac Surg 2012;93(4):1027–32.
4. Shigemura N, Akashi A, Funaki S, et al. Long-term outcomes after a variety of video-assisted thoracoscopic lobectomy approaches for clinical stage IA lung cancer: a multi-institutional study. J Thorac Cardiovasc Surg 2006;132(3):507–12.

5. Berry MF, D'Amico TA. Complications of thoracoscopic pulmonary resection. Semin Thorac Cardiovasc Surg 2007;19(4):350–4.

6. Cheng D, Downey RJ, Kernstine K, et al. Video-assisted thoracic surgery in lung cancer resection: a meta-analysis and systematic review of controlled trials. Innovations (Phila) 2007;2(6):261–92.

7. West D, Rashid S, Dunning J. Does video-assisted thoracoscopic lobectomy produce equal cancer clearance compared to open lobectomy for non-small cell carcinoma of the lung? Interact Cardiovasc Thorac Surg 2007;6(1):110–6.

8. Fischer GW, Cohen E. An update on anesthesia for thoracoscopic surgery. Curr Opin Anaesthesiol 2010;23(1):7–11.

9. Lohser J. Evidence-based management of one-lung ventilation. Anesthesiol Clin 2008;26(2):241–72.

10. Ishikawa S, Lohser J. One-lung ventilation and arterial oxygenation. Curr Opin Anaesthesiol 2011;24(1):24–31.

11. Fredman B. Physiologic changes during thoracoscopy. Anesthesiol Clin North America 2001;19(1):141–52.

12. Ko R, McRae K, Darling G, et al. The use of air in the inspired gas mixture during two-lung ventilation delays lung collapse during one-lung ventilation. Anesth Analg 2009;108(4):1092–6.

13. Brock H, Rieger R, Gabriel C, et al. Haemodynamic changes during thoracoscopic surgery the effects of one-lung ventilation compared with carbon dioxide insufflation. Anaesthesia 2000;55(1):10–6.

14. Ishikawa S, Shirasawa M, Fujisawa M, et al. Compressing the non-dependent lung during one-lung ventilation improves arterial oxygenation, but impairs systemic oxygen delivery by decreasing cardiac output. J Anesth 2010;24(1):17–23.

15. Tusman G, Böhm SH, Sipmann FS, et al. Lung recruitment improves the efficiency of ventilation and gas exchange during one-lung ventilation anesthesia. Anesth Analg 2004;98(6):1604–9.

16. Unzueta C, Tusman G, Suarez-Sipmann F, et al. Alveolar recruitment improves ventilation during thoracic surgery: a randomized controlled trial. Br J Anaesth 2012;108(3):517–24.

17. Cinnella G, Grasso S, Natale C, et al. Physiological effects of a lung-recruiting strategy applied during one-lung ventilation. Acta Anaesthesiol Scand 2008; 52(6):766–75.

18. Garutti I, Martinez G, Cruz P, et al. The impact of lung recruitment on hemodynamics during one-lung ventilation. J Cardiothorac Vasc Anesth 2009;23(4):506–8.

19. Hansen LK, Koefoed-Nielsen J, Nielsen J, et al. Are selective lung recruitment maneuvers hemodynamically safe in severe hypovolemia? An experimental study in hypovolemic pigs with lobar collapse. Anesth Analg 2007;105(3):729–34.

20. Slinger PD, Hickey DR. The interaction between applied PEEP and auto-PEEP during one-lung ventilation. J Cardiothorac Vasc Anesth 1998;12(2):133–6.

21. Bardoczky GI, d'Hollander AA, Cappello M, et al. Interrupted expiratory flow on automatically constructed flow-volume curves may determine the presence of intrinsic positive end-expiratory pressure during one-lung ventilation. Anesth Analg 1998;86(4):880–4.

22. Roberts DH, Lepore JJ, Maroo A, et al. Oxygen therapy improves cardiac index and pulmonary vascular resistance in patients with pulmonary hypertension. Chest 2001;120(5):1547–55.

23. Carlsson AJ, Bindslev L, Hedenstierna G. Hypoxia-induced pulmonary vasoconstriction in the human lung. The effect of isoflurane anesthesia. Anesthesiology 1987;66(3):312–6.

24. Klima UP, Lee MY, Guerrero JL, et al. Determinants of maximal right ventricular function: role of septal shift. J Thorac Cardiovasc Surg 2002;123(1):72–80.

25. Vlahakes GJ, Turley K, Hoffman JI. The pathophysiology of failure in acute right ventricular hypertension: hemodynamic and biochemical correlations. Circulation 1981;63(1):87–95.

26. Slinger P, Scott WA. Arterial oxygenation during one-lung ventilation. A comparison of enflurane and isoflurane. Anesthesiology 1995;82(4):940–6.

27. Russell WJ, James MF. The effects on arterial haemoglobin oxygen saturation and on shunt of increasing cardiac output with dopamine or dobutamine during one-lung ventilation. Anaesth Intensive Care 2004;32(5):644–8.

28. Groves BM, Reeves JT, Sutton JR, et al. Operation Everest II: elevated high-altitude pulmonary resistance unresponsive to oxygen. J Appl Physiol 1987; 63(2):521–30.

29. Ross AF, Ueda K. Pulmonary hypertension in thoracic surgical patients. Curr Opin Anaesthesiol 2010;23(1):25–33.

30. Rich GF, Lowson SM, Johns RA, et al. Inhaled nitric oxide selectively decreases pulmonary vascular resistance without impairing oxygenation during one-lung ventilation in patients undergoing cardiac surgery. Anesthesiology 1994;80(1): 57–62.

31. Moutafis M, Liu N, Dalibon N, et al. The effects of inhaled nitric oxide and its combination with intravenous almitrine on Pao2 during one-lung ventilation in patients undergoing thoracoscopic procedures. Anesth Analg 1997;85(5): 1130–5.

32. Schwarzkopf K, Klein U, Schreiber T, et al. Oxygenation during one-lung ventilation: the effects of inhaled nitric oxide and increasing levels of inspired fraction of oxygen. Anesth Analg 2001;92(4):842–7.

33. Sticher J, Scholz S, Böning O, et al. Small-dose nitric oxide improves oxygenation during one-lung ventilation: an experimental study. Anesth Analg 2002;95(6): 1557–62.

34. Haché M, Denault A, Bélisle S, et al. Inhaled epoprostenol (prostacyclin) and pulmonary hypertension before cardiac surgery. J Thorac Cardiovasc Surg 2003;125(3):642–9.

35. Max M, Kuhlen R, Dembinski R, et al. Effect of aerosolized prostacyclin and inhaled nitric oxide on experimental hypoxic pulmonary hypertension. Intensive Care Med 1999;25(10):1147–54.

36. Khan TA, Schnickel G, Ross D, et al. A prospective, randomized, crossover pilot study of inhaled nitric oxide versus inhaled prostacyclin in heart transplant and lung transplant recipients. J Thorac Cardiovasc Surg 2009;138(6):1417–24.

37. Haché M, Denault AY, Bélisle S, et al. Inhaled prostacyclin (PGI2) is an effective addition to the treatment of pulmonary hypertension and hypoxia in the operating room and intensive care unit. Can J Anaesth 2001;48(9):924–9.

38. Della Rocca G, Coccia C, Pompei L, et al. Inhaled aerosolized prostaglandin E1, pulmonary hemodynamics, and oxygenation during lung transplantation. Minerva Anestesiol 2008;74(11):627–33.

39. De Wet CJ, Affleck DG, Jacobsohn E, et al. Inhaled prostacyclin is safe, effective, and affordable in patients with pulmonary hypertension, right heart dysfunction, and refractory hypoxemia after cardiothoracic surgery. J Thorac Cardiovasc Surg 2004;127(4):1058–67.

40. Moutafis M, Dalibon N, Liu N, et al. The effects of intravenous almitrine on oxygenation and hemodynamics during one-lung ventilation. Anesth Analg 2002;94(4): 830–4.

41. Silva-Costa-Gomes T, Gallart L, Vallès J, et al. Low- vs high-dose almitrine combined with nitric oxide to prevent hypoxia during open-chest one-lung ventilation. Br J Anaesth 2005;95(3):410–6.

42. Doering EB, Hanson CW, Reily DJ, et al. Improvement in oxygenation by phenylephrine and nitric oxide in patients with adult respiratory distress syndrome. Anesthesiology 1997;87(1):18–25.

43. Watanabe A, Koyanagi T, Nakashima S, et al. How to clamp the main pulmonary artery during video-assisted thoracoscopic surgery lobectomy. Eur J Cardiothorac Surg 2007;31(1):129–31.

44. Kamiyoshihara M, Nagashima T, Ibe T, et al. A tip for controlling the main pulmonary artery during video-assisted thoracic major pulmonary resection: the outside-field vascular clamping technique. Interact Cardiovasc Thorac Surg 2010;11(5):693–5.

45. Cohen E, Eisenkraft JB, Thys DM, et al. Oxygenation and hemodynamic changes during one-lung ventilation: effects of CPAP10, PEEP10, and CPAP10/PEEP10. J Cardiothorac Anesth 1988;2(1):34–40.

46. Badner NH, Goure C, Bennett KE, et al. Role of continuous positive airway pressure to the non-ventilated lung during one-lung ventilation with low tidal volumes. HSR Proc Intensive Care Cardiovasc Anesth 2011;3(3):189–94.

47. Kim SH, Jung KT, An TH. Effects of tidal volume and PEEP on arterial blood gases and pulmonary mechanics during one-lung ventilation. J Anesth 2012;26(4):568–73.

48. El-Tahan MR, El Ghoneimy YF, Regal MA, et al. Comparative study of the non-dependent continuous positive pressure ventilation and high-frequency positive-pressure ventilation during one-lung ventilation for video-assisted thoracoscopic surgery. Interact Cardiovasc Thorac Surg 2011;12(6):899–902.

49. Russell WJ. Intermittent positive airway pressure to manage hypoxia during one-lung anaesthesia. Anaesth Intensive Care 2009;37(3):432–4.

50. Ku CM, Slinger P, Waddell TK. A novel method of treating hypoxemia during one-lung ventilation for thoracoscopic surgery. J Cardiothorac Vasc Anesth 2009;23(6):850–2.

51. Sanchez-Lorente D, Gómez-Caro A, Jimenez MJ, et al. Apnoeic oxygenation on one-lung ventilation in functionally impaired patients during sleeve lobectomy. Eur J Cardiothorac Surg 2011;39(4):77–9.

52. Slimani J, Russell WJ, Jurisevic C. An evaluation of the relative efficacy of an open airway, an oxygen reservoir and continuous positive airway pressure 5 cm H2O on the non-ventilated lung. Anaesth Intensive Care 2004;32(6):756–60.

53. Pfitzner J, Peacock MJ, McAleer PT. Gas movement in the nonventilated lung at the onset of single-lung ventilation for video-assisted thoracoscopy. Anaesthesia 1999;54(5):437–43.

54. Pfitzner J, Peacock MJ, Daniels BW. Ambient pressure oxygen reservoir apparatus for use during one-lung anaesthesia. Anaesthesia 1999;54(5):454–8.

55. Baraka A, Lteif A, Nawfal M, et al. Ambient pressure oxygenation via the nonventilated lung during video-assisted thoracoscopy. Anaesthesia 2000;55(6):602–3.

56. Rozenberg B, Katz Y, Isserles SA, et al. Near-sitting position and two-lung ventilation for endoscopic transthoracic sympathectomy. J Cardiothorac Vasc Anesth 1996;10(2):210–2.

57. Bonavina L, Laface L, Abate E, et al. Comparison of ventilation and cardiovascular parameters between prone thoracoscopic and Ivor Lewis esophagectomy. Updates Surg 2012;64(2):81–5.

58. Gentili A, Lima M, De Rose R, et al. Thoracoscopy in children: anaesthesiological implications and case reports. Minerva Anestesiol 2007;73(3):161–71.
59. Ender J, Brodowsky M, Falk V, et al. High-frequency jet ventilation as an alternative method compared to conventional one-lung ventilation using double-lumen tubes during minimally invasive coronary artery bypass graft surgery. J Cardiothorac Vasc Anesth 2010;24(4):602–7.
60. Buise M, van Bommel J, van Genderen M, et al. Two-lung high-frequency jet ventilation as an alternative ventilation technique during transthoracic esophagectomy. J Cardiothorac Vasc Anesth 2009;23(4):509–12.
61. Misiolek H, Knapik P, Swanevelder J, et al. Comparison of double-lung jet ventilation and one-lung ventilation for thoracotomy. Eur J Anaesthesiol 2008;25(1): 15–21.
62. Suzuki Y, Katori K, Mayama T, et al. Anesthetic management for thoracoscopic partial lobectomy in a patient with one lung. Masui 2002;51(8):921–3 [in Japanese].
63. Knüttgen D, Zeidler D, Vorweg M, et al. Unilateral high-frequency jet ventilation supporting one-lung ventilation during thoracic surgical procedures. Anaesthesist 2001;50(8):585–9 [in German].
64. Knüttgen D, Zeidler D, Doehn M. Secondary lung surgery following contralateral pneumonectomy. Anaesthesiological considerations. Anaesthesist 2003;52(1): 42–6 [in German].
65. Godet G, Bertrand M, Rouby JJ, et al. High-frequency jet ventilation vs continuous positive airway pressure for differential lung ventilation in patients undergoing resection of thoracoabdominal aortic aneurysm. Acta Anaesthesiol Scand 1994;38(6):562–8.
66. Williams EA, Quinlan GJ, Goldstraw P, et al. Postoperative lung injury and oxidative damage in patients undergoing pulmonary resection. Eur Respir J 1998; 11(5):1028–34.
67. Misthos P, Katsaragakis S, Theodorou D, et al. The degree of oxidative stress is associated with major adverse effects after lung resection: a prospective study. Eur J Cardiothorac Surg 2006;29(4):591–5.
68. Yuluğ E, Tekinbas C, Ulusoy H, et al. The effects of oxidative stress on the liver and ileum in rats caused by one-lung ventilation. J Surg Res 2007;139(2):253–60.
69. Hemmerling TM, Bluteau MC, Kazan R, et al. Significant decrease of cerebral oxygen saturation during single-lung ventilation measured using absolute oximetry. Br J Anaesth 2008;101(6):870–5.
70. Iwata M, Inoue S, Kawaguchi M, et al. Jugular bulb venous oxygen saturation during one-lung ventilation under sevoflurane- or propofol-based anesthesia for lung surgery. J Cardiothorac Vasc Anesth 2008;22(1):71–6.
71. Murkin JM, Adams SJ, Novick RJ, et al. Monitoring brain oxygen saturation during coronary bypass surgery: a randomized, prospective study. Anesth Analg 2007; 104(1):51–8.

Advancements in Robotic-Assisted Thoracic Surgery

Brad Steenwyk, MD*, Ralph Lyerly III

KEYWORDS

- Robotic • Thoracic • Lobectomy • Thymectomy • Ivor Lewis
- Esophagogastrectomy

KEY POINTS

- The robotic instruments translate the surgeon's hand movements from the robotic console without need for counteractive adaptation.
- Robotic arms #1 and #2 represent the surgeon's right and left hands, which allows for bimanual dissection and other coordinated movements. A third robotic arm is used to attach a camera, which the surgeon is able to directly control. With the optional fourth arm, a third device (such as a retractor) can be used simultaneously while still being controlled by the surgeon.

Robotic-assisted thoracic surgery (RATS) has become increasingly used as a technique to facilitate less invasive thoracic surgery. As surgical approaches change, it is necessary to understand the impacts these changes have to modify the perioperative care to optimize operative success, safety, and patient satisfaction.

The minimally invasive platform for surgical technique has been in progress for many years. The first thoracoscopy was performed by the Irish physician Francis Richard Cruise in 1865. However, it was the Swedish physician H.C. Jacobeus who first described a detailed description of endoscopic techniques using a cystoscope for the diagnosis and treatment of pleural diseases as early as 1910, thus becoming known as the father of thoracoscopy.[1] This device consisted of a long tube with a light at the distal end, and provided only direct line of sight. It had significant limitations in image magnification, operator-only visualization of the surgical field, and limited functionality of surgical instruments.

VIDEO-ASSISTED THORACOSCOPIC SURGERY

With the addition of video imaging systems using xenon-powered 300 W cold light, smaller fiber optic tubes to enhance light transmission, zero to 30° viewing telescopes,

Disclosure: There are no financial or other conflicts to be disclosed.
Department of Anesthesiology, University of Alabama School of Medicine, JT845, 619 South 19th Street, Birmingham, AL 35249, USA
* Corresponding author.
E-mail address: bsteenwy@uab.edu

Anesthesiology Clin 30 (2012) 699–708
http://dx.doi.org/10.1016/j.anclin.2012.08.010   **anesthesiology.theclinics.com**
1932-2275/12/$ – see front matter © 2012 Published by Elsevier Inc.

and cameras with three-chip image processors, the limitations of poor visual field and operator-only viewing were decreased.[2,3] In addition, accompanying instrument functionality was refined and improved significantly. Video-assisted thoracoscopic surgery (VATS) became commonplace in the early 1990s and has progressed to be a valid and commonly chosen option for the treatment of certain pleural space diseases (eg, pneumothorax, chylothorax, hemothorax, empyema), esophageal diseases, mediastinal lesions, and in benign and malignant pulmonary disease (minor [wedge or segmentectomy] or major [lobar]). Proponents of VATS cite smaller wounds, less postsurgical pain, less blood loss, shorter patient hospital stays, and improved survival in patients with non–small-cell lung cancer with comparable or improved surgical results over open thoracotomy techniques.[4–7]

VATS is, however, limited by several significant issues. The two-dimensional image contributes to lack of depth perception. Ergonomically, the surgeon's hands have to move in large motions, counteractive to the direction of the instrument's tip. Movement of the tip is generated by hand motion and that movement, along with any tremor, is accentuated at the device tip. This can make dissection or maneuvering around vulnerable tissues difficult, dangerous, and potentially jeopardize the success of the operation (eg, lymph node and vessel dissections). Also, with VATS, the instruments pivot at the point of insertion in the chest wall, and excess motion and rubbing of the intercostal nerves can contribute to pain at the portal site.

RATS

The robotic platform was introduced, in part, to remedy some of these issues. The da Vinci surgical robotic system (Intuitive Surgical, Sunnyvale, CA, USA) consists of an operating console for the surgeon and a bedside chassis with three or four robotic arms. The console offers high-definition, three-dimensional optics for clear, magnified viewing, and ergonomic controls for the surgeon's hands. An accompanying line of surgical instruments attach to the robotic arms. These devices are jointed, offering superior maneuverability with 7° of freedom in movement of the instrument tip and 360° of rotation. The robotic instruments translate the surgeon's hand movements from the robotic console without need for counteractive adaptation. Robotic arms #1 and #2 represent the surgeon's right and left hands, which allows for bimanual dissection and other coordinated movements. Another robotic arm is used to attach a camera, which the surgeon is able to control directly. With the optional fourth arm, a third device (such as a retractor) can be used simultaneously while still being controlled by the surgeon. Effectively, this provides the operator the ability to navigate through and operate in the confined spaces of the chest, as well as perform more delicate maneuvers, via the minimally invasive approach.

The robotic platform requires a trained assistant at the patient's bedside to facilitate the surgery. The assistant's responsibilities include changing robotic instruments, introducing and removing sutures, and firing the stapler on pulmonary vessels.

DRAWBACKS TO RATS

Similar to robotic applications in other surgical subspecialties, there are several significant hurdles that have made universal use of this device difficult: cost and training. In regard to cost, the capital cost of acquiring the four-arm robot with two consoles is more than $2,000,000. The maintenance contract approaches $100,000 per year. The instruments are about $2000 each and are limited to 10 uses. The noncapital costs include team-training costs, as well as increased operating room times during the learning process.

Park and Flores[8] compared relative costs for thoracotomy lobectomy, VATS lobectomy, and RATS lobectomy. The average VATS lobectomy cost $1479, the RATS lobectomy averaged at $3981, while the average for thoracotomy lobectomy was reported to be $8368. Interestingly, the surgical fees for either minimally invasive approach were $515 less than thoracotomy. Also, the increase of relative cost from VATS to RATS was noted to be almost completely due to day-of-surgery costs. That study did not amortize the capital cost of the robot into the findings; however, based on their capital expenses and projected usage, it would have added $1715 per case. Although RATS lobectomy was significantly more expensive than VATS lobectomy, it was still less than thoracotomy approach. Most cost benefit from both minimally invasive techniques occurred from the decreased hospital stay.

In regard to training, it is currently at the discretion of individual hospitals to define the criteria for credentialing a surgeon for RATS. Recommendations suggested by teams that have successfully incorporated robotics into their practice include preceptorship, observation, and simulation.[9,10] After basic online training designed to orient the team on the robot's functional and safety features, onsite training should be performed, including setting up the robot and console familiarization. A software package allows for training and documentation of robotic skills by teaching basic exercises and monitoring surgical skill and speed. Cadaveric training is required, as there is no software program that allows for full simulation of thoracic surgeries. Before the first case, the surgeon and team should observe an experienced team performing surgery to allow for questions and discussion. After the team is fully prepared, the key is to provide a steady supply of cases to generate experience, repetition, and feedback.

DESCRIPTION OF OPERATIVE APPROACHES FOR THORACIC SURGERY
Completely Portal Robotic Lobectomy with Four Robotic Arms

The positioning for robotic approach using completely portal robotic lobectomy with four robotic arms (CPRL-4) for tumor or other pathologic conditions located superior to the inferior pulmonary vein is described (**Fig. 1**)[11]:

1. The patient is in the lateral decubitus position and single-lung ventilation of the nonoperative lung is used.
2. The pleural space is entered over the top of rib 7 with a 5-mm port in the midaxillary line.
3. A 5-mm VATS camera is used to verify entry into the pleural space and isothermic carbon dioxide is insufflated to drive the diaphragm inferiorly.

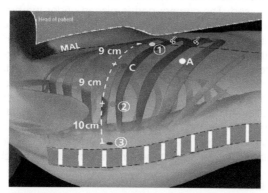

Fig. 1. CPRL-4. The circled numbers represent the robotic arms used. A, 15 mm access port; C, camera port. (*From* Cerfolio RJ, Bryant AS, Skylizard L, et al. Initial consecutive experience of completely portal robotic pulmonary resection with 4 arms. J Thorac Cardiovasc Surg 2011;142(4):740–6; with permission.)

4. A paravertebral block is performed with a 21g needle from ribs 3 to 11.
5. The second incision, which will be the most posterior, is then made two ribs below the major fissure and as posterior in the chest as possible (anterior to the spinal process of the vertebral body).
6. A 5-mm trocar is placed for robotic arm #3.
7. The incision and insertion of an 8-mm trocar for robotic arm #2 will be made 10 cm anterior to that incision along the same rib (usually rib 8).
8. A fourth incision site is marked 9 cm anterior to this port along the same rib, which will serve as the robotic camera port.
9. The site for the access port is identified at the most anterior and inferior aspect of the chest just above the diaphragm.
10. The access port is used by the assistant for access and removal of devices and tissue specimens.
11. The VATS camera will be replaced with a trocar for robotic arm #1.
12. The robot will be driven over the patients shoulder at a 15° angle and attached to the ports.

The approach for inferior and posterior mediastinal pathologic conditions can be more difficult.[12] The robotic viewpoint will be unable to expose the area inferior to the inferior pulmonary vein with the previously described approach. The lesion to be resected should lie in between the camera port and the robot. To this end, then, there are two options:

1. Dock the robot alongside the operating room table, parallel to the patient, behind the patient's torso. CPRL-4 trocar placements are used. This option is commonly used for inferior esophageal leiomyomas, inferior posterior mediastinal tumors, esophageal myotomy for achalasia, or diaphragmatic plication.
2. Place all the trocars in the midaxillary line and drive the robot in dorsally over the patient's spine. This allows for exposure to the very low and posterior mediastinum and diaphragm with greater ease of robotic docking. It is the preferred approach for robotic Ivor Lewis esophagogastrectomy operations and diaphragmatic tumors.

The approach for anterior mediastinal masses (eg, thymectomy) commonly involves only three incisions (a fourth incision for a working port is used by some surgeons).[13,14] The patient is either placed supine with a slight bump under the chest and the whole bed is angled slightly or positioned operative side up at 30°. Either the left or the right thorax can be accessed. The camera port is placed under the breast crease in the midaxillary line. The left robotic arm port is placed generally in the second or third intercostal space in the midaxillary region (the patient's anatomy will dictate the ideal location because the highest incision should not be above the level of the right internal mammary vein junction with the superior vena cava). If a right-sided technique is used, the right robotic arm port is placed above the diaphragm (intercostal space 8 or 9). If a left-sided technique is used, the right robotic arm port is placed in the fifth intercostal space in the midaxillary region. The benefit to the left-sided approach is that there may be enhanced visualization of the phrenic nerve; however, there is more room in the right thorax for instrumentation and maneuvering. Keeping the robotic arms at least 8 cm apart minimizes the chance that the arms will collide with each other.

ANESTHESIA FOR RATS

Adapting the anesthetic for RATS is most similar to that for VATS or open thoracostomies, but there are unique considerations that can save time and/or improve patient safety (see later discussion).

Preoperative Considerations

Preoperative considerations differ little from those routinely used for VATS or open thoracotomy. Specifically, one must always be prepared for conversion to either of these techniques. Pulmonary function and cardiac testing should be performed according to current guidelines for intrathoracic, noncardiac surgery. Laboratory testing should account for patient-specific considerations as well as the potential for significant blood loss. The myasthenia gravis patient should be assessed and assigned according to the Myasthenia Gravis Foundation of America Clinical Classification[14] and the anesthetic procedure planned accordingly.[15] Special considerations should be given for patients with vertebral disease, especially if they have radiculopathy or loss of function, tominimize position-induced neuromuscular compromise in the lateral decubitus position. Preoperative consideration of postoperative pain control methods should replicate those of VATS procedures.

Monitoring Considerations

There are no specific monitoring modalities required for RATS other than the standard American Society of Anesthesiologists monitoring for the anesthetized patients. Choice of invasive monitoring (eg, central venous catheters, pulmonary artery catheters, arterial catheters) should be based on patient-specific needs. Special consideration should be entertained to account for the experience of the surgical team and expected duration of the surgical procedure. Transesophageal echocardiography is logistically more difficult when the robot is docked over the patient's head but it can be performed.

Logistical Considerations

The large footprint of the robot chassis and broad reach of the robotic arms have proven to be a logistical consideration for room layout. To facilitate exposure, the patient is often turned 90° from the anesthesia provider. Often the head and hands are obscured by the robot, which makes access to them difficult after the robot is docked. Hence, vascular access and lung isolation is best obtained before final patient positioning.

Limitations of Access

The robotic arms, monitors, and surgical personnel will occupy the zone around the patient (**Fig. 2**). Extensions for intravenous (IV) tubing are necessary, and injection ports or stopcocks need to be in an accessible location. Long monitoring lines and anesthesia circuits (or extensions added to a regular length circuit) allow the patient to be several feet away from the anesthesia console. Bundling the lines, IVs, and anesthesia circuit in a singular, easily visible fashion minimizes the risk of accidental dislodgment by surgical personnel as they move around the patient.

VENOUS RETURN IMPAIRMENT

The use of carbon dioxide (CO_2) insufflation in the thorax is generally well tolerated, but can present specific risks, such as venous gas embolism, decreased venous return to the right atrium, or acute cardiovascular collapse (most commonly hypotension, bradycardia, and/or arterial desaturation). For thoracoscopy, it is recommended that CO_2 insufflation should be started only after the pleural cavity has been open to ambient air for 30 to 60 seconds and to start insufflation slowly (1 L/min) to avoid cardiovascular collapse.[16] The effects of insufflation must be accounted for if the central venous pressure is being monitored. As a precaution, de-airing of all IV lines should be performed to minimized risk of systemic air embolus through a patent foramen ovale.

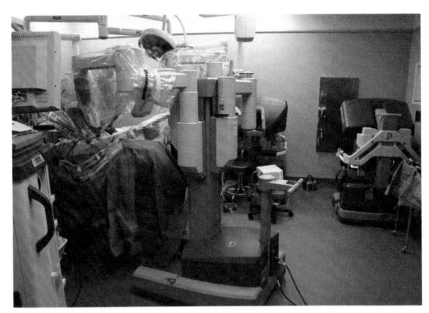

Fig. 2. Robot docked at head of patient.

Patient positioning also contributes to decreased venous return. For maximal robotic arm range and maneuverability, the patient is positioned in a lateral decubitus position (right or left, depending on the surgery), flexed, then tilted so the thorax is the highest point. This position places the lower extremities below the level of the heart and can impair venous return (**Fig. 3**).

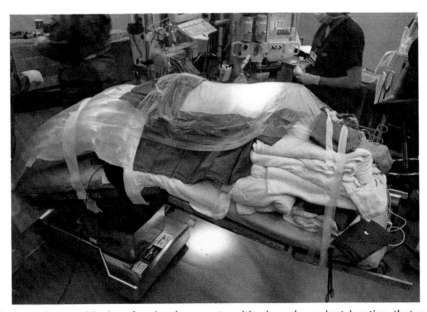

Fig. 3. Patient positioning showing lower extremities in a dependent location that may impair venous return to the heart.

Occasionally, malposition of the internal retractor may unintentionally compress cardiac or major vascular structures, resulting in hemodynamic instability with accompanying EKG changes (**Fig. 4**).

Fluid management in thoracic surgery has long been an area of debate secondary to concern for pulmonary edema.[17] Certainly that debate is beyond the scope of this article, but practitioners may encounter the need to augment vasoconstriction and/or venoconstriction pharmacologically while the patient's position and CO_2 insufflation in the thorax hinder venous return, especially if volume restriction is used.

PATIENT IMMOBILITY

As with any RATS, patient immobility is an absolute must. The robotic arms will not accommodate patient movement. Movement of the patient's thorax while robotic instruments are docked could lead to tearing or puncturing of the intrathoracic organs and vasculature with devastating consequences. Pharmacologic paralysis is routinely used, albeit judiciously, in patients with myasthenia gravis. Standard train-of-four neuromuscular twitch monitoring is useful but can be cumbersome to access while the robot is docked. Special precautions to ensure no bed movement should be used, such as turning the power to the bed off or removing the bed controller.

POSITIONING NEUROPATHY

Several factors can contribute to positioning neuropathy. Ischemia of the nerve due to external compression can occur from inadequate padding or positioning, as well as from inadvertent robotic arm pressure if it is allowed to rest on the patient. Additionally, peripheral nerves are intolerant of stretch, so care must be taken to exclude hyperextension of the shoulder or brachial plexus.

PROPHYLAXIS CONSIDERATIONS

Pharmacologic prophylaxis against deep vein thrombosis is achieved by preoperative low-molecular-weight heparin subcutaneous injection. The application of thromboembolic-deterrent antiembolic hosing and intermittent compression devices on the lower extremities is intended to prevent venous pooling in the lower extremities.

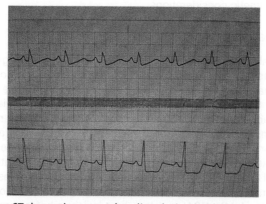

Fig. 4. EKG showing ST depression versus baseline during inadvertent retraction of the left atrium during RATS.

Antibiotic prophylaxis should be administered per current Society of Thoracic Surgery guidelines (www.sts.org).[18]

SINGLE-LUNG VENTILATION

The preferred method to achieve single-lung ventilation with adequate operative lung egress is via a double-lumen endotracheal tube. When placed with fiberoptic scope guidance, it also allows for evaluation of the airway for anomalies or debris. Insufflation of the thorax with CO_2 can lead to malpositioning of the bronchial cuff. It is important to be observant for any lung insufflation while operative devices are in the chest because trauma to the lung parenchyma can occur.

BLADDER CATHETERIZATION

Routine catheterization need not be performed just because a case is robotically assisted. Instead, consideration for coexisting disease, expected case length, volume requirements, and presence of an epidural for postoperative pain management must be taken into account. Intrinsic to any procedure is risk of injury or infection, so the risks versus the benefits must be taken into account.

TEMPERATURE MANAGEMENT

Hypothermia can be prevented or diminished with expeditious patient positioning, isothermic carbon dioxide, reasonable operating room temperatures, and a forced-air warming blanket placed over the abdomen and lower extremities. To minimize airborne dispersion of bacteria, the warm air should not be blown into the blanket until the patient is satisfactorily prepped and draped. Nasopharyngeal or core temperature monitoring via bladder catheter (if present) is preferred. Likewise, if a pulmonary artery catheter is used and is positioned in the nonoperative pulmonary artery, it can serve as a reliable source.

LEARNING CURVE

With adequate case volume and a dedicated team effort, one can expect to reduce operative times and rates of conversion to VATS or open thoracotomy. This may affect choice of monitoring modalities, vascular access, postoperative pain control strategies, or other anesthetic considerations.

EMERGENCY PLANNING

As with all surgical procedures, plans should be in place for management of hemorrhage or cardiovascular instability. In regard to RATS, undocking of the robot is an additional step that must be accounted for before complete access to the patient can be conveniently obtained. The robotic team should be proficient in undocking the robot, preferably in less than 60 seconds. All team members must understand management plans for immediate cardiopulmonary resuscitation and/or advanced cardiac life support. Specifically, external defibrillation should not be attempted while the robot is docked in the thorax. Additionally, external defibrillation will likely be unsuccessful until two-lung ventilation is reinstituted with decompression of the iatrogenic pneumothorax.[19] The placement of a large antimicrobial incision drape, such as an Ioban (3M, St. Paul, MN, USA) over the chest incisions before breach of the sterile field can help preserve surgical site sterility.

SUMMARY

Advancements in RATS present potential advantages for patients as well as new challenges for the anesthesia and surgery teams. It has become increasingly used as a technique to facilitate less invasive thoracic surgery. As surgical approaches change, it is necessary to understand the impacts these changes have to modify the perioperative care to optimize operative success, safety, and patient satisfaction.

REFERENCES

1. Moisiuc F, Colt H. Thoracoscopy: origins revisited. Respiration 2007;74:344–55.
2. Berber E, Siperstein AE. Understanding and optimizing laparoscopic videosystems. Surg Endosc 2001;15:781–7.
3. Rivas H, Cacchione R, Allen JW. Understanding and optimizing laparoscopic videosystems. Surg Endosc 2002;16:1376.
4. Mahtabifard A, DeArmond DT, Fuller CB, et al. Video-assisted thoracoscopic surgery for stage I lung cancer. Thorac Surg Clin 2007;17:223–31.
5. Whitson BA, Groth SS, Duval SS, et al. Surgery for early-stage non-small cell lung cancer: a systematic review of the video-assisted thoracoscopic surgery versus thoracotomy approaches to lobectomy. Ann Thorac Surg 2008;86:2008–18.
6. Yan TD, Black D, Bannon PG, et al. Systematic review and meta-analysis of randomized and nonrandomized trials on safety and efficacy of video-assisted thoracic surgery lobectomy for early-stage non-small-cell lung cancer. J Clin Oncol 2009;27:2553–62.
7. Flores RM, Ihekweasu UN, Rizk N, et al. Patterns of recurrence and incidence of second primary tumors after lobectomy by means of video-assisted thorascopic surgery (VATS) versus thoracotomy for lung cancer. J Thorac Cardiovasc Surg 2011;141:59–64.
8. Park B, Flores R. Cost comparison of robotic, video-assisted thoracic surgery and thoracotomy approaches to pulmonary lobectomy. Thorac Surg Clin 2008;18: 297–300.
9. Landry C, Grubbs E, Lee J, et al. From scalpel to console: a suggested model for surgical skill acquisition. Bull Am Coll Surg 2010;95(8):20–4.
10. Cerfolio RJ, Bryant AS, Minnich DJ. Starting a robotic program in general thoracic surgery: why, how, and lessons learned. Ann Thorac Surg 2011;91:1729–37.
11. Cerfolio RJ, Bryant AS, Skylizard L, et al. Initial consecutive experience of completely portal robotic pulmonary resection with 4 arms. J Thorac Cardiovasc Surg 2011;142(4):740–6.
12. Cerfolio RJ, Bryant AS, Minnich DJ. Operative techniques in robotic thoracic surgery for inferior or posterior mediastinal pathology. J Thorac Cardiovasc Surg 2012;143(5):1138–43.
13. Goldstein SD, Yang SC. Assessment of robotic thymectomy using the Myasthenia Gravis Foundation of America guidelines. Ann Thorac Surg 2010;89:1080–6.
14. Jaretski A III, Barohn RJ, Ernstoff RM, et al. Myasthenia gravis: recommendations for clinical research standards. Ann Thorac Surg 2000;70:327–34.
15. Abel M, Eisenkraft J. Anesthetic implications of myasthenia gravis. Mt Sinai J Med 2002;69(1–2):31–7.
16. Harris RJ, Benveniste G, Pfitzner J. Cardiovascular collapse caused by carbon dioxide insufflation during one-lung anaesthesia for thoracoscopic dorsal sympathectomy. Anaesth Intensive Care 2002;30:86–9.
17. Slinger P. Post-pneumonectomy pulmonary edema: is anesthesia to blame? Curr Opin Anaesthesiol 1999;12(1):49–54.

18. Engelman R, Shahian D, Shemin R, et al. The Society of Thoracic Surgeons Practice Guideline Series: antibiotic prophylaxis in cardiac surgery, part II: antibiotic choice. Ann Thorac Surg 2007;83:1569–76.
19. Hatton KW, Kilinski LC, Ramaiah C, et al. Multiple failed external defibrillation attempts during robot-assisted internal mammary harvest for myocardial revascularization. Anesth Analg 2006;103(5):1113–4.

Anesthesia for Tracheal Resection and Reconstruction

Ion A. Hobai, MD, PhD[a,b],*, Sanjeev V. Chhangani, MD, MBA[a,b],
Paul H. Alfille, MD[a,b]

KEYWORDS

- Tracheal stenosis • Tracheal tumors • Endotracheal intubation
- Total intravenous anesthesia • Bronchoscopy

KEY POINTS

- Tracheal resection and reconstruction is the treatment of choice for most patients with tracheal stenosis or tracheal tumors.
- In the presence of tracheal pathology, induction of anesthesia and endotracheal intubation need to be meticulously planned and executed.
- Close communication with the surgical team is required throughout the case, and particularly during the open airway phase of the operation.
- An extubation that is initiated too early or too late, or the injudicious use of postoperative pain medications may result in immediate loss of the airway patency, and may require either a reintubation under difficult circumstances, or performance of emergent tracheostomy.

INTRODUCTION

Anesthesia for tracheal resection and reconstruction (TRR) is a challenging undertaking because of the compromised airway and the need to share the airway with the surgeon while maintaining respiratory function. Unique to this operation is the preoperative assessment and plan for induction in the presence of tracheal pathology, the coordination with the surgeon during airway excision and anastomosis, the management of emergence, and postoperative care.[1–4] Here, we first explore the common and simpler proximal tracheal resection, and then discuss special considerations for distal tracheal pathology.

Disclosures: None of the authors have any direct financial interests in the subject matter or materials discussed in the article or with a company making a competing product.
[a] Department of Anesthesia, Critical Care and Pain Medicine, Massachusetts General Hospital, 55 Fruit Street, GRB 444, Boston, MA 02114, USA; [b] Harvard Medical School, 651 Huntington Avenue, Boston, MA 02115, USA
* Corresponding author. Department of Anesthesia, Critical Care and Pain Medicine, Massachusetts General Hospital, 55 Fruit Street, GRB 444, Boston, MA 02114.
E-mail address: ihobai@partners.org

Anesthesiology Clin 30 (2012) 709–730
http://dx.doi.org/10.1016/j.anclin.2012.08.012
1932-2275/12/$ – see front matter © 2012 Elsevier Inc. All rights reserved.

There are no controlled studies comparing various methods of anesthetic management and airway control for TRR operations. With only a few centers having extensive experience in the procedure, even the experienced anesthesiologist may be unfamiliar with the nuances of successful management. This monograph distills TRR management techniques culled at Massachusetts General Hospital from more than 30 years of clinical experience. Note that there is renewed interest in artificial "engineered" airway tissue,[5] as well as tracheal transplantation.[6] We can expect that anesthetic management will evolve with changes in surgical practice.

ANATOMY AND PHYSIOLOGY
Anatomy of Upper Airway and Trachea

The airway can be functionally divided into upper and lower airway. The upper airway includes the nose, pharynx, and larynx. The lower airway includes the trachea, bronchi, and distal bronchial segments ending in the alveoli. The larynx guards the lower airway during breathing and swallowing and is an important structure for speech. The thyroid, cricoid cartilages, and hyoid bone form external landmarks of the larynx.[7]

The adult lower airway extends from the true vocal cords to the level of carina (**Fig. 1**A). The first 2 cm to the cricoid cartilage forms the subglottic airway. The narrowest plane of the upper airway is located at the level of the vocal cords. The trachea is a tubular structure consisting of incomplete cartilages (16–20 in number) and fibromuscular membrane and lined by mucosa. Tracheal cartilage is an incomplete ring anterolaterally with posterior deficiency bridged by a flat muscular wall. The posterior wall of the trachea bulges into the lumen and this is exaggerated in expiration and coughing and can be observed during bronchoscopy.

The adult trachea is approximately 10 to 11 cm long and descends from the larynx (sixth cervical vertebra) to carina (fifth thoracic vertebra), where it divides into right and left main bronchi. Approximately one-third of the total tracheal length is extrathoracic (above the suprasternal notch) and the remaining two-thirds is intrathoracic. The trachea is primarily a midline structure with its point of bifurcation slightly to the right. Normally, trachea is quite mobile and its length can rapidly change with respiration and neck movement. With deep inspiration, the carina may descend to the level of the sixth thoracic vertebra. Clinically, this is visible as "tracheal tugging" and may create difficulty gaining control of tracheal stoma in a patient with acute respiratory distress. Depending on neck flexion or extension, the trachea can become either more mediastinal or cervical, respectively. The use of neck extension and flexion, in particular, is an important aspect of managing surgical exposure and postoperative healing in TRR.

The external diameter of trachea is approximately 2 cm in adult males, and 1.5 cm in adult females. The trachea in children is smaller, and more mobile and deeply placed. The transverse shape of the tracheal lumen may be round, lunate, or flattened. The right main bronchus is wider, shorter (2.5 cm), and more vertical than the left. The right main bronchus quickly divides into right upper lobe bronchus, and continues as bronchus intermedius, which divides into right middle and lower lobe bronchi. The right upper lobe take-off may be displaced at the level of the carina or lower end of trachea. This may create difficulty with right lung isolation. The left main bronchus is narrower and less vertical than the right and 5 cm in length. It divides into left upper and lower lobe bronchi.

The trachea has a rich vascular supply and lymphatic drainage. Despite its extensive blood supply, the tracheal mucosa is sensitive to pressure from internal forces, such

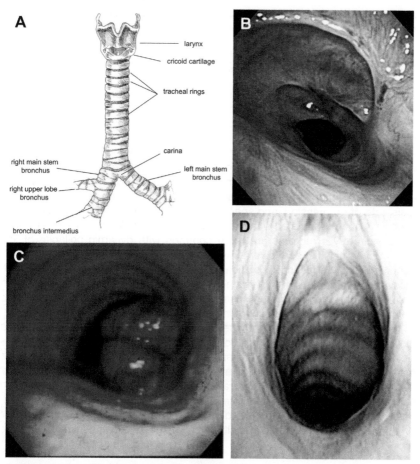

Fig. 1. (*A*) Anatomy of trachea and larynx. (*Illustration by* Ioana Hobai). (*B–D*) Bronchoscopy views of a case of postintubation tracheal stenosis (*B*), tracheal tumor (*C*), as well as a typical postoperative view (*D*). (*Courtesy of* John C. Wain MD, Division of Thoracic Surgery, Massachusetts General Hospital, Boston, MA.)

as those exerted by an endotracheal tube and its cuff pressure. The presence of microangiopathies associated with diabetes mellitus and radiation can compromise vascular supply and anastomotic healing. The tracheal blood supply approaches laterally and is composed of branches of the inferior thyroid, subclavian, innominate, internal thoracic, first intercostal, and bronchial arteries. Maintaining the blood supply to the trachea, by avoiding circumferential dissection, is a principal tenet of TRR operations.

The larynx and trachea are innervated by vagus nerve through the superior and recurrent laryngeal nerves. The recurrent laryngeal nerves lie closely in the groove between the trachea and the esophagus and are subject to involvement in tracheal pathology and permanent or temporary injury by surgical manipulation.

Physiology of Airway Obstruction

The signs and symptoms of significant upper airway obstruction (eg, stridor or dyspnea) correlate with the reduction in intraluminal diameter and resistance to air flow across the area of narrowing. In uncompromised airways, flow is laminar and depends strongly on airway diameter. The Hagen–Poiseuille equation for laminar tube flow is:

$$AirFlow = PressureDrop \times \frac{\Pi \times radius^4}{8 \times viscosity \times length}$$

Flow can be maintained by increasing the pressure gradient, at the expense of increased work of breathing and decreased ability to exercise. As the airway diameter decreases, small additional changes from swelling, secretions, or bleeding are poorly tolerated.

Respiratory symptoms first become apparent with exertion when tracheal lumen (internal diameter) is reduced to approximately 50% or 8 mm.[8] Inspiratory stridor appears at rest, when the tracheal lumen is further reduced to 5 to 6 mm.[9,10] The severity of presentation and the degree of compensation depends on the location of stenosis, rate of progression, and specific etiology of obstruction. Inspiratory airway obstruction is often associated with fixed obstruction of the larynx and upper trachea, whereas expiratory symptoms are more common with dynamic collapse of lower trachea (tracheomalacia) and lower airway tumors.

Pulmonary function testing, specifically flow-volume loops, has been used in the diagnosis and characterization of tracheal pathology. The classical teaching is that fixed stenosis (the more common case) attenuates both inspiratory and expiratory peak flows. Dynamic collapse occurs in different phases depending on the location of the lesion. Extrathoracic compromise occurs in inspiration, when airway pressure is below atmospheric pressure. Intrathoracic compromise occurs in expiration when thoracic pressure is above tracheal pressure. In contrast, the emphysematous pattern of small airway collapse occurs in expiration and later in exhalation.[11–13] Spontaneous ventilation is better tolerated with intrathoracic lesions because thoracic pressure drops below tracheal pressure during inspiration. In actual practice, the role of flow-volume loops has been deemphasized. Imaging has improved and careful clinical observation and questioning can elicit much of the relevant dynamic respiratory components.

SURGICAL INDICATIONS

Most patients that require TRR present with tracheal obstruction, the most common etiology of which is represented by inflammatory (postintubation) tracheal stenosis (~75%),[14] followed by primary (~15%) or secondary (~8%) tracheal tumors.[14] Other rare etiologies are presented in **Table 1**.

Postintubation Tracheal Stenosis (Fig. 1B)

Despite great progress in its prevention, including the introduction of low-pressure, high-volume endotracheal tube (ETT) cuffs, postintubation tracheal stenosis still occurs,[15] and represents the most common cause of tracheal pathology. Postintubation tracheal stenosis can follow even the briefest periods of intubation.[16] Etiologically, it is a consequence of the initial injury of the tracheal mucosa from the ETT (or tracheostomy tube) cuff, followed by a chronic inflammatory reaction, with granuloma formation. Symptoms usually appear between 1 and 3 months after extubation,[15] and include first exertional dyspnea and then dyspnea at rest. Airway narrowing leads to difficulty of clearing secretions; for this reason, acute decompensations are common, and should be treated seriously, because they may turn fatal without warning.

Table1
Causes of tracheal obstruction

Benign	Malignant	Infectious	Non-infectious
Congenital	Primary tracheal	• Papillomas	Inflammatory
• Vascular rings	tumors	• Tuberculosis	• Amyloidosis
• Aortic aneurysm	• Adenoid carcinoma	• Rhinoscleroma	• Wegener's
• Tracheogenic cyst	• Squamous cell	• Viral	granulomatosis
• Congenital tracheal	carcinoma	tracheobronchitis	• Relapsing
stenosis or malacia	• Neurofibroma	• Bacterial	polychondritis
	• Chondroma	tracheitis	
Acquired	• Chondroblastoma		Miscellaneous
• Foreign body	• Hemangioma		• Aortic aneurysm
• Blood clots	• Carcinoid		• Retrosternal
• Mucus plug			goiter
• Post-surgical	Metastatic tumors		• Mediastinal
○ Lung transplant	(origin)		adenopathy
○ Sleeve resection	• Thyroid		• Mediastinal
(trachea or	• Larynx		fibrosis
bronchus)	• Lung		
○ Tracheostomy	• Esophagus		
• Traumatic	• Breast		
○ Post-intubation	• Lymphoma		
○ Burn/inhalation			
○ Airway hematoma			
○ Laceration			

Primary Tracheal Tumors (Fig. 1C)

Primary tracheal tumors are rare (less than 0.5% of total cancers) and in adults most are malignant. Histologically, the most prevalent tracheal tumors are squamous cell carcinomas (50%–70%), adenoid cystic carcinomas (10%–15%), and mucoepidermoid carcinomas.[17–20] The rare benign tracheal lesions include hemangioma, hamartoma, neurogenic tumors, granular cell tumors, and squamous papillomas.[21–23] The mean age at presentation is approximately 60 years.

The prognosis of unresected tracheal tumors is poor, with a 5-year survival of 5% to 7%.[24] Patients who undergo surgical resection, sometimes followed by postoperative radiotherapy, may have a 5-year survival rate of 47%, and a 10-year survival rate of 37%.[25] Prognosis is determined mostly by the surgical stage at presentation and histopathological type.[17] In terms of surgical stage, patients with distant metastasis have a 5-year survival of 4%, compared with 26% for patients with regionally invasive disease, and 47% for those with localized disease. As far as the cancer type is concerned, squamous cell carcinomas convey significantly worse prognosis, with a 5-year survival of 13%, compared with 74% for adenoid cystic carcinoma.[17]

PREOPERATIVE EVALUATION
Clinical Evaluation

In the evaluation of a patient with tracheal obstruction, the most important information is clinical. The development and aggravation of exertion dyspnea and subsequently of dyspnea at rest needs to be ascertained, and usually corresponds to a narrowing of the tracheal diameter below 8 mm.[15] The pattern of dyspnea (inspiratory *vs.* expiratory) can indicate the location of stenosis, as discussed above. It is also important to assess the patient's ability to breathe in the supine position; if this is impeded, induction of anesthesia should be undertaken in a position in which the patient's breathing is easiest.

On physical examination, the degree of air-flow obstruction can be assessed by performing a "birthday candle test": asking the patient to inspire maximally and then blow forcefully against the examiner's hand (like "blowing the birthday candles"). Feeling the power of the expired air flow is remarkably indicative of the existence and severity of airway obstruction. Certainly, a routine examination of the upper airway should not be forgotten, with the goal of predicting the difficulty of intubation.

Finally, the surgical notes from the most recent bronchoscopy should be reviewed. However, one needs to be aware that tracheal obstruction, either caused by inflammation (as in benign postintubation stenosis) or tumors, can worsen quickly, over weeks or even days, so the information obtained in surgical notes may not be actual at the time of presentation for surgery.

Imaging Studies

Among imaging studies, a dedicated computed tomography (CT) examination is the most informative. Routine chest radiographs are typically not diagnostic. The standard CT scan of the chest is not sensitive enough to provide details of tracheal pathology. Therefore, a high-resolution CT of the neck and upper thorax (which may include 3-dimensional airway reconstruction) is the most helpful[26] in both the initial assessment of the lesion and in follow-up.

Compared with a good CT examination, other modalities are used infrequently. Magnetic resonance imaging offers little additional detail, and is cumbersome and potentially risky to a patient with airway obstruction. Dynamic flow-volume loop spirometry can offer objective information about the physiologic consequences of the airway lesion, but this is rarely of critical value, if one is provided with a good imaging study and meticulous clinical assessment of the airway.

Coexisting Medical Conditions

As is the case with most surgical procedures, coexisting medical conditions will affect and complicate anesthesia management. The requirements added by various coexisting conditions are similar to those for a general anesthetic case, and will not be covered here.

Specific to a TRR operation, there are 3 relative contraindications.

First, patients with severe pulmonary dysfunction who are ventilator dependent should not undergo a TRR operation, because the need for prolonged postoperative intubation will likely compromise the anastomosis. These patients are best served by performing a tracheostomy, weaning from the ventilator, and subsequently performing a TRR combined with tracheostomy closure.

Second, patients who are steroid dependent should likewise be weaned off steroids, because these drugs are thought to interfere with wound healing and increase the likelihood of airway dehiscence. A history of previous neck and chest radiation therapy is also considered a relative contraindication,[27] as it may predispose to anastomosis dehiscence.

It should be considered, though, that TRR (**Fig. 1**D) is not a life-saving operation, and, in patients with significant comorbidities, it should be replaced by a laryngo-tracheal resection, combined with a tracheostomy.

INTRAOPERATIVE MANAGEMENT
Operating Room Setup

Apart from the usual operating room setup, the equipment that needs to be available for a TRR operation includes (1) an assortment of small-diameter ETTs (from 4.0 to

6.5); (2) a sterile, spiral steel reinforced ETT (for ventilation across the surgical field); (3) a pediatric bronchoscope (in case the ETT needs to be checked, or in case of inadvertent extubation); and (4) adult and pediatric size rigid bronchoscopes.

Intravenous Access and Monitors

One or 2 midsize (20–18 gauge, ga) peripheral intravenous (IV) catheters should be sufficient, as blood loss is usually minimal. Placement of a second IV line is prudent, because the arms will be tucked, and access to the IV site may be limited during the case.

In addition to the standard American Society of Anesthesiologists monitors, an intra-arterial catheter is placed, preferably in the left radial artery, for hemodynamic and arterial blood gas monitoring. An arterial line is particularly useful in case of jet ventilation, to monitor the partial pressure of arterial CO_2 ($PaCO_2$), in the absence of a reliable end-tidal CO_2 pressure ($ETCO_2$) monitoring. Also, in the case that hilar releases are needed, direct measurements of the arterial pressure are required to monitor hemodynamic changes associated with retraction of the heart.

We do not usually insert a central venous line (CVL) for TRR surgery. In the rare patient in whom a CVL may be needed (such as those with severe cardiomyopathy, for example, in which the need for potent vasoactive drugs is anticipated) a subclavian or femoral approach is preferred, as the internal jugular approach would be in close proximity to the surgical field.

Commonly an anesthesia depth monitor is used (such as SEDLine, from Masimo, Irvine, CA, or BIS, from Covidien, Dublin, Ireland), since these cases are typically performed under total IV anesthesia. Contrary to the usual inhalation anesthesia, in which the end-tidal concentration of the anesthetic agent is an effective means of monitoring the depth of anesthesia, and to minimize the risk of awareness,[28] in the case of total IV anesthetics, no such feedback is available, and justifies the use of a dedicated monitoring system.

A train-of-four monitor is also used, to ensure complete neuromuscular blockade during the case. Tracheal manipulation can induce a cough reflex, which needs to be prevented since it can could jeopardize the precise dissection and suturing needed. Also, the patient must regain full muscular strength for extubation, and the recovery from neuromuscular blockade needs to be directly measured.

A urinary catheter is usually inserted, as these cases are commonly more than 3 hours long.

Patient Positioning

The patient is typically placed in supine position with arms tucked and the neck extended. To help with neck extension, an inflatable ("thyroid") bag is placed under the shoulders. The head needs to rest on the gel head rest and not be suspended. Cases of postoperative quadriplegia have been reported, and attributed to unnatural strain of the neck during the operation.[29]

Induction of Anesthesia

For patients without significant tracheal obstruction, the usual IV induction is an acceptable choice. For example, administration of propofol (2 mg/kg), fentanyl (2 μg/kg), and cisatracurium (0.15 mg/kg) would provide satisfactory anesthesia and muscle relaxation before intubation.

Rigid bronchoscopy

TRR operations are usually preceded by a careful endoscopic evaluation of the airway, by means of a rigid bronchoscopy. Four distinct parameters need to be assessed, and should be communicated by the surgeon explicitly before resection begins: (1) the location and extent of the lesion to be resected, (2) the health and function of the vocal cords, (3) any areas of inflammation of the trachea, including signs of aspiration, and (4) any areas of tracheomalacia. If none of these worrying signs are present, and the lesion appears resectable, then the patient is intubated with the largest size ETT possible (**Fig. 2**A). In case the stenosis is tight, it can be cored out or dilated at this time to allow endotracheal intubation.[30]

Brief Account of the Surgical Procedure

Proximal tracheal lesions are approached via a small transverse cervical incision. The trachea is then dissected and mobilized, ensuring not to jeopardize the blood supply, or the recurrent laryngeal nerve that lies laterally. Complete muscle paralysis is critical at this point, because coughing during dissection can result in injuries that may make the lesion unresectable.

Next, the trachea is incised (see **Fig. 2**B and C) carefully, so as not to puncture the cuff of the ETT that lies inside. The ETT is then withdrawn under direct vision (see **Fig. 2**D), until it is positioned above the lesion (at this time a large leak will make ventilation impossible). Other incisions are made at this time, including one at the distal end of the lesion to gain access at the distal trachea below the would-be anastomosis. Traction sutures are placed around one ring, and allow dissection of the posterior tracheal wall from the esophagus. A first tentative incision at the level that is thought to be the end of the lesion may be followed by others, if the lesion end is more distal. This is done patiently and meticulously, because one can always remove more rings, but cannot reattach healthy rings that have been inadvertently resected. At times, there are no completely healthy rings to be found, and the experienced surgeon will know when to stop resecting, even if that means placing the final anastomosis in an area with some residual inflammation. This carries a known risk of re-stenosis, but it is preferable to resecting too much trachea, and ending up with a tenuous anastomosis at risk of dehiscence. Traction sutures are placed around the first ring of the distal trachea, to identify it and help intubation.

The distal trachea is intubated with a sterile (preferably reinforced) ETT, and connected to a sterile breathing circuit across the surgical field (**Fig. 3**A). Effective ventilation across the field is verified by assessing lung inflation and $ETCO_2$. (If the $ETCO_2$ suddenly disappears, in the presence of what looks like effective ventilation, it is probably because of compression of the CO_2 sampling tubing by surgical instruments under the drapes). Blood is carefully suctioned from the operative field, to minimize seepage into the trachea and lungs.

The segment to be resected is dissected circumferentially and then removed (see **Fig. 2**B). To verify that approximation of the trachea can be achieved without undue tension, a brief test of neck flexion is performed at this time, and, if the margins can be brought together satisfactorily, the neck is returned to the extended position.

From this moment, the operation will feature alternating times of surgical work and ventilation. Sutures are placed through the posterior wall of the trachea, and then through the anterior rings (see **Fig. 2**C). Ventilation can be achieved either in the same time, or, if the bulk of the ETT does not allow precise suturing, between periods of surgical work. Ventilation is mostly manual and aims to bring the patient in a zone of relative hypocapnia, to create a buffer zone in case extended periods of apnea may be needed.

After all the sutures are placed, it is time to reintubate with the oral ETT (**Fig. 4**). This is achieved most easily in a retrograde fashion, in which a flexible rubber catheter (usually a urethral catheter) is passed from the incision retrogradely into the hypopharynx (see **Fig. 4**A), from where it is retrieved by the anesthesiologist. The end of

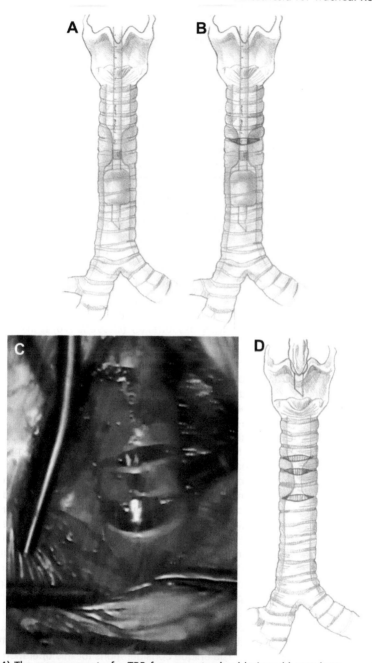

Fig. 2. (*A*) The management of a TRR for upper tracheal lesions (shown here as a stenosis between the fourth and sixth tracheal rings) begins with endotracheal intubation across the lesion. This is best achieved by a direct laryngoscopy approach, using a small (5.0–6.0) ETT, over a stylet. After intubation, the lungs are ventilated and recruited meticulously, to prepare for the immediately following periods of apnea. (*Illustration by* Ioana Hobai.) (*B*) An incision is made at the level of the lesion, carefully as not to damage the ETT. (*Illustration by* Ioana Hobai.) (*C*) A photograph of the surgical field, showing the incised trachea, with the ETT inside. (*D*) Under direct vision, the ETT is retracted above the lesion, and then removed. (*Illustration by* Ioana Hobai.)

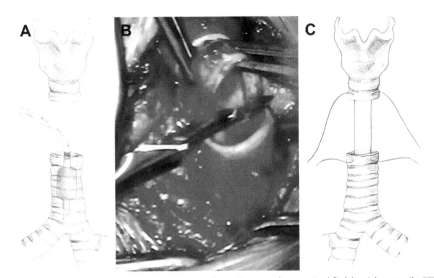

Fig. 3. (*A*) The distal end of the trachea is intubated across the surgical field, with a sterile ETT. Ventilation is performed during or between times dedicated to surgical work, leading to the completion of the resection (*B*) and placing of sutures (*C*). (*Illustrations by* Ioana Hobai.)

the catheter is then sutured to the distal end of an ETT (see **Fig. 4**B, C and D), that is then guided inside the trachea by pulling the catheter back into the surgical field.

At this time the neck is flexed again (this time definitively), to bring the cut ends of the trachea together, by placing blankets under the patient's head. The ETT is then advanced across the incision (**Fig. 5**A), into the distal trachea and the tracheal sutures are tied. This has to be done carefully, with the sutures away from the ETT, because entangling of the 2 is known to be possible (as improbable as it may seem), and will lead to rupture of the anastomosis during extubation.

After the trachea is closed (see **Fig. 5**B), a test is performed to assess that the anastomosis is leak proof. This is done by flooding the operative field with saline, deflating the ETT cuff and applying 30 cm of water pressure to the breathing circuit. If no bubbles are seen, then the incision is closed, after placing 1 or 2 small suction drains in the pretracheal space.

Before extubation, a "guardian" suture is placed from the skin over the manubrium to the submental crease to keep the neck flexed. The guardian suture should not be as tight as to maintain the neck in an uncomfortable position. The goal is to prevent hyperextension, not to force hyperflexion.

Emergence and Extubation

The time of emergence and extubation is a critical stage of the operation, and the time when most complications occur. The unique considerations for this operation are the following:

1. Maintaining neck flexion
2. Assessing and managing tracheal bleeding and obstruction
3. Laryngeal swelling
4. Vocal cord dysfunction

The course of the extubation period may be protracted. At the ready should be tools for airway rescue: various endotracheal tubes, a flexible bronchoscope, and

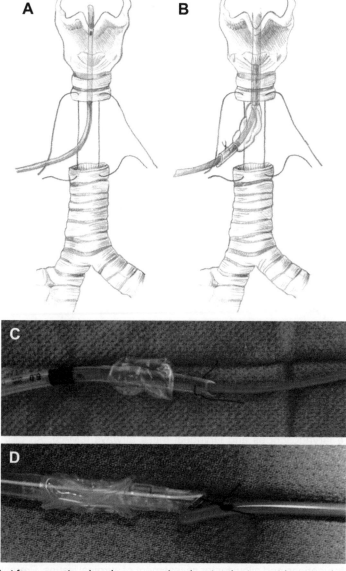

Fig. 4. (*A*) After resection has been completed, reintubation with an oral ETT is best achieved in a retrograde fashion. A flexible rubber catheter is first passed from the incised trachea into the larynx and then pharynx, from where it is retrieved. (*Illustration by* Ioana Hobai.) (*B*) The catheter is sutured to a new ETT, which is then guided back into the trachea. (*Illustration by* Ioana Hobai.) (*C*) For a secure catheter-ETT assembly, one needs to ensure that enough length of the catheter is passed inside the ETT, and that the suture is tight. (*D*) If not, the tip of the catheter might come out of the ETT during guiding into the trachea, leaving the tip of the ETT exposed and misaligned. Such an assembly is unlikely to pass easily though the cords, and will become stuck on the arytenoids during intubation.

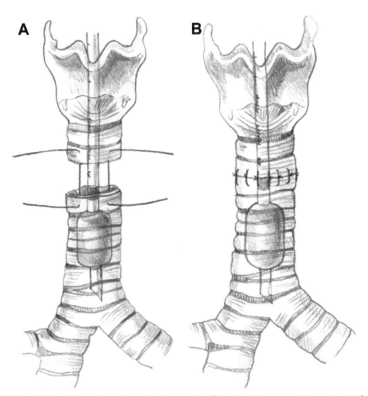

Fig. 5. (*A*) By flexing the patient's neck, the ends of the trachea are approximated, and the ETT is passed distal to the anastomosis, with the cuff placed as distal as possible, away from the anastomosis line. (*B*) The sutures are closed. (*Illustrations by* Ioana Hobai.)

appropriate laryngoscopes and laryngeal mask airways (LMAs). An LMA is often a good tool to both facilitate ventilation and provide a conduit for the flexible scope. Immediately after extubation, breathing needs to be assessed. The range of response to problems spans reassurance and observation, to respiratory assistance, to bronchoscopic assessment and airway toilet, to emergent intubation or tracheotomy. With experience, assessment of the airway and selection of the best intervention will come naturally.

In general, the goal is to extubate the patient after surgery in the operating room. An anesthetic technique that provides an alert and comfortable patient will minimize the need for interventions and allow faster assessment of surgical issues. Premature extubation, before the patient is fully awake, may be followed by the patient becoming unresponsive and apneic, and necessitating reintubation. Reintubation of a freshly extubated TRR patient, with the neck in flexion and a tenuous anastomosis, is a dire proposition. Conversely, agitation during emergence, with uncontrollable extensions of the neck, or vigorous coughing, will also endanger the fresh anastomosis.

There are several techniques to optimize the immediate postoperative period. Good oropharyngeal suctioning, antiemetics, and an elevated head of the bed all assist in keeping the upper airway clear. An oral or nasal airway can be placed before emergence. If airway swelling is anticipated, typically with high lesions or extensive manipulation, nebulized epinephrine can reduce swelling. Humidified gas is helpful throughout the recovery period.

Post extubation respiration distress should be assessed systematically. Lack of gas movement signals obstruction or insufficient respiratory drive. The latter is easy to counter with mask or LMA ventilatory assistance and management of the anesthetic problem. Obstruction requires emergent fiberoptic examination and either clearing of obstructing mucus and blood, or surgical correction of anastomotic issues. Guiding a small endotracheal tube over the fiberscope allows ventilation while the problem is addressed. Vocal cord dysfunction or swelling may simply require time to abate.

If air movement seems adequate but the patient subjectively experiences respiratory impairment, the assessment is more nuanced. Reassurance and observation are indicated, especially to follow the direction of respiratory function. Following oxygenation and obtaining a chest radiograph will help in analysis.

Any anesthetic technique that accomplishes these emergence goals is acceptable. Neuromuscular function must be completely restored. Agents that allow rapid emergence with mildly blunted airway reflexes (eg, low-dose remifentanil, dexmedetomidine, sevoflurane) can be used. A common mistake is excessive narcotic administration. Neck incisions are surprisingly not painful, and tracheal reflexes seem attenuated by the surgery.

Two common techniques are used for the end game. Either the endotracheal tube is removed once the patient wakes and demonstrates good respiratory drive (again in sitting position, suctioned airway, and rescue precautions at the ready), or an LMA can be placed with the patient still anesthetized and used not only for the emergence, but for a concluding fiberoptic examination and airway clearance.

Immediately after extubation, the patient's phonation should be assessed to exclude a possible injury of the recurrent laryngeal nerve. One member of the operative team should be designated to ensure the patient keeps the neck flexed, as the distractions of emergence and transfer can allow this state to lapse. The patient is usually positioned sitting up, and given supplemental oxygen by mask, and is continuously reminded to keep the neck flexed, and refrain from violent movements.

POSTOPERATIVE CARE

Patients are transferred to an intensive care setting for careful observation of their breathing. Avoidance of respiratory depression is paramount. None or only small amounts of intravenous opioids are usually needed to alleviate the mild degree of pain from the neck incision. Feeding is resumed on postoperative day 1 or 2, beginning with liquids, paying attention to signs of aspiration.

After 1 postoperative day, the uncomplicated patient can be transferred to a regular hospital floor, with experienced nursing care. Patients are commonly kept in the hospital for 7 days, after which a flexible bronchoscopy (or tracheoscopy) is performed to assess the anastomosis. For this, either sedation with local anesthesia is used, or general anesthesia with an LMA airway. If no problems are identified, the patient is discharged home.

COMPLICATIONS

Historically, the operative mortality rate of a TRR operation ranged from 7% to 11%.[24,25,31] Currently, experienced centers can perform this operation with a mortality as low as 3%.[24]

Operative complications can be divided into early, evident immediately after extubation (such as respiratory failure, from various etiologies, and vocal cord paralysis) or delayed (such as anastomosis dehiscence and hemoptysis).

Postextubation Respiratory Failure

One of the most feared complications after extubation is respiratory failure.

Should this occur, it is imperative that etiologic diagnosis and pharmacologic treatment are achieved immediately, and, followed, if not effective, by surgically reestablishing the airway.

To reestablish adequate ventilation, first, the cause of respiratory failure should be established. Three major mechanisms are possible: persistent narcosis (with insufficient respiratory drive, ie, extubation too early), insufficient reversal of the neuromuscular blockade (NMB), and, in the worst case, airway obstruction. Distinguishing among these 3 mechanisms should be easily achieved by a careful clinical observation.

An *overnarcotized patient* (one that is extubated too early and still affected by the opioid-induced respiratory depression) will show the unique feature of being apneic and calm. At the opposite spectrum, a truly suffocating patient (due either to airway obstruction or incomplete NMB reversal) is usually agitated, frightened, tachycardic, and hypertensive. The two conditions are most easily distinguished on this basis. The sensation of suffocation is one of the most terrifying human experiences,[32] and, after seeing only one such patient, the expression of sheer terror in their eyes is a picture that will never be forgotten, and never be confused with the sedated appearance of the overnarcotized patient.

Treatment of the overnarcotized patient is by opioid reversal with naloxone (0.4 mg IV bolus), in addition to establishing the airway and manual ventilation by the aid of a mask airway, or, if necessary, insertion of an LMA. Reintubation or a tracheostomy should not be necessary, in the absence of an unobstructed airway.

Contrary to the overnarcotized patient, a patient with *insufficient reversal* of the NMB will be agitated, moving uncontrollably, but weak. Insufficient muscle force will be evident in the weakness of the grip, or of the arm movements. The management of the patient with incomplete NMB reversal includes a number of distinct actions. First, it should be remembered that the respiratory depression of these patients is mainly due to the upper airway collapse.[33] Thus, the first therapeutic maneuver should be opening of the upper airway, by jaw thrust, insertion of an oral or nasal airway, or, in the most severe cases, reinduction and insertion of an LMA. After the airway becomes patent, manual ventilation can be achieved, and the patient can be sedated to wait for full recovery of the muscle force. If noninvasive methods of ventilation are not effective, reintubation or performing a surgical airway is necessary.

As mentioned previously, the presence of an *airway obstruction*, in an otherwise awake and strong patient is also easy to recognize. After a TRR, airway obstruction can be attributable to either insufficient patency of the vocal cords (most commonly owing to vocal cord edema) or to an obstruction at the level of the anastomosis (by a blood clot, or a mucosal flap). Differentiating between the 2 is difficult without a bronchoscopy, and usually unnecessary, as both are managed with reintubation.

Immediate reintubation after a TRR operation is a daunting proposition, one in which feelings of personal failure should not inhibit a swift and skillful intubation. A bronchoscopic approach is preferred for a number of reasons. Foremost, with the neck in flexion, direct laryngoscopy may be difficult. Moreover, bronchoscopy will allow the examination of vocal cords and of the tracheal anastomosis, before insertion of the ETT, as well as the precise positioning of the ETT with the cuff away from the anastomosis line.

In my experience (I.A.H.) a combined direct/fiberoptic approach is preffered, using direct laryngoscopy with a Mac blade to achieve the best view possible (usually at least the tip of the epiglottis), after which the laryngoscope handle is given to an assistant, and the tip of the bronchoscope is placed under direct vision at the tip of the epiglottis and used only to negotiate the glottis and enter the trachea.

Regardless of the technique, reintubation should be performed with a small (5.5–6.5) ETT, either uncuffed or, more commonly, with the cuff not inflated. The tube should be positioned with the tip above or well below the anastomosis, because the presence of an inflated cuff over the anastomosis will lead to dehiscence.

If reintubation is difficult, a small tracheotomy should be performed, below the anastomosis. This will not be an easy task, in a fresh surgical field, and especially in the case of a distal anastomosis, so, if envisaged, it should be initiated early, before complications of hypoxia occur.

This last aspect cannot be overemphasized. Although the above management may appear logical and algorithmic, in the real world it is almost never so. In the short time that is usually available to act, actions become based on instinct and intuition, rather than a fully informed, logical reasoning. The diagnosis must be made in seconds, not minutes, and before the saturation drops. Reestablishing the airway, too, has to be done quickly, and usually there is not enough time to test whether the least-invasive methods are efficient. In a rapidly desaturating patient, one will not have enough time to adequately try the effectiveness of mask ventilation, then an LMA, and then fiberoptic intubation, and, in this case, a swift execution of a more invasive technique (such as reintubation, or even a tracheostomy) may be safer. Like in all critical situations in the operating room, a cold head and calm demeanor, as well as a collegial teamwork with the surgical and nursing staff, are the most critical determinants of successful management,[34] and also, more often than not, the most difficult to achieve.

Vocal Cord Paralysis

The vocal cords are innervated by the recurrent laryngeal nerve, which lies closely alongside the lateral wall of the trachea and can be invaded by a tracheal tumor, or compromised during surgical dissection. Therefore, vocal cord competence should be carefully documented preoperatively, especially in patients with tracheal tumors. If vocal cord paralysis occurs as a result of surgical manipulation, it will manifest itself immediately after extubation as the inability to speak loudly. The paralyzed, abducted cords may also create a resistance to air flow, and manifest as dyspnea. It is important to realize that in patients with vocal cord paralysis, air flow will be impeded more in the case of forced breathing, which is usually the case in patients who are suffocating and panicking. This is one of the very few cases in which the patient's ability to breathe will be improved after judicious administration of sedatives.

In addition to the risk of airway obstruction, vocal cord paralysis may also predispose patients to recurrent aspiration (see later in this article). On the positive side, nerve dysfunction that occurs as a result of surgical manipulation is usually temporary and can be expected to improve with time (albeit slowly, over months or a few years). If voice remains affected, or if aspiration is a problem, vocal cord injections can ameliorate their function.

Hemoptysis

Postoperative hemoptysis usually means erosion of an artery adjacent to the anastomosis. Prompt reintervention is usually necessary. If anything more than a minimal amount of blood is coughed, the patients need immediate reintubation, usually by a fiberoptic approach. In the case of hemoptysis, the ETT cuff should be positioned at the level of the anastomosis, and may offer some compression of the bleeding vessel, until surgical exploration and repair.

Recurrent Aspiration

A number of factors may conspire to induce a recurrent aspiration after a TRR operation. This is especially common in patients with invasive tracheal tumors that undergo extensive resections. In these patients, a shortened trachea may show limited mobility, with limited elevation during deglutition. Vocal cord paralysis from damage of the recurrent laryngeal nerve is another factor. Finally, chronic aspiration commonly occurs after laryngeal releases, especially of the suprathyroid type.

If the danger of aspiration pneumonitis is avoided, recovery of the deglutition reflexes usually occurs spontaneously, although slowly (over a number of months). A temporary gastrostomy tube may be necessary for feeding during this period.

DEPARTURES FROM THE BASIC CASE
Induction and Intubation of the Critically Obstructed Airway

Unique to tracheal surgery is the focus on lower airway pathology. Classical algorithms for assessing and managing "the difficult airway" stop after the vocal cords are passed.[35] In patients with tracheal pathology, merely entering the airway may be insufficient. As such, the management of the obstructed airway is one of the most challenging interventions anesthesiologists may be called on.

Patients with critical airway obstruction are often anxious, sitting upright, and breathing with audible stridor. Many are oxygen dependent and should be well preoxygenated before anesthesia and sedation begins. Alternatively, using a mixture of helium and oxygen (Heliox[36]) may improve airflow and reduce work of breathing (at the obvious expense of decreasing the alveolar oxygen pressure).[37] Severe coughing episodes can result in sudden and severe airway obstruction and must be avoided.

Premedication with anxiolytics must be avoided or performed with extreme caution, as a decrease in respiratory effort can easily proceed to complete airway obstruction. Glycopyrrolate (0.2 mg, IV) is useful in providing drying effect on airway secretions as well as counteracting the vagotonic effects of remifentanil and airway manipulation.

In the management of the obstructed airway there are 2 critical decision points that need to be considered beforehand. One is the choice between an IV or an inhalation induction of anesthesia, each with its benefits and perils. The second is the choice between a fiberoptic and a direct laryngoscopic intubation.

A careful decision must be made between choosing an IV or inhalation induction. For lesions that produce a fixed airway obstruction, a conventional IV anesthetic, followed by a fast-acting muscle relaxant (succinylcholine or rocuronium) is the most appropriate. In patients with variable intrathoracic obstruction, however, one must be aware of the possibility that changing from spontaneous (negative pressure) ventilation to assisted (positive pressure) ventilation may lead to an aggravation of the obstruction and complete airway collapse. In these patients, the most prudent approach is to attempt an inhalational anesthetic (sevoflurane breath down), which maintains spontaneous ventilation. Once the patient is anesthetized (unresponsive), gentle manual ventilation can be attempted. If the patient can be effectively ventilated by mask, then muscle relaxation can be administered and the trachea intubated in the usual fashion. If, however, mask ventilation is not effective, spontaneous ventilation must be maintained and the patient intubated while breathing spontaneously. Common complications of the inhalation induction are vomiting and coughing; if these occur, alternative choices, described later, must be considered.

A second decision point is choosing between a direct laryngoscopy versus a fiberoptic approach. In my experience (I.A.H.), a direct laryngoscopy, followed by intubation with a small ETT over a stylet is the first choice. This allows testing ETTs of various sizes, so the largest ETT that can pass though the stenosis is finally used. Also (compared with the bronchoscope) the stylet gives enough stiffness to allow intubation through a tight stenosis.

Compared with direct laryngoscopy, a fiberoptic intubation technique has 2 main disadvantages. First, the size of the ETT to be used must be determined beforehand and cannot be changed easily, as changing the ETT in the middle of the procedure implies withdrawal of the fiberoptic bronchoscope and the need to regain the view of the glottis. Second, the small (pediatric) bronchoscopes needed to accommodate the small-size ETT implies that the bronchoscopes are also very flexible. The lack of stiffness may not allow passing the ETT over the bronchoscope through the stenosis, with the ETT and bronchoscope curling up above the stenosis. Of course, the advantage of the fiberoptic approach is that it allows the visual inspection of the stenotic airway, right before the intubation.

Backup plans for endotracheal intubation should be planned carefully. The following possible strategies should be considered carefully:

1. Performing a rigid bronchoscopy and ventilating through the bronchoscope,
2. Using jet ventilation, either supraglottic or transtracheal, and,
3. Performing a surgical airway below the stenosis.
4. Waking the patient up and aborting the procedure is also a theoretical alternative, but its feasibility should not be assumed, as it may not be a viable option in a patient with an uncorrected tracheal obstruction that has been worsened by multiple intubation attempts.
5. Emergency initiation of cardiopulmonary bypass is a final rescue option.

Alternative Ventilation Strategies

Jet ventilation (JV) may be used during TRR either initially, to provide effective ventilation in patients with critically obstructed airways, or intraoperatively, for ventilation across the surgical field. In this latter case, the smaller diameter of a JV catheter may allow better exposure in the surgical field, compared with an ETT, at the expense of a less closely monitored ventilation (in the absence of a reliable tidal volume and $ETCO_2$ measurement) and also of a significant splashing with blood and secretions from the airway. A detailed discussion of the use of JV in airway surgery can be found elsewhere.[1]

The use of an LMA as an airway device until the trachea is opened is another possibility, especially in patients with critical airway obstruction, in which spontaneous ventilation is preferable.

Carinal Resection

Carinal resection, especially if performed with right pneumonectomy, is a much riskier variant of the TRR, fraught with serious complications and mortality.[38] A detailed discussion of the anesthetic management[39] of these cases is beyond the scope of this article; here only a brief discussion of airway management is presented.

Before opening the airway, intubation can be achieved using an SLT with the tip placed either above the lesion (in which case a high airflow resistance can be expected, **Fig. 6**A) or below the lesion (with the risk of ventilating preferentially only one lung).

After opening of the airway, ventilation can be achieved through a number of different strategies. In the simplest form, a single lung ventilation approach can be used. Initially, the left main stem bronchus (MSB) is opened and intubated across the field (see **Fig. 6**B). Ventilation of the left lung can be performed easily while the

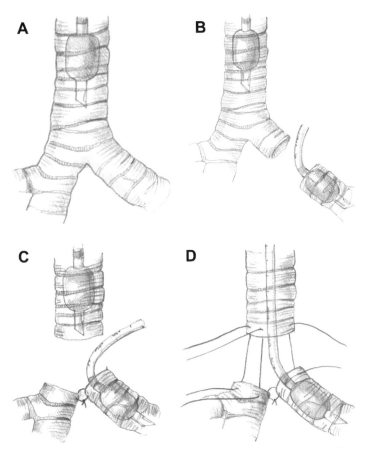

Fig. 6. Carinal resection. (*A*) If the carinal lesion obstructs airflow, it should be cored out during the rigid bronchoscopy stage, before intubation with the ETT. (*B*) Usually, the left main stem bronchus is incised first, and ventilated across the field with a second, sterile ETT. (*C*) Resection of the carina is completed. (*Illustrations by* Ioana Hobai.) (*D*) Ventilation of the left lung can then be accomplished by using the oral ETT, advanced into the bronchus, to allow the sutures be closed.

trachea and right main stem bronchus are being incised and sutures are placed (see **Fig. 6C**). Ventilation of the left lung is then performed intermittently, while sutures are placed across the tracheal and left MSB stumps, either across the field (as before) or by using the oral ETT (see **Fig. 6D**). In this last case, an extra-long, small-cuffed ETT needs to be used. Such tubes are available commercially, if not, they can be fashioned either from 2 single-lumen ETTs connected together, or from a double-lumen tube, by removing the tracheal lumen and cuff.[39] In patients who do not tolerate single-lung ventilation, the operative (right, in this example) lung can be ventilated as well, or provided with continuous positive airway pressure, using a second single-lumen ETT.

Other alternative strategies can be used in difficult cases. Jet ventilation of 1 of 2 lungs[40] can also be used. The use of cardiopulmonary bypass was also advocated[41]; however, this is marred by the bleeding complications associated with systemic heparinization.

In addition to the challenge of airway management, a few other specific aspects are the following:

1. Postoperative pain management. Carinal resections are usually approached through a right thoracotomy incision. The postoperative pain is significant (as opposed to the mild pain caused by a transverse cervical incision for upper tracheal lesions), and justifies the use of an epidural catheter or other regional techniques. In patients in whom this is contraindicated or refused, relying on systemic opioids for postoperative pain control is fraught with the risk of inducing respiratory depression.
2. Especially in patients who undergo a pneumonectomy, postoperative intubation may be necessary for 12 to 24 hours, as discussed later in this article.
3. Post-pneumonectomy pulmonary edema may occur even after uneventful cases, and is commonly fatal. Administration of IV hydration during the case is limited (usually to <1 L), although its causative role has not been demonstrated unequivocally.[42]

Extended resections

In patients with extensive lesions, up to one-half of the total tracheal length may be removed, if procedures to gain laryngeal (for high lesions) or hilar (for low lesions) release are performed.[43,44]

A so-called "suprathyroid release" procedure, involving the thyrohyoid muscle, membrane, and ligament, is commonly associated with postoperative dysphagia and aspiration and has been largely abandoned. The more common "suprahyoid release" involves cutting the mylohyoid, geniohyoid, and genioglossus muscles, cutting the lesser cornua of the hyoid bone and performing an anterior division of the hyoid bone. This procedure can provide a laryngeal descent of 2 to 3 cm.[43,44]

Lower tracheal lesions may require a hilar release, which is best approached via a right thoracotomy.[38] Dissecting the right hilar ligaments may require compressing and displacing the heart, with concomitant decreases in venous return and pulse pressure. These episodes are temporary, but should be carefully managed so as not to cause a critical decrease in cardiac perfusion, with development of arrhythmias or other signs of ischemia. Having an arterial line to monitor the pulse pressure on a beat-to-beat basis is mandatory to achieve close and timely communication with the surgical team.

Postoperative intubation

Commonly after carinal resection, especially after prolonged operations, postoperative ventilation may be necessary for 12 to 24 hours. This is necessary because a patient's ability to cough and clear secretions is commonly impaired. If this is the case, patients are intubated with a small ETT, placed above the anastomosis line. Extubation is performed in the intensive care unit on postoperative day 1 or 2, as soon as the usual extubation criteria are met. If extubation is unsuccessful, it is critical to understand the specific causes of its failure, and have these attended to until improved. Another extubation trial is then attempted 4 to 5 days later, this time in the operating room. If again unsuccessful, it is better that a tracheostomy be performed.

SUMMARY

Providing anesthesia for a TRR operation remains one of the most challenging tasks for thoracic anesthesiologists. Serious complications may result from even minor errors of judgment, at multiple critical times. A casual approach during induction and intubation of a patient with tracheal obstruction may result in life-threatening hypoxemia. Reflex coughing in a patient in whom the NMB is inadvertently allowed to fade may jeopardize a tenuous tracheal anastomosis. An extubation that is initiated too early or too late, or the injudicious use of postoperative pain medications may result in immediate loss of the airway patency, and may require either a reintubation under difficult circumstances, or the performance of emergent tracheostomy.

However, TRR is an operation that is performed safely in a growing number of centers. This article aimed to share some of our experience in the management of TRR anesthesia, in the hope that this will help improve its management and allow this therapeutic option to be offered to an ever increasing number of patients worldwide.

REFERENCES

1. McRae K. Anesthesia for airway surgery. Anesthesiol Clin North America 2001; 19(3):497–541, vi.
2. Sandberg W. Anesthesia and airway management for tracheal resection and reconstruction. Int Anesthesiol Clin 2000;38(1):55–75.
3. Pinsonneault C, Fortier J, Donati F. Tracheal resection and reconstruction. Can J Anaesth 1999;46(5 Pt 1):439–55.
4. Geffin B, Bland J, Grillo HC. Anesthetic management of tracheal resection and reconstruction. Anesth Analg 1969;48(5):884–90.
5. Jungebluth P, Moll G, Baiguera S, et al. Tissue-engineered airway: a regenerative solution. Clin Pharmacol Ther 2011;91(1):81–93.
6. Delaere PR. Tracheal transplantation. Curr Opin Pulm Med 2012;18(4):313–20.
7. Fung D, Devitt J. Anatomy, physiology, and innervation of larynx. Anesth Clin North Am 1995;13:259–76.
8. Al-Bazzaz F, Grillo H, Kazemi H. Response to exercise in upper airway obstruction. Am Rev Respir Dis 1975;111(5):631–40.
9. Geffin B, Grillo HC, Cooper JD, et al. Stenosis following tracheostomy for respiratory care. JAMA 1971;216(12):1984–8.
10. Lavelle TF Jr, Rotman HH, Weg JG. Isoflow-volume curves in the diagnosis of upper airway obstruction. Am Rev Respir Dis 1978;117(5):845–52.
11. Vander Els NJ, Sorhage F, Bach AM, et al. Abnormal flow volume loops in patients with intrathoracic Hodgkin's disease. Chest 2000;117(5):1256–61.
12. Gamsu G, Borson DB, Webb WR, et al. Structure and function in tracheal stenosis. Am Rev Respir Dis 1980;121(3):519–31.
13. Acres JC, Kryger MH. Clinical significance of pulmonary function tests: upper airway obstruction. Chest 1981;80(2):207–11.
14. Grillo HC, Zannini P, Michelassi F. Complications of tracheal reconstruction. Incidence, treatment, and prevention. J Thorac Cardiovasc Surg 1986;91(3):322–8.
15. Grillo HC, Donahue DM, Mathisen DJ, et al. Postintubation tracheal stenosis. Treatment and results. J Thorac Cardiovasc Surg 1995;109(3):486–92 [discussion: 92–3].
16. Yang KL. Tracheal stenosis after a brief intubation. Anesth Analg 1995;80(3): 625–7.
17. Urdaneta AI, Yu JB, Wilson LD. Population based cancer registry analysis of primary tracheal carcinoma. Am J Clin Oncol 2011;34(1):32–7.
18. Manninen MP, Antila PJ, Pukander JS, et al. Occurrence of tracheal carcinoma in Finland. Acta Otolaryngol 1991;111(6):1162–9.
19. Licht PB, Friis S, Pettersson G. Tracheal cancer in Denmark: a nationwide study. Eur J Cardiothorac Surg 2001;19(3):339–45.
20. Honings J, van Dijck JA, Verhagen AF, et al. Incidence and treatment of tracheal cancer: a nationwide study in the Netherlands. Ann Surg Oncol 2007;14(2):968–76.

21. Macchiarini P. Primary tracheal tumours. Lancet Oncol 2006;7(1):83–91.
22. Gaissert HA, Grillo HC, Shadmehr MB, et al. Uncommon primary tracheal tumors. Ann Thorac Surg 2006;82(1):268–72 [discussion: 72–3].
23. Ahn Y, Chang H, Lim YS, et al. Primary tracheal tumors: review of 37 cases. J Thorac Oncol 2009;4(5):635–8.
24. Gaissert HA, Grillo HC, Shadmehr MB, et al. Long-term survival after resection of primary adenoid cystic and squamous cell carcinoma of the trachea and carina. Ann Thorac Surg 2004;78(6):1889–96 [discussion: 96–7].
25. Regnard JF, Fourquier P, Levasseur P. Results and prognostic factors in resections of primary tracheal tumors: a multicenter retrospective study. The French Society of Cardiovascular Surgery. J Thorac Cardiovasc Surg 1996;111(4): 808–13 [discussion: 13–4].
26. LoCicero J 3rd, Costello P, Campos CT, et al. Spiral CT with multiplanar and three-dimensional reconstructions accurately predicts tracheobronchial pathology. Ann Thorac Surg 1996;62(3):811–7.
27. Mathisen DJ. Complications of tracheal surgery. Chest Surg Clin N Am 1996;6(4): 853–64.
28. Avidan MS, Zhang L, Burnside BA, et al. Anesthesia awareness and the bispectral index. N Engl J Med 2008;358(11):1097–108.
29. Dominguez J, Rivas JJ, Lobato RD, et al. Irreversible tetraplegia after tracheal resection. Ann Thorac Surg 1996;62(1):278–80.
30. Colt HG, Harrell JH. Therapeutic rigid bronchoscopy allows level of care changes in patients with acute respiratory failure from central airways obstruction. Chest 1997;112(1):202–6.
31. Maziak DE, Todd TR, Keshavjee SH, et al. Adenoid cystic carcinoma of the airway: thirty-two-year experience. J Thorac Cardiovasc Surg 1996;112(6): 1522–31 [discussion: 31–2].
32. Hirsh M, Barry J, Klaidman D. A tortured debate. Amid feuding and turf battles, lawyers in the White House discussed specific terror-interrogation techniques like 'water-boarding' and 'mock burials'. Newsweek 2004;143(25):50–3.
33. Herbstreit F, Peters J, Eikermann M. Impaired upper airway integrity by residual neuromuscular blockade: increased airway collapsibility and blunted genioglossus muscle activity in response to negative pharyngeal pressure. Anesthesiology 2009;110(6):1253–60.
34. Sax HC. Building high-performance teams in the operating room. Surg Clin North Am 2012;92(1):15–9.
35. Practice guidelines for management of the difficult airway: an updated report by the American Society of Anesthesiologists Task Force on Management of the Difficult Airway. Anesthesiology 2003;98(5):1269–77.
36. Palange P, Valli G, Onorati P, et al. Effect of heliox on lung dynamic hyperinflation, dyspnea, and exercise endurance capacity in COPD patients. J Appl Physiol 2004;97(5):1637–42.
37. Milner QJ, Abdy S, Allen JG. Management of severe tracheal obstruction with helium/oxygen and a laryngeal mask airway. Anaesthesia 1997;52(11): 1087–9.
38. Mitchell JD, Mathisen DJ, Wright CD, et al. Clinical experience with carinal resection. J Thorac Cardiovasc Surg 1999;117(1):39–52 [discussion: 3].
39. Alfille P. Anesthesia for tracheal surgery. In: Grillo H, editor. Surgery of the trachea and bronchi. Hamilton (CA): BC Decker Inc; 2004. p. 453–70.
40. Perera ER, Vidic DM, Zivot J. Carinal resection with two high-frequency jet ventilation delivery systems. Can J Anaesth 1993;40(1):59–63.

41. Peterffy A, Konstantinov IE. Resection of distal tracheal and carinal tumours with the aid of cardiopulmonary bypass. Scand Cardiovasc J 1998;32(2):109–12.
42. Bigatello LM, Allain R, Gaissert HA. Acute lung injury after pulmonary resection. Minerva Anestesiol 2004;70(4):159–66.
43. Heitmiller RF. Tracheal release maneuvers. Chest Surg Clin N Am 1996;6(4): 675–82.
44. Heitmiller RF. Tracheal release maneuvers. Chest Surg Clin N Am 2003;13(2): 201–10.

Anesthetic Management for Esophageal Resection

J. Michael Jaeger, MD, PhD[a,b,c,d], Stephen R. Collins, MD[c],
Randal S. Blank, MD, PhD[e],*

KEYWORDS

- Esophagectomy • Esophageal cancer • Anesthesia • Intraoperative management
- Postoperative management • Perioperative complications

KEY POINTS

- Factors that show promise for the improvement of perioperative outcomes include protective ventilatory strategies, thoracic epidural analgesia, goal-directed fluid therapy approaches to optimize tissue oxygen delivery, and attention to issues that may reduce anastomotic complications.
- Although it may be difficult to show a measurable benefit from any one intervention, a multimodal management approach that encompasses multiple aspects of perioperative care may provide the best hope for improving outcomes after esophagectomy.

INTRODUCTION

Esophageal resection has traditionally been considered the best option for localized esophageal cancer, either with or without a combination of neoadjuvant or adjuvant radiotherapy and/or chemotherapy.[1] Esophageal cancer has been well described since the beginning of the nineteenth century. It currently ranks as the seventh leading cause of cancer-related deaths worldwide.[2] Malignant tumors of the esophagus are classified by histologic type (squamous cell carcinoma or adenocarcinoma) and differ by cause, incidence, risk factors, and affected populations. Squamous cell carcinoma accounts for most (95%) esophageal cancers worldwide; however, the epidemiology of esophageal cancer has changed over the last several decades in the Western world, with adenocarcinoma currently accounting for more than half of all new cases

Disclosures: The authors have no conflicts of interest.
[a] TCV Surgical ICU, University of Virginia Health System, PO Box 800710, Charlottesville, VA 22908-0710, USA; [b] Division of Critical Care Medicine, University of Virginia Health System, PO Box 800710, Charlottesville, VA 22908-0710, USA; [c] Department of Anesthesiology, University of Virginia Health System, PO Box 800710, Charlottesville, VA 22908-0710, USA; [d] Department of Surgery, University of Virginia Health System, PO Box 800710, Charlottesville, VA 22908-0710, USA; [e] Thoracic Anesthesia, Department of Anesthesiology, University of Virginia Health System, PO Box 800710, Charlottesville, VA 22908-0710, USA
* Corresponding author.
E-mail address: rsb8p@virginia.edu

Anesthesiology Clin 30 (2012) 731–747
http://dx.doi.org/10.1016/j.anclin.2012.08.005
1932-2275/12/$ – see front matter © 2012 Elsevier Inc. All rights reserved.
anesthesiology.theclinics.com

of esophageal cancer.[3] The pathogenesis of esophageal adenocarcinoma is linked to gastroesophageal reflux disease (GERD) and the development of (Barrett esophagus) metaplasia, which progresses to dysplasia.[4] The outcome for patients with esophageal adenocarcinoma remains poor, with 5-year survival rates of around 49% for local-staged tumors and 2.8% for distant-staged tumors.[2] Operative mortality after esophagectomy has improved in the past few decades but remains as high as 8% to 9% at high-volume centers.[5]

Esophagectomy is also performed for a variety of nonmalignant disorders of the esophagus including hiatal hernias, severe GERD refractory to medical management, esophageal strictures and diverticula, and dysmotility disorders such as achalasia. Although the anesthetic and perioperative approaches remain similar, this article focuses on management aspects in patients undergoing esophagectomy for esophageal cancer.

The first successful esophageal resection was performed in 1913 by Frank Torek.[6] Later, Ohsawa[7] of Japan and Marshall[8] in the United States performed the first successful one-stage transthoracic esophagectomies with reconstruction. In 1933, the first successful transhiatal approach to esophagectomy for carcinoma was performed,[9] thus eliminating the need for thoracotomy. This transhiatal approach was performed only sporadically over the following decades but resurged after a recent report provided an operative benchmark standard.[10] Common approaches currently include transthoracic esophagectomy, combining a laparotomy and right thoracotomy with an esophagogastric anastomosis in the mediastinum (Ivor-Lewis technique) or in the neck (McKeown or 3-field technique); transhiatal esophagectomy, using a laparotomy incision and blunt thoracic esophageal dissection with anastomosis in the neck; or newer minimally invasive techniques using laparoscopy and/or thoracoscopy. Early reports highlighted outcome advantages such as decreased pulmonary complications and decreased intensive care unit (ICU) length of stay with the transhiatal approach.[11] However, a meta-analysis of multiple comparative studies showed no difference in long-term (5-year) survival rates between the transhiatal and transthoracic approaches,[12] and the investigators suggested that tumor characteristics might be a more important factor than the surgical approach in determining long-term survival, a conclusion supported by several recent studies.[5,13,14]

The choice of surgical approach to esophageal resection in a given patient is typically guided by several factors including individual surgeon skill and preference, tumor location, and prior surgery in, or radiation to, the thorax. Little high-quality evidence exists to guide decision making in this regard. The transhiatal approach avoids a thoracotomy incision and some of the associated pulmonary morbidity but may not be practical or safe in patients with a history of prior mediastinal surgery. The transthoracic approach facilitates extensive lymphadenopathy during resection; however, there is an attendant risk of intrathoracic anastomotic leak as well as pulmonary morbidity in this approach.[15]

Efforts to further decrease morbidity include minimally invasive techniques that have made possible en-bloc esophagectomy without laparotomy or thoracotomy (minimally invasive esophagectomy [MIE]). Potential benefits include limiting the physiologic stress associated with open esophagectomy and shorter hospital stay, but such advantages have not been clearly established. One of the largest series on MIE in 222 patients undergoing esophagectomy for high-grade dysplasia or cancer reported morbidity and mortality results equivalent to the best reported results from conventional open approaches with a median hospital stay of 7 days, anastomotic leak rate of 11.7%, and operative mortality of 1.4%. Although MIE has been deemed safe and feasible in a more recent systemic review,[16] a lack of high-quality comparative studies with conventional techniques preclude direct comparisons. Morbidity and mortality may perhaps best be linked to surgeon and hospital volume,[17–22] as shown in multiple studies. Improved outcomes in the last few decades in patients undergoing esophagectomy may also be related to institutional utilization of multimodal management[23,24] with defined strategies (eg, restrictive intraoperative fluid management, thoracic epidural analgesia, early tracheal extubation) and standardized clinical care pathways,[25] as discussed recently by Low.[26]

Perioperative management of patients presenting for esophagectomy presents a multitude of challenges for surgeons, anesthesiologists, and intensive care specialists. It seems likely that both intraoperative and postoperative strategies may lead to improved outcomes in these patients. This article focuses on perioperative management of the patient needing esophagectomy and reviews the factors that contribute to perioperative morbidity and mortality.

PULMONARY MORBIDITY

Pulmonary complications remain a significant concern in the patient undergoing esophagectomy and constitute the most common cause of postoperative death in patients with cancer undergoing esophageal resection.[27] Specific complications include atelectasis, aspiration pneumonia, hypoxia, pulmonary edema, pulmonary embolism, and acute respiratory distress syndrome (ARDS), which may occur in up to 10% of patients undergoing esophagectomy and result in a mortality of up to 50%.[28] Risk factors for the development of pulmonary complications include advanced age, preexisting pulmonary dysfunction, cigarette smoking, operative duration, and proximal tumor location; conflicting evidence exists regarding the possible role of induction chemoradiotherapy.[27,28] One of the most frequently seen surgical complications after esophagectomy is a leak at the esophagogastric anastomosis. This potentially devastating complication may occur in up to 14% of patients[14,29] and has a significant role in the development of pulmonary complications. In 1 retrospective series,[30] an anastomotic leak was found in 42% of those patients who developed ARDS. A recent review[28] highlights important factors associated with the development of pulmonary complications after esophagectomy and suggests that several interventions may be needed to influence measurable outcomes in such patients. However, few randomized trials are available to guide anesthetic management.

VENTILATORY MANAGEMENT

Prevention of lung injury remains an important challenge in the perioperative management of the patient needing esophagectomy. Esophagectomy elicits a profound inflammatory response[31] which in turn seems to predict pulmonary morbidity.[30,32] Moreover, transthoracic esophagectomy requires one-lung ventilation (OLV), which subjects the lungs to additional hazards including ventilation-induced lung injury, oxygen toxicity, atelectasis, and, perhaps, ischemia-reperfusion injury. The use of nonphysiologic ventilation strategies such as large tidal volumes and high inflation pressures without the addition of positive end-expiratory pressure (PEEP) can cause systemic inflammation and lung injury even in patients without lung disease.[33] Injury severity may also be linked to the duration of mechanical ventilation.

Although there is no clear causality between the inflammatory response and the development of lung injury, more protective ventilatory strategies have been shown to reduce the severity of lung injury during mechanical ventilation.[33] These strategies include low tidal volume ventilation, application of PEEP, and low ventilatory pressures (inspiratory plateau pressures <35 cm H_2O) through the use of pressure-controlled ventilation and permissive hypercapnia. Application of such strategies has been shown to improve outcomes in patients with ARDS as shown in a landmark Acute Respiratory Distress Syndrome Network (ARDSNet) trial[34] and discussed in more recent reviews.[35] The direct applicability of these data to the stable perioperative patient undergoing OLV is not clear and no specific evidence-based recommendations exist. Similar protective ventilation strategies are generally advocated for thoracic surgical patients requiring OLV and are supported by studies that show increased inflammatory and injurious effects of OLV[36] and the mitigation of these effects with protective ventilation strategies. One recent randomized trial[37] found that patients undergoing esophagectomy with a protective ventilation strategy during OLV (tidal volumes of 5 mL/kg and PEEP 5 cm H_2O) showed a dramatically reduced systemic inflammatory systemic and improved pulmonary gas exchange.

THORACIC EPIDURAL ANALGESIA

Thoracic epidural analgesia (TEA) remains the standard clinical approach for postoperative pain control in patients undergoing transthoracic esophagectomy at most institutions.[38] It has been shown to improve postoperative pulmonary function[39] and reduce pulmonary complications.[40,41] Its full effects on immune function and the stress response during esophagectomy are unclear[42]; however, in multiple studies, TEA has been shown to provide superior analgesia compared with intravenous opioid analgesia,[43,44] to reduce pulmonary complications,[41,45,46] to facilitate immediate or early extubation,[24] and to reduce time in intensive care.[47] A disadvantage of TEA is the resultant sympathectomy-induced hypotension which can lead to excessive fluid administration or vasopressor use. However, TEA is an important component of standardized clinical pathways that have shown improved recovery and reduced costs in patients needing esophagectomy.[23,25] Improved pain control after thoracotomy is thought to facilitate more effective cough, physiotherapy, and earlier mobilization during recovery.[48]

TEA may have other advantages in patients needing esophagectomy by improving gastric conduit flow by its effects on splanchnic perfusion. Ischemia at the gastric conduit anastomosis is thought to be a major cause of anastomotic failure and leak.[48] In an animal model,[49] TEA with 0.5% bupivacaine improved gastric microcirculation within the newly formed gastric tube. In a prospective clinical study,[50] gastric mucosal blood flow was measured in patients after esophagectomy and improved at the anastomosis in those patients with a TEA infusion of ropivacaine and sufentanil. It seems that TEA has benefits beyond those of pain management and the facilitation of pulmonary rehabilitation.

INTRAOPERATIVE FLUID MANAGEMENT

The overriding goal in fluid management of major surgical patients including those undergoing esophagectomy is to optimize tissue blood flow and oxygen delivery. An important secondary goal is the avoidance of excessive fluid administration, which may result in tissue edema, delay the return of normal gastrointestinal function, impair wound healing, and increase cardiac and/or pulmonary morbidity including pulmonary edema and cardiac/respiratory failure.[51] No practice consensus exists in regards to perioperative fluid therapy, and different fluid regimens and end points used in various studies make it challenging to draw conclusions. Recent studies have focused on restrictive fluid regimens despite a lack of standardization of this term. Prospective studies comparing restrictive versus liberal fluid strategies generally favor the former approach in major surgical procedures.[52,53] Retrospective studies of patients undergoing esophagectomy[54–56] have shown that there is an association between greater cumulative fluid balance in the perioperative period and increased morbidity such as pneumonia, respiratory failure, and delayed extubation.

Intravenous fluid is often the first strategy used by many practitioners to treat hypotension or a perceived decrement in tissue blood flow (eg, urine output). This approach may need revision.[24] Caution must be exercised in the administration of excessive fluids because the lung on the operative side has been traumatized to an extent by factors including surgical manipulation, prolonged atelectasis, and ischemia/reperfusion injury. In addition, the dependent lung is subjected to a protracted period of mechanical ventilation during these cases. Goal-directed fluid therapy (GDFT) is a recent attempt to optimize tissue blood flow and oxygen delivery in patients undergoing major surgical procedures. Hemodynamic goals used in such approaches include cardiac output (CO), stroke volume (SV), stroke volume variation (SVV), or pulse pressure variation (PPV). Minimally invasive devices are now available to guide therapy using these parameters[57] and more are likely to be forthcoming. Other traditional monitoring parameters such as central venous pressure or pulmonary capillary wedge pressure have not been found to reflect circulating blood volume in patients undergoing esophagectomy[58] and are not useful for predicting fluid responsiveness. Reports have shown that GDFT in major surgery has been linked to reduced vasopressor use[59] and reduced length of hospital stay and other morbidity measures.[60–62] Two recent studies[63,64] of patients undergoing esophagectomy have reported that the FloTrac/Vigileo system (Edwards Lifesciences, Irving, CA) is an accurate predictor of hypovolemia and is useful for improving hemodynamic stability during surgery.

Experimental studies of gastrointestinal surgery in several animal models have also examined the impact of specific fluid regimens.[65–68] Prospective trials of GDFT have shown that colloids may be superior to crystalloids in some settings.[69] Kimberger and colleagues[65] studied the effects of intraoperative GDFT (lactated Ringer solution [LR] or hetastarch [HES] 130/0.4 bolus) versus a restrictive regimen with LR in a porcine colonic anastomosis model. The GDFT target was mixed venous oxygen saturation greater than 60%. Intestinal tissue oxygen tension was assessed by polarographic tissue oxygen tension sensors placed between the serosa and mucosal layers; microcirculatory blood flow was assessed by laser Doppler flowmetry. A GDFT colloid regimen produced the largest increases in perianastomotic microcirculatory blood flow and tissue oxygen tension compared with either the restrictive or the GDFT crystalloid groups, despite a higher average positive fluid balance. Although not yet shown, an analogous improvement in blood flow and oxygen delivery to the esophagogastric anastomosis could represent a particularly important therapy for the optimization of anastomotic healing, integrity, and postoperative anastomotic outcomes.

THE ESOPHAGOGASTRIC ANASTOMOSIS AND GASTRIC CONDUIT PERFUSION

The gastric conduit has an altered vascular physiology that remains incompletely understood. It is clear from numerous animal models and clinical studies[49,50,70–73] that the native blood supply is compromised significantly by the gastric dissection, including arterial division and the gastroplasty procedure itself. It is thus not surprising that perfusion of the gastric conduit and the anastomotic region in particular may be tenuous in patients undergoing esophagectomy with esophagogastric anastomoses.

The normal blood supply of the esophagus is derived at its most cephalad portion by contributions of the inferior thyroid artery with smaller accessory branches from the common carotid, subclavian, and superficial cervical arteries. In the caudad direction, collateral branches from the bronchial arteries and variable esophageal contributions from the aorta are the primary sources of nutrition. In addition, significant branches ascending from the short gastric arteries, the celiac artery, and inferior phrenic arteries complete the vascular network supplying blood to the native esophagus. Throughout the esophagus, particularly the thoracic portion, these small arteries subsequently branch into a rich intramural network of arterioles and capillaries that supply nourishment to the esophagus but result in watershed areas between the major vascular source vessels,[74] especially in the intrathoracic esophagus. Where the site of the neoesophageal anastomosis occurs with regard to these watershed areas is completely unknown. It therefore seems that resultant perfusion might also be limited in part by a suboptimal selection of the anastomotic site.

The importance of venous drainage and the possible role of venous congestion in impairing circulation at the anastomotic site has also received considerable experimental attention. Esophageal capillary blood flows into an elaborate submucosal venous plexus. This blood subsequently drains into a periesophageal venous plexus from which the esophageal veins originate. In the native esophagus, the cervical esophagus drains into the inferior thyroid veins. In the thoracic region, the esophageal veins variably drain into the bronchial, the azygos, or hemiazygos veins; the diaphragmatic portion the drainage is predominantly into the left gastric vein. Conduit stretch can result in excessive tension that may in turn compromise venous drainage. To date, the responses to nitroglycerin or sodium nitroprusside infusions are inconclusive.[75,76] In a clinical study,[77] 1 group of researchers used a recirculating gas tonometry probe to continuously monitor intraconduit mucosal pH (and, by inference, adequacy of perfusion within the gastric conduit) and showed an immediate decline in perfusion (an increase in the difference between mucosal pH and blood pH) from the time of admission to the ICU, which lasted an average of more than 84 hours. CO, mean systemic arterial pressure, and systemic vascular resistance were largely unchanged during this period of observation. In addition, these patients had an uneventful recovery from their esophagectomy (ie, no complications from the gastric conduit anastomosis). This study strongly suggests that gastric conduit microcirculatory blood flow is compromised in the perioperative period.

VASOPRESSOR THERAPY

The use of vasopressor agents in patients needing esophagectomy, either during or after surgery, is controversial because of concern for vasopressor-induced decrements in gastric conduit blood flow. A retrospective review[78] of postoperative patients with a variety of gastrointestinal anastomoses showed a significant association between the development of an anastomotic leak (in 10% of patients) and more than 72 hours of vasopressor use (23% of those patients with anastomotic leaks). In a porcine model of esophagectomy,[79] severe hypoperfusion of the gastric conduit was shown when blood pressure was maintained using a norepinephrine infusion. However, this experimental study may not have clinical relevance to routine patients after esophagectomy because it used an acute hemorrhage model to decrease blood pressure and a potent vasopressor alone to normalize it.

More recent studies in porcine models of gastric conduits suggest that maintenance of a normal mean arterial blood pressure with vasopressors in an otherwise euvolemic state may improve blood flow locally at the anastomosis as measured by laser Doppler flowmetry.[73,76] Perhaps more relevant may be the discovery that raising the mean arterial blood pressure more than 70 mm Hg with vasopressors had no appreciable benefit in microcirculatory blood flow.[73] In a study of epidural-induced hypotension in patients needing esophagectomy,[80] the use of intravenous epinephrine restored both hemodynamic parameters and anastomotic blood flow.

At present, the impact of vasopressor use in patients undergoing esophagectomy remains inconclusive, but it seems that, in the fluid-replete patient, the use of low-dose vasopressor/inotropes such as norepinephrine or epinephrine to optimize both blood pressure and tissue blood flow is preferable to hypotension or the risks of substantial volume overload.

ANASTOMOTIC LEAK

Esophageal anastomotic leak is a significant cause of morbidity and mortality after esophagectomy. Although reports vary, leakage rates occur with an incidence as high as 14%; associated mortality ranges from less than 5% to 35%.[81] The location of the anastomosis (cervical vs thoracic) does not seem to affect the leak rate,[82] although it may affect resultant morbidity. Surgical technique and vascularity of the gastric conduit may contribute to the rate of anastomotic leak; other factors that have been implicated include tumor stage, intraoperative bleeding, respiratory complications, and low serum albumin concentration.[83] Anastomotic failure and leakage can lead to severe damage of surrounding tissue. Leakage of digestive fluids and seeding of the perianastomotic region with bacteria, yeast, and fungi can produce a vigorous and dangerous inflammatory response. This risk applies particularly to mediastinal anastomoses because the resulting mediastinitis may remain undetected for a prolonged time and ultimately cause significant injury.[84] Detection is typically more rapid and treatment more easily accomplished for leaks from cervical anastomoses because of their superficial location. Morbidity and mortality from conduit leaks can be considerable and site dependent, with reported mortalities of 8.5% to 35% for intrathoracic leaks and 6.7% to 10% for cervical leaks.[5,13,29,85–88] Recognition and treatment of a leak from the gastric conduit can be difficult. Intrathoracic anastomotic leaks typically present as empyema or mediastinitis with high fevers, leukocytosis, chest pain, dyspnea, cardiac arrhythmias, and hypotension. The surgical team and intensivist must maintain a high index of suspicion. Ipsilateral or bilateral pleural effusions (frequently loculated) can develop and thoracostomy tube drainage with Gram stain and culture of fluid are diagnostic. A modified barium swallow study may reveal a fistulous tract or small leak but may be nondiagnostic and confirmation with endoscopy is suggested.[85,87,89,90] Intra-abdominal free air with peritonitis is present if dehiscence of any subdiaphragmatic gastric remnant occurs. Small anastomotic leaks, particularly those in the cervical region, can be treated conservatively with drainage and broad-spectrum prophylactic antibiotics. However, if the leak is large or intrathoracic in location, an intervention is required. Endoscopically placed stents are commonly used to prevent further leakage and allow for healing.[91,92] Esophageal stents remain in place for about 3 weeks to allow for healing of the conduit in the absence of any contact with gastroduodenal fluid. Esophageal stents can migrate distally and require recovery and subsequent redeployment.[91] Alternate approaches include the endoscopic placement of vacuum-assisted sponge-tipped nasogastric tubes.[93,94]

Although many anastomotic leaks can be managed nonoperatively using the techniques described,[89] an operative approach may be required in severe cases, particularly those within the mediastinum. If dehiscence with empyema becomes apparent early in the postoperative course, immediate thoracic re-exploration with excision of the primary anastomosis and construction of a new conduit may be warranted. This technique can be successful if pleural infection is not well established and sufficient conduit length remains to avoid tension on the new anastomosis. As an alternative, it may be necessary to excise the primary anastomosis, exteriorize the esophageal stump (cervical esophagostomy), close the gastric stoma, reduce the stomach into the abdomen, and perform a gastrostomy for drainage. A colon or jejunal interposition may be performed later to reestablish alimentary continuity. Attention to adequate nutrition to promote healing cannot be overstated. Spontaneous healing typically requires up to 3 months.

OTHER INTRATHORACIC COMPLICATIONS: ATELECTASIS, PNEUMONIA, PLEURAL EFFUSIONS, AND CHYLOTHORAX

Risk factors for pulmonary and other intrathoracic complications include advanced age, operative duration, tumor location, blood transfusion,[27] preoperative pulmonary function, tobacco abuse,[95,96] and surgical approach.[97] The most common respiratory complications are atelectasis and hypoxemia. If poor pulmonary function necessitates the continuation of mechanical ventilation in the postoperative period, protective ventilatory strategies should be used with the following goals: minimize ventilator-induced injury, avoid patient-ventilator dyssynchrony during emergence from sedation, provide sufficient PEEP to prevent pulmonary edema formation while avoiding significant hemodynamic compromise, and allow adequate work of the respiratory muscles to limit disuse complications.

Most patients with normal preoperative pulmonary function can be extubated in the operating room at emergence. Once extubated, pulmonary toilet is imperative with hourly use of incentive spirometry, deep breathing, and coughing maneuvers to facilitate recruitment of atelectatic regions, clearance of pulmonary secretions, and prevention of pneumonia. However, the use of positive airway pressure modalities, especially continuous positive airway pressure or biphasic positive airway pressure masks, cannot be recommended because these modalities can contribute to distension of the gastric conduit even in the presence of a nasogastric drainage tube. TEA remains the current standard for pain control after transthoracic esophagectomy and is thought to reduce pulmonary morbidity by enabling pulmonary rehabilitation maneuvers as well as mobilization after emergence and extubation.[96,98] Mobilization of the patient out of bed by postoperative day 1 is an important goal in postoperative care. Aspiration precautions with head of bed increase greater than 30° should be strictly followed after surgery. Glottic function may be compromised, particularly after a cervical anastomoses, potentially increasing the risk of aspiration, a well-known complication following esophagectomy.[99–102] Optimal oral hygiene may minimize the accumulation of oral bacteria. However, it is generally recommended that the patient not swallow oral rinse solution until after the conduit has been evaluated, typically on or around postoperative day 4 or 5.

Because mild to moderate pulmonary edema is common in the first few days following esophagectomy, oxygen supplementation is frequently necessary. Reintubation is rarely required. The use of high-flow nasal cannulae (>6 L/min) and any positive-pressure breathing-assist device (CPAP, BiPAP) should be discouraged because of the potential for over-distension of the gastric conduit. To minimize the risk of intravascular volume depletion, the use of diuretics should be avoided as far as possible. Instead, close monitoring of total fluid intake as well as thoracostomy tube, nasogastric tube, and urine output should allow fluid intake to be adjusted appropriately.

Pleural effusions are generally minor and drained by a thoracostomy tube on the operative side if a thoracotomy was performed. On occasion, a pleural effusion may develop on the contralateral side and should be monitored carefully for evidence of an anastomotic leak or a chyle leak from a thoracic duct injury. Postesophagectomy chylothorax is uncommon, with an incidence of less than 4%; if it persists in the face of conservative treatment, thoracic duct ligation is required, significantly increasing the risk of attendant morbidity and length of hospital stay.[103] Thoracic duct injury should be suspected if daily thoracostomy tube drainage output exceeds 400 mL, especially if the drainage is cloudy. Fluid can be analyzed for triglyceride content. Conservative treatment consists of avoidance of fat in the diet, eliminating lipid infusions if total parenteral nutrition is used, and cessation of propofol if used for sedation in order to reduce production and flow.[104]

Pneumonia is the most feared complication after gastric conduit anastomotic leak because it has been implicated in postesophagectomy in-hospital mortality.[27,105,106] Many postoperative pneumonias in patients needing esophagectomy are related to aspiration. Pulmonary aspiration can occur during induction of anesthesia, during surgery, or after surgery. Postoperative aspiration occurs most commonly, probably because of diminished airway protective reflexes, left recurrent laryngeal nerve injury,[107] oropharyngeal deglutitive dysfunction,[100] or delayed gastric emptying.[108] Most cases of aspiration pneumonia in this population are evaluated with flexible bronchoscopy and bronchoalveolar lavage to obtain a specimen for Gram stain and aerobic bacterial culture. Fungal cultures may also be prudent if the hospital course has been protracted or the patient is immunosuppressed. Broad-spectrum antibiotic coverage can be initiated but rapidly discontinued or narrowed as the Gram stain and culture results become available. Other sources of pneumonia include bronchoesophageal fistulas secondary to conduit anastomotic dehiscence, which can produce severe injuries to the lung and require prolonged antibiotic coverage for both aerobes and fungi until resolution. Successful treatment may require esophageal or bronchial stenting or surgical repair.

CARDIAC ARRHYTHMIAS

Cardiac arrhythmias are common in the postoperative period following major thoracic surgery in general and esophagectomy in particular.[109,110] Postoperative new-onset supraventricular tachycardia (SVT) presents in 13% to 40% of patients needing esophagectomy.[111–114] Atrial fibrillation (AF) constitutes most of these cases and may cause significant hypotension requiring ICU admission.[111,114] Peak incidence of AF occurs within 48 hours after surgery.[114] Numerous studies have implicated AF as a sign of other underlying disorders that frequently are the cause of serious morbidity in this population. Pulmonary complications were found in 40% of those developing new AF.[112] More importantly, AF was associated with a high likelihood of anastomotic leak[114] (28.1% vs 6.45%; $P<.01$). Other investigators have found significant associations of SVT with conduit leaks[112] and sepsis.[112,113] Current strategies to prevent postesophagectomy arrhythmias include β-adrenergic antagonists and amiodarone. Tisdale and colleagues[115] used an amiodarone infusion for the first 96 hours after esophagectomy as AF prophylaxis and reported a 62.5% relative risk reduction.

VENOUS THROMBOEMBOLISM

Like other malignancies, esophageal cancer predisposes patients to a higher than normal risk of venous thromboembolism in the perioperative period (4%–20%). This complication is associated with high mortality.[116] The incidence of thromboembolism in patients with esophageal cancer undergoing neoadjuvant chemotherapy with or without surgery was determined in 1 study to be 13%.[117] Cisplatin and 5-fluorouracil may incite venous thromboembolism by virtue of their effects on endothelium and the coagulation system. To reduce the risks of thromboembolism and its sequelae, most clinicians recommend the use of intraoperative pneumatic leg compression devices and perioperative anticoagulant prophylaxis and stress the importance of early ambulation after surgery.

NUTRITION AND GASTROINTESTINAL FUNCTION

Esophageal cancer may cause severe debilitation because it often prevents the consumption of adequate nutrition to counter catabolism. Even benign disorders of the esophagus including strictures and motility disorders can result in significant weight loss. Nutrition may also be adversely affected by a reduced appetite caused by chemotherapy, as well as the effects of fatigue, dysphagia, or depression. When malnutrition is severe, the surgeon may place a feeding jejunostomy tube for enteral nutrition weeks in advance of a scheduled esophageal resection in order to improve the patient's physical and immune status. Otherwise a jejunostomy tube is placed during laparotomy/laparoscopy for esophagogastric resection. Enteral feeding is initiated on postoperative day 2 at a rate consistent with intraluminal epithelium maintenance (trophic feeds). It may be necessary to delay enteral feeding and initiate parenteral nutrition if prolonged ileus, anastomotic leak, aspiration, or chylothorax supervene.[118]

The gastric conduit should be tested for integrity about a week after surgery using a modified barium swallow study and/or endoscopy. Once integrity of the gastric conduit is assured, the patient is allowed sips of clear liquids. However, to permit healing and promote adequate anastomotic strength, most of the nutritional requirement is provided via the jejunostomy tube for a minimum of several weeks. Over this period the oral diet can be advanced to full liquids and a mechanical soft diet if tolerated. The patient is taught to avoid overloading the conduit by adopting a pattern of multiple small meals and alternating meals with fluid consumption.

Several additional postoperative complications are also possible. Strictures can develop at the anastomotic site as a consequence of scarring and healing. These strictures often present as dysphagia and generally are delayed and unlikely to present during the original hospitalization.[119] Treatment consists of periodic and careful serial dilatations with Maloney dilators. The postvagotomy dumping syndrome is variable but has been reported to occur to some degree in up to 50% of patients.[119,120] Symptoms such as nausea, diaphoresis, cramping, cardiac palpitations, and diarrhea are associated with an early form presenting within an hour or less of eating.[119] This is to be distinguished from a late form that develops several hours later and is characterized by tremors, loss of consciousness, or somnolence. Although the true cause of these different forms remains unclear, resolution can usually be accomplished with alterations in diet or changes in timing or pattern of eating. In addition, delayed gastric emptying occurs in 10% to 50% of patients after esophagectomy.[120] Presenting symptoms occur rapidly while eating and include early satiety, postprandial discomfort, dysphagia, or regurgitation. Pyloroplasty performed as part of the gastric conduit formation and attention to an adequate diaphragmatic hiatus for the conduit seem to prevent the problem; however, results are mixed.[121] Furthermore, extensive pyloroplasty increases the chance of duodenal-gastric reflux that tends to affect patients later in the course of their recovery. Some cases of delayed gastric emptying resolve with the use of prokinetic drugs to enhance motility.

SUMMARY

The anesthetic and perioperative management of patients requiring esophagectomy remain challenging. In practice, these patients require close attention to numerous aspects of intraoperative and postoperative care in order to optimize outcomes. Factors that show promise for the improvement of perioperative outcomes include protective ventilatory strategies, TEA, GDFT approaches to optimize tissue oxygen delivery, and attention to factors that might reduce anastomotic complications. Although it may be difficult to show a measurable benefit from any one intervention, a multimodal management approach that encompasses multiple aspects of perioperative care may provide the best hope for improving outcomes after esophagectomy.

REFERENCES

1. Mariette C, Piessen G, Triboulet JP. Therapeutic strategies in oesophageal carcinoma: role of surgery and other modalities. Lancet Oncol 2007;8:545–53.
2. American Cancer Society. Cancer facts & figures. Atlanta, (GA): American Cancer Society; 2012.
3. Holmes RS, Vaughan TL. Epidemiology and pathogenesis of esophageal cancer. Semin Radiat Oncol 2007;17(1):2–9.
4. Anderson LA, Watson RG, Murphy SJ, et al. Risk factors for Barrett's oesophagus and oesophageal adenocarcinoma: results from the FINBAR study. World J Gastroenterol 2007;13(10):1585–94.
5. Connors RC, Reuben BC, Neumayer LA, et al. Comparing outcomes after transthoracic and transhiatal esophagectomy: a 5-year prospective cohort of 17,395 patients. J Am Coll Surg 2007;205:735–40.
6. Torek F. The first successful resection of the thoracic portion of the esophagus for carcinoma. Surg Gynecol Obstet 1913;16:614–7.
7. Ohsawa T. Surgery of the esophagus. Arch Jpn Chir 1933;10:605–8.
8. Marshall SF. Carcinoma of the esophagus: successful resection of lower end of esophagus with re-establishment of esophageal gastric continuity. Surg Clin North Am 1938;18:643.
9. Turner GG. Excision of thoracic esophagus for carcinoma with construction of extrathoracic gullet. Lancet 1933;2:1315–6.
10. Orringer MB, Marshall BM, Iannettoni MD. Transhiatal esophagectomy: clinical experience and refinements. Ann Surg 1999;230:392–400.
11. Hulscher JB, van Sandick JW, de Boer AG, et al. Extended transthoracic resection compared with limited transhiatal resection for adenocarcinoma of the esophagus. N Engl J Med 2002;347(21):1662–9.
12. Hulscher JB, Tijssen J, Obertop H, et al. Transthoracic versus transhiatal resection for carcinoma of the esophagus: a meta-analysis. Ann Thorac Surg 2001;72:306–13.
13. Chang AC, Ji H, Birkmeyer NJ, et al. Outcomes after transhiatal and transthoracic esophagectomy for cancer. Ann Thorac Surg 2008;85:424–9.
14. Orringer MB, Marshall B, Chang AC, et al. Two thousand transhiatal esophagectomies: changing trends, lessons learned. Ann Surg 2007;246:363–74.
15. de Hoyos A, Litle VR, Luketich JD. Minimally invasive esophagectomy. Surg Clin North Am 2005;85:631–47.
16. Gemmill EH, McCulloch P. Systematic review of minimally invasive resection for gastro-oesophageal cancer. Br J Surg 2007;94:1461–7.
17. Rouvelas I, Jia C, Viklund P, et al. Surgeon volume and postoperative mortality and oesophagectomy for cancer. Eur J Surg Oncol 2007;33:162–8.
18. Migliore M, Choong CK, Lim E, et al. A surgeon's case volume of oesophagectomy for cancer strongly influences the operative mortality rate. Eur J Cardiothorac Surg 2007;32:375–80.
19. Verhoef C, van de Weyer R, Schaapveld M, et al. Better survival in patients with esophageal cancer after surgical treatment in university hospitals: a plea for performance by surgical oncologists. Ann Surg Oncol 2007;14:1678–87.

20. Wouters MW, Wijnhoven BP, Karim-Kos HE, et al. High-volume versus low-volume for esophageal resections for cancer: the essential role of case-mix adjustments based on clinical data. Ann Surg Oncol 2008;15:80–7.

21. Hollenbeck BK, Dunn RL, Miller DC, et al. Volume-based referral for cancer surgery: informing the debate. J Clin Oncol 2007;25:91–6.

22. Al-Sarira AA, David G, Willmott S, et al. Oesophagectomy practice and outcomes in England. Br J Surg 2007;94:585–91.

23. Brodner G, Pogatzki E, van Aken H, et al. A multimodel approach to control postoperative pathophysiology and rehabilitation in patients undergoing abdominothoracic esophagectomy. Anesth Analg 1998;86:228–34.

24. Neal JM, Wilcox RT, Allen HW, et al. Near-total esophagectomy: the influence of standardized multimodal management and intraoperative fluid restriction. Reg Anesth Pain Med 2003;28:328–34.

25. Low DE, Kunz S, Schembre D, et al. Esophagectomy – it's not just about mortality anymore: standardized perioperative clinical pathways improve outcomes in patients with esophageal cancer. J Gastrointest Surg 2007;11:1395–402.

26. Low DE. Evolution in perioperative management of patients undergoing oesophagectomy. Br J Surg 2007;94:655–6.

27. Law S, Wong KH, Kwok KF, et al. Predictive factors for postoperative pulmonary complications and mortality after esophagectomy for cancer. Ann Surg 2004; 240(5):791–800.

28. McKevith JM, Pennefather SH. Respiratory complications after oesophageal surgery. Curr Opin Anaesthesiol 2010;23:34–40.

29. Atkins BZ, Shah AS, Hutcheson KA, et al. Reducing hospital morbidity and mortality following esophagectomy. Ann Thorac Surg 2004;78:1170–6.

30. Tandon S, Batchelor A, Bullock R, et al. Perioperative risk factors for acute lung injury after elective oesophagectomy. Br J Anaesth 2001;86:633–8.

31. Kooguchi K, Kobayashi A, Kitamura Y, et al. Elevated expression of inducible nitric oxide synthase and inflammatory cytokines in the alveolar macrophages after esophagectomy. Crit Care Med 2002;30:71–6.

32. Katsuta T, Saito T, Shigemitsu Y, et al. Relation between tumor necrosis factor alpha and interleukin 1beta producing capacity of peripheral monocytes and pulmonary complications following oesophagectomy. Br J Surg 1998;85:548–53.

33. Slinger P. Perioperative lung injury. In: Slinger P, editor. Principles and practice of anesthesia for thoracic surgery. New York: Springer; 2011. p. 143–51.

34. Ventilation with lower tidal volumes as compared with traditional tidal volumes for acute lung injury and the acute respiratory distress syndrome. The Acute Respiratory Distress Syndrome Network. N Engl J Med 2000;342(18):1301–8.

35. Yilmaz M, Gajic O. Optimal ventilator settings in acute lung injury and acute respiratory distress syndrome. Eur J Anaesthesiol 2008;25:89–96.

36. Gothard J. Lung injury after thoracic surgery and one-lung ventilation. Curr Opin Anaes 2006;19:5–10.

37. Michelet P, D'Journo XB, Roch A, et al. Protective ventilation influences systemic inflammation after esophagectomy: a randomized controlled study. Anesthesiology 2006;105:911–9.

38. Blank R, Huffmyer J, Jaeger J. Anesthesia for esophageal surgery. In: Slinger P, editor. Principles and practice of anesthesia for thoracic surgery. New York: Springer; 2011. p. 415–43.

39. Ballantyne JC, Carr DB, deFerranti S, et al. The comparative effects of postoperative analgesic therapies on pulmonary outcome: cumulative meta-analysis of randomized, controlled trials. Anesth Analg 1998;86(3):598–612.

40. Popping DM, Elia N, Marret E, et al. Protective effects of epidural analgesia on pulmonary complications after abdominal and thoracic surgery: a meta-analysis. Arch Surg 2008;143:990–9.
41. Cense HA, Lagarde SM, de Jong K, et al. Association of no epidural analgesia with postoperative morbidity and mortality after transthoracic esophageal cancer resection. J Am Coll Surg 2006;202:395–400.
42. Yokoyama M, Itano Y, Katayama H, et al. The effects of continuous epidural anesthesia and analgesia on stress response and immune function in patients undergoing radical esophagectomy. Anesth Analg 2005;101:1521–7.
43. Rudin A, Flisberg P, Johansson J, et al. Thoracic epidural analgesia or intravenous morphine analgesia after thoracoabdominal esophagectomy: a prospective follow-up of 201 patients. J Cardiothorac Vasc Anesth 2005;19:350–7.
44. Flisberg P, Tornebrandt K, Walther B, et al. Pain relief after esophagectomy: thoracic epidural analgesia is better than parenteral opioids. J Cardiothorac Vasc Anesth 2001;15:282–7.
45. Watson A, Allen PR. Influence of thoracic epidural analgesia on outcome after resection for esophageal cancer. Surgery 1994;115(4):429–32.
46. Tsui SL, Law S, Fok M, et al. Postoperative analgesia reduces mortality and morbidity after esophagectomy. Am J Surg 1997;173(6):472–8.
47. Smedstad KG, Beattie WS, Blair WS, et al. Postoperative pain relief and hospital stay after total esophagectomy. Clin J Pain 1992;8:149–53.
48. Ng JM. Perioperative anesthetic management for esophagectomy. Anesthesiol Clin 2008;26:293–304.
49. Lázár G, Kaszaki J, Ábrahám S, et al. Thoracic epidural anesthesia improves the gastric microcirculation during experimental gastric tube formation. Surgery 2003;134:799–805.
50. Michelet P, Roch A, D'Journo XB, et al. Effect of thoracic epidural analgesia on gastric blood flow after oesophagectomy. Acta Anaesthesiol Scand 2007;51:587–94.
51. Holte K, Sharrock NE, Kehlet H. Pathophysiology and clinical implications of perioperative fluid excess. Br J Anaesth 2002;89(4):622–32.
52. Brandstrup B, Tonnesen H, Beier-Holgersen R, et al. Effects of intravenous fluid restriction on postoperative complications: comparisons of two perioperative fluid regimens: a randomized assessor-blinded multicenter trial. Ann Surg 2003;238(5):641–8.
53. Nisanevich V, Felsentein I, Almogy G, et al. Effect of intraoperative fluid management on outcome after intraabdominal surgery. Anesthesiology 2005;103(1):25–32.
54. Wei S, Tian J, Song X, et al. Association of perioperative fluid balance and adverse surgical outcomes in esophageal cancer and esophagogastric junction cancer. Ann Thorac Surg 2008;86(1):266–72.
55. Kita T, Mammoto T, Kishi Y. Fluid management and postoperative respiratory disturbances in patients with transthoracic esophagectomy for carcinoma. J Clin Anesth 2002;14(4):252–6.
56. Casado D, López F, Martí R. Perioperative fluid management and major respiratory complications in patients undergoing esophagectomy. Dis Esophagus 2010;23:523–8.
57. Cannesson M. Arterial pressure variation and goal-directed fluid therapy. J Cardiothorac Vasc Anesth 2010;24:487–97.
58. Oohashi S, Endoh H. Does central venous pressure or pulmonary capillary wedge pressure reflect the status of circulating blood volume in patients after extended transthoracic esophagectomy? J Anesth 2005;19:21–5.

59. Goepfert MS, Reuter DA, Akyol D, et al. Goal-directed fluid management reduces vasopressor and catecholamine use in cardiac surgery patients. Intensive Care Med 2007;33(1):96–103.

60. Gan TJ, Soppitt A, Maroof M, et al. Goal-directed intraoperative fluid administration reduces length of hospital stay after major surgery. Anesthesiology 2002; 97(4):820–6.

61. Pearse R, Dawson D, Fawcett J, et al. Early goal-directed therapy after major surgery reduces complications and duration of hospital stay: a randomized, controlled trial. Crit Care 2005;9(6):R687–93.

62. Donati A, Loggi S, Preiser JC, et al. Goal-directed intraoperative therapy reduces morbidity and length of hospital stay in high-risk surgical patients. Chest 2007;132(6):1817–24.

63. Kobayashi M, Ko M, Kimura T, et al. Perioperative monitoring of fluid responsiveness after esophageal surgery using stroke volume variation. Expert Rev Med Devices 2008;5:311–6.

64. Kobayashi M, Koh M, Irinoda T, et al. Stroke volume variation as a predictor of intravascular volume depression and possible hypotension during the early postoperative period after esophagectomy. Ann Surg Oncol 2009;16:1371–7.

65. Kimberger O, Arnberger M, Brandt S, et al. Goal-directed colloid administration improves the microcirculation of healthy and perianastomotic colon. Anesthesiology 2009;110:496–504.

66. Marjanovic G, Villain C, Juettner E, et al. Impact of different crystalloid volume regimes on intestinal anastomotic stability. Ann Surg 2009;249:181–5.

67. Marjanovic G, Villain C, Timme S, et al. Colloid vs. crystalloid infusions in gastrointestinal surgery and their different impact on the healing of intestinal anastomoses. Int J Colorectal Dis 2010;25:491–8.

68. Hotz B, Hotz HG, Arndt M, et al. Fluid resuscitation with human albumin or hydroxyethyl starch – are there differences in the healing of experimental intestinal anastomoses? Scand J Gastroenterol 2010;45:106–14.

69. Moretti EW, Robertson KM, El-Moalem H, et al. Intraoperative colloid administration reduces postoperative nausea and vomiting and improves postoperative outcomes compared with crystalloid administration. Anesth Analg 2003;96(2): 611–7.

70. Schilling M, Redaelli C, Mauerer C, et al. Gastric microcirculatory changes during gastric tube formation: assessment with laser Doppler flowmetry. J Surg Res 1996; 62:125–9.

71. Boyle NH, Pearce A, Hunter D, et al. Intraoperative scanning laser Doppler flowmetry in the assessment of gastric tube perfusion during esophageal resection. J Am Coll Surg 1999;188:498–502.

72. Schroder W, Stippel D, Beckurts KTE, et al. Intraoperative changes in mucosal pCO_2 during gastric tube formation. Langenbecks Arch Surg 2001;386: 324–7.

73. Klijn E, Niehof S, de Jonge J, et al. The effect of perfusion pressure on gastric tissue blood flow in an experimental gastric tube model. Anesth Analg 2010; 110:541–6.

74. Liebermann-Meffert DM, Luescher U, Neff U, et al. Esophagectomy without thoracotomy: is there a risk of intramediastinal bleeding? Ann Surg 1987;206: 184–92.

75. Buise M, van Bommel J, Jahn A, et al. Intravenous nitroglycerin does not preserve gastric microcirculation during gastric tube reconstruction: a randomized controlled trial. Crit Care 2006;10:R131–5.

76. van Bommel J, De Jonge J, Buise MP, et al. The effects of intravenous nitroglyc-erine and norepinephrine on gastric microvascular perfusion in an experimental model of gastric tube reconstruction. Surgery 2010;148:71–7.
77. Schroder W, Stippel D, Gutschow C, et al. Postoperative recovery of microcircu-lation after gastric tube formation. Langenbecks Arch Surg 2004;389:267–71.
78. Zakrison T, Nascimento BA, Tremblay LN, et al. Perioperative vasopressors are associated with an increased risk of gastrointestinal anastomotic leakage. World J Surg 2007;31:1627–34.
79. Theodorou D, Drimousis PG, Larentzakis A, et al. The effect of vasopressors on perfusion of gastric graft after esophagectomy. An experimental study. J Gastrointest Surg 2008;12:1497–501.
80. Al-Rawi OY, Pennefather SH, Page RD, et al. The effect of thoracic epidural bu-pivacaine and an intravenous adrenaline infusion on gastric tube blood flow during esophagectomy. Anesth Analg 2008;106:884–7.
81. Sarela A, Tolan D, Harris K, et al. Anastomotic leakage after esophagectomy for cancer: a mortality-free experience. J Am Coll Surg 2008;206:516–23.
82. Blewett C, Miller J, Young J, et al. Anastomotic leaks after esophagectomy for esophageal cancer: a comparison of thoracic and cervical anastomoses. Ann Thorac Cardiovasc Surg 2001;7:75–8.
83. Tabatabai A, Hashemi M, Mohajeri G, et al. Incidence and risk factors predis-posing anastomotic leak after transhiatal esophagectomy. Ann Thorac Med 2009;4(4):197–200.
84. Urschel JD. Esophagogastrostomy anastomotic leaks complicating esophagec-tomy: a review. Am J Surg 1995;169:634–40.
85. Whooley BP, Law S, Alexandrou A, et al. Critical appraisal of the significance of intrathoracic anastomotic leakage after esophagectomy for cancer. Am J Surg 2001;181:198–203.
86. Rentz J, Bull D, Harpole D, et al. Transthoracic versus transhiatal esophagec-tomy: a prospective study of 945 patients. J Thorac Cardiovasc Surg 2003; 125:1114–20.
87. Cooke DT, Lin GC, Lau CL, et al. Analysis of cervical esophagogastric anasto-motic leaks after transhiatal esophagectomy: risk factors, presentation, and detection. Ann Thorac Surg 2009;88:177–85.
88. Morita M, Nakanoko T, Fujinaka Y, et al. In-hospital mortality after a surgical resection for esophageal cancer: analyses of the associated factors and histor-ical changes. Ann Surg Oncol 2011;18:1757–65.
89. Griffin SM, Lamb PJ, SM Dresner, et al. Diagnosis and management of a mediastinal leak following radical oesophagectomy. Br J Surg 2001;88: 1346–51.
90. Crestanello JA, Deschamps C, Cassivi SD, et al. Selective management of intra-thoracic anastomotic leak after esophagectomy. J Thorac Cardiovasc Surg 2005;129:254–60.
91. Feith M, Gillen S, Schuster T, et al. Healing occurs in most patients that receive endoscopic stents for anastomotic leakage; dislocation remains a problem. Clin Gastroenterol Hepatol 2011;9:202–10.
92. Freeman RK, Vyverberg A, Ascioti AJ. Esophageal stent placement for the treat-ment of acute intrathoracic anastomotic leak after esophagectomy. Ann Thorac Surg 2011;92:204–8.
93. Ahrens M, Schulte T, Egberts J, et al. Drainage of esophageal leakage using endoscopic vacuum therapy: a prospective pilot study. Endoscopy 2010;42: 693–8.

94. Wedemeyer J, Brangewitz M, Kubicka S, et al. Management of major postsurgical gastroesophageal intrathoracic leaks with an endoscopic vacuum-assisted closure system. Gastrointest Endosc 2010;71:382–6.

95. Ferguson MK, Calauro AD, Prachand V. Prediction of major pulmonary complications after esophagectomy. Ann Thorac Surg 2011;91:1494–501.

96. Zingg U, Smithers BM, Gotley DC, et al. Factors associated with postoperative pulmonary morbidity after esophagectomy for cancer. Ann Surg Oncol 2011;18:1460–8.

97. Bakhos CT, Fabian T, Oyasiji TO, et al. Impact of surgical technique on pulmonary morbidity after esophagectomy. Ann Thorac Surg 2011;93:221–7.

98. Joshi GP, Bonnet F, Shah R, et al. A systematic review of randomized trials evaluating regional techniques for postthoracotomy analgesia. Anesth Analg 2008;107:1026–40.

99. Heitmiller RF, Jones B. Transient diminished airway protection after transhiatal esophagectomy. Am J Surg 1991;162:442–6.

100. Easterling CS, Bousamra M, Lang IM, et al. Pharyngeal dysphagia in postesophagectomy patients: correlation with deglutitive biomechanics. Ann Thorac Surg 2000;69:989–92.

101. Martin RE, Letsos P, Taves DH, et al. Oropharyngeal dysphagia in esophageal cancer before and after transhiatal esophagectomy. Dysphagia 2001;16:23–31.

102. Berry MF, Atkins BZ, Tong BC, et al. A comprehensive evaluation for aspiration after esophagectomy reduces the incidence of postoperative pneumonia. J Thorac Cardiovasc Surg 2010;140:1266–71.

103. Shah RD, Luketich JD, Schuchert MJ, et al. Postesophagectomy chylothorax: incidence, risk factors, and outcomes. Ann Thorac Surg 2012;93:897–904.

104. Karagianis J, Sheean PM. Managing secondary chylothorax: the implications for medical nutrition therapy. J Am Diet Assoc 2011;111:600–4.

105. Avendano CE, Flume PA, Silvestri GA, et al. Pulmonary complications after esophagectomy. Ann Thorac Surg 2002;73:922–6.

106. Kinugasa S, Tachibana M, Yoshimura H, et al. Postoperative pulmonary complications are associated with worse short- and long-term outcomes after extended esophagectomy. J Surg Oncol 2004;88:71–7.

107. Gockel I, Kneist W, Keilmann A, et al. Recurrent laryngeal nerve paralysis (RLNP) following esophagectomy for carcinoma. Eur J Surg Oncol 2005;31:277–81.

108. Lee HS, Kim MS, Lee JM, et al. Intrathoracic gastric emptying of solid food after esophagectomy for esophageal cancer. Ann Thorac Surg 2005;80:443–7.

109. Hollenberg SM, Dellinger RP. Noncardiac surgery: postoperative arrhythmias. Crit Care Med 2000;28(Suppl):N145–50.

110. Malhotra SK, Kaur RP, Gupta NM, et al. Incidence and types of arrhythmias after mediastinal manipulation during transhiatal esophagectomy. Ann Thorac Surg 2006;82:298–302.

111. Amar D, Burt ME, Bains MS, et al. Symptomatic tachydysrhythmias after esophagectomy: incidence and outcome measures. Ann Thorac Surg 1996;61:1506–9.

112. Murthy SC, Law S, Whooley BP, et al. Atrial fibrillation after esophagectomy is a marker for postoperative morbidity and mortality. J Thorac Cardiovasc Surg 2003;126:1162–7.

113. Stippel DL, Taylan C, Schroder W, et al. Supraventricular tachyarrhythmia as early indicator of a complicated course after esophagectomy. Dis Esophagus 2005;18:267–73.

114. Stawicki SP, Prosciak MP, Gerlach AT, et al. Atrial fibrillation after esophagectomy: an indicator of postoperative morbidity. Gen Thorac Cardiovasc Surg 2011;59:399–405.

115. Tisdale JE, Wroblewski HA, Wall DS, et al. A randomized, controlled study of amiodarone for prevention of atrial fibrillation after transthoracic esophagectomy. J Thorac Cardiovasc Surg 2010;140:45–51.

116. Khorana AA, Francis CW, Culakova E. Thromboembolism is a leading cause of death in cancer patients receiving outpatient chemotherapy. J Thromb Haemost 2007;5:632–4.

117. Rollins KE, Peters CJ, Safranek PM, et al. Venous thromboembolism in oesophagogastric carcinoma: incidence of symptomatic and asymptomatic events following chemotherapy and surgery. Eur J Surg Oncol 2011;37:1072–7.

118. Kight CE. Nutrition considerations in esophagectomy patients. Nutr Clin Pract 2008;23:521–8.

119. Parekh K, Iannettoni MD. Complications of esophageal resection and reconstruction. Semin Thorac Cardiovasc Surg 2007;19:79–88.

120. Poghosyan T, Gaujoux S, Chirica M, et al. Functional disorders and quality of life after esophagectomy and gastric tube formation for cancer. J Visc Surg 2011; 148:e327–35.

121. Urschel JD, Blewett CJ, Young JE, et al. Pyloric drainage (pyloroplasty) or no drainage in gastric reconstruction after esophagectomy: a meta-analysis of randomized controlled trials. Dig Surg 2002;19:160–4.

Perioperative Management of the Pregnant Patient with an Anterior Mediastinal Mass

George W. Kanellakos, MD, FRCPC

KEYWORDS

- Mediastinal mass • Pregnancy • Anesthetic considerations • Tracheal compression
- Superior vena cava syndrome • Mediastinal mass syndrome
- Perioperative management • Cardiopulmonary bypass

KEY POINTS

- Airway collapse upon induction is a rare finding in the adult population and maintenance of spontaneous respiration does not guarantee stability.
- Detailed preoperative cardiovascular evaluation is essential in predicting hemodynamic stability post induction and the use of cardiopulmonary bypass.
- Ventilation-perfusion mismatch caused by compression of a bronchus and the contralateral pulmonary artery has been shown to be fatal, and treatments need to be tailored on an individual basis by critically evaluating structures that are affected to predict stability after induction.
- Mediastinal mass syndrome is defined as immediate right heart failure secondary to vascular compression when positive pressure ventilation is initiated.

OBJECTIVES

This article describes the perioperative risks of pregnant patients with anterior mediastinal masses, and demonstrates the importance of a multidisciplinary approach for the management of high-risk patients. Such an approach challenges the conventional teaching of risks associated with mediastinal masses in the adult population.

SYMPTOMS

The patient is a 33-year-old woman, 28 weeks' gestation, who presented to thoracic surgery with increasing shortness of breath. The pregnancy was otherwise normal, with normal fetal size and development. Her medical history was unremarkable until 4 months previously when she developed cough, asthma, and eventually orthopnea. Routine treatments for upper respiratory tract infection and asthma were attempted without success.

Thoracic Anesthesia, Dalhousie Department of Anesthesia, Pain Management and Perioperative Medicine, Queen Elizabeth II Health Sciences Center, 10 West Victoria, 1276 South Park Street, Halifax, Nova Scotia B3H 2Y9, Canada
E-mail address: George.Kanellakos@dal.ca

Anesthesiology Clin 30 (2012) 749–758
http://dx.doi.org/10.1016/j.anclin.2012.07.010   **anesthesiology.theclinics.com**
1932-2275/12/$ – see front matter © 2012 Elsevier Inc. All rights reserved.

Diagnostic imaging studies were performed and revealed a large anterior mediastinal mass. Computed tomography (CT), cardiac magnetic resonance imaging (MRI), and echocardiography revealed a large anterior mediastinal mass, the findings being presented in **Box 1**. **Figs. 1** and **2** are CT-scan slices representing some of the findings. The interpretation of the CT scan can be challenging, especially when there is structural rotation of the carina. The coronal plane in **Fig. 2** depicts a significantly different view of the carina compared with the transverse planes in **Fig. 1**. Percutaneous biopsies (at least 10–15) were taken and a diagnosis of benign leiomyoma was made, indicating surgical resection as the treatment of choice. Multiple pathologists reviewed the samples and no evidence of leiomyosarcoma was found. The patient's respiratory status improved significantly with steroid therapy to the point where she could leave the hospital to attend to her family's activities, and she no longer has orthopnea.

PERIOPERATIVE MANAGEMENT

The case raises many principles of anesthetic care that are difficult to balance. Very few anesthesiologists have regular exposure to cases like this, which adds to the uncertainty.[1–4] Guidance from the literature is problematic because it is a collection of case reports offering examples of masses that were treated successfully and unsuccessfully.[4] Textbooks are no longer the gold standard because they are often outdated and tend to focus on theoretical principles that are difficult to translate into clinical practice. In addition, what is typically written in textbooks is unrealistic in most hospital settings. Of utmost importance with this type of case is thorough preoperative planning from a multidisciplinary approach.[5–8] **Box 2** lists the

---

Box 1
CT, MRI, and echocardiographic findings

Mass Location:
- Origin of mass not easily determined
- Mass occupies almost entire right chest, measuring 19 × 17 × 15 cm

Airway:
- No evidence of invasion of lung or other structures
- Mild displacement of the trachea to the left
- 50% narrowing of the distal trachea (1.3 cm down to 0.8 cm down to 0.6 cm at the carina)
- Left mainstem bronchus compressed, internal lumen close to 0.5 cm
- Right mainstem bronchus severely compressed and then opening up again
- Obliteration of the right upper lobe, right middle lobe partial obstruction, patent right lower lobe

Vascular (Venous and Arterial):
- Superior vena cava (SVC) severely flattened but patent with no signs of SVC syndrome
- Significant right pulmonary artery compression, normal main and left pulmonary arteries
- Minor left and right atrial compression posteriorly, no hemodynamic compromise

Cardiac:
- Normal heart function and valves
- No pericardial or pleural effusions

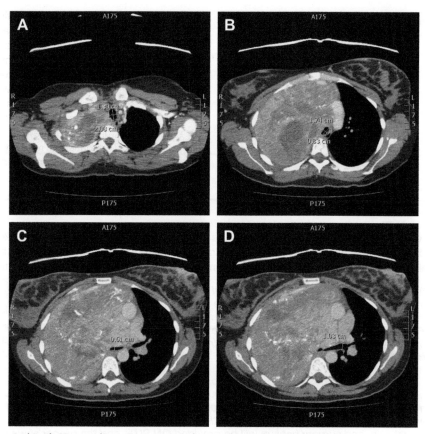

Fig. 1. (*A–D*) CT-scan slices representing the presence of mediastinal mass.

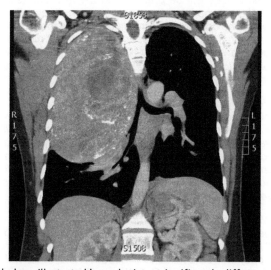

Fig. 2. The coronal plane illustrated here depicts a significantly different view of the carina compared with the transverse planes in **Fig. 1**.

Box 2
Perioperative multidisciplinary team

- Anesthesiology (thoracic, cardiac, and obstetric specialists)
- Thoracic surgery
- Cardiac surgery
- Intensive care
- Neonatology
- Obstetrics
- Nursing (surgery, obstetrics, neonatology)
- Social work

---

recommended multidisciplinary team to be involved in the perioperative setting. The subsequent plan was agreed upon, with scenarios distributed to all members of the multidisciplinary team to maintain clear communication:

An attempt will be made to optimize fetal maturity to 32 weeks while observing if maternal deterioration develops from the tumor mass. She is to be transferred to the obstetric hospital where she will be rounded on daily by the thoracic team. This location was chosen to facilitate the fastest obstetric response in the event of a crash cesarean section (C-section) (in addition, all other wards were uncomfortable with antenatal patient care).

Scenario 1: Successfully makes it to 32 weeks

She will be transferred to a CARDIAC surgery operating room (where cardiopulmonary bypass [CPB] backup is available) and the obstetric anesthesia team will assist in a normal C-section delivery with a titrated epidural. Thoracic, cardiac, anesthesia, and surgery backup will be provided ON SITE, and the proper airway equipment (reinforced endotracheal tube [ETT] and rigid bronchoscope) will be available. Obstetric nurses will be present and the neonatal resuscitation team will take care of the newborn and arrange transfer. It is anticipated that this team will need to use the operating room adjacent to the room used for C-section. The intensive care unit (ICU) will have been consulted but most likely the mother will be recovered in a step-down unit. If stable, she will be transferred to the thoracic ward on postoperative day #1 or #2. Mediastinal mass resection will commence approximately 1 week after C-section.

Scenario 2: Fetal distress before 32 weeks

While at the obstetric hospital, an urgent/emergent C-section will be arranged by the in-house anesthesiologist. Thoracic surgery/anesthesia will be called and the proper airway equipment (reinforced ETT and rigid bronchoscope) will be available, if needed. The obstetricians are aware that a crash general anesthetic is not the preferred choice. Post-op, the patient would be stabilized and transferred to the thoracic step-down unit (or ICU). Mediastinal mass resection will commence 1 week after C-section.

Scenario 3: Maternal decompensation

Thoracic surgery and anesthesia will be called immediately and the rapidity of intervention will be assessed. The proper airway equipment (reinforced ETT and rigid bronchoscope) will be available, if needed. The fetus will be monitored and when the mother is stable, a C-section will be planned. The subsequent timing of mediastinal mass surgery will be discussed.

Preoperative airway plan:

The course of anesthesia management of her airway will likely depend on who is on call. The group of individuals on call will be kept to a minimum and an agreement has been reached on a general approach. The CT scan was reviewed in detail with a chest radiologist. This is where the measurements of the trachea, distal trachea, carina, left mainstem bronchus (LMB) listed above came from. A reinforced endobronchial tube would work well and can be directed into the LMB past the tumor. The reinforced tube is helpful in that it won't compress with manipulation or warmth and it is malleable enough to facilitate LMB placement. Large intravenous access above and below the diaphragm with appropriate invasive lines will be placed.

ANESTHETIC MANAGEMENT

Mediastinal masses have multiple causes, including thymoma, thyroid, teratoma, and lymphoma.[9,10] Signs and symptoms are numerous but usually include cough, chest pain, dyspnea, hoarseness, orthopnea, superior vena cava (SVC) syndrome, syncope, and dysphagia. The structures that may be affected in the superior, anterior, and middle mediastinum include the SVC, tracheal bifurcation, pulmonary arteries, aortic arch, atria, and ventricles. The anesthetic considerations that consequently can be derived are listed in **Box 3**.

The presence of a fetus significantly elevates the risks imposed by a mediastinal mass. A reduced functional residual capacity coupled with swelling and increased blood volume can significantly diminish the respiratory reserve in pregnant patients.[2] Aortocaval compression is even more likely to be problematic in the presence of a mediastinal mass that has SVC involvement. Finally, the acute blood loss at the time of delivery poses a significant insult to cardiovascular stability in a patient with SVC syndrome, and could lead to refractory hypotension.

Airway Evaluation

The decision of how to induce this patient was discussed at length, and is of primary importance to anesthesiologists. The traditional principle of maintaining spontaneous

---

Box 3
Anesthetic considerations of mediastinal masses

- Airway compromise (compression of trachea and/or mainstem bronchi)
- Armored endotracheal tube
- Maintenance of spontaneous respiration on induction
- Decreased cardiac output due to vascular compression (veins, atria, right ventricle, pulmonary artery)
- SVC syndrome (including consideration of line placement)
- Pericardial effusion
- CT-scan evaluation (location of tumor, degree of compression)
- Lateral or prone position may alleviate instability
- Echocardiography for hemodynamic compromise
- Invasive monitors
- Massive blood loss
- CPB availability

respiration on induction is based on prevention of airway collapse[6,11] secondary to decreased muscle tone. Fatal airway collapse that requires cardiopulmonary backup primarily reflects observations from the pediatric population.[12–15] Infant airways easily collapse even without the presence of tumor, but can be predicted if tracheal compression exceeds 50%.[16] It is more likely that spontaneous ventilation would maintain adequate preload than prevention of airway collapse.[17] Airway collapse is a rare finding in adult patients[18] but decompensation can occur, and has been reported in situations where compression of the trachea is severe (>50%).[19] Contrary to traditional teaching, the mechanism is not likely airway collapse but rather hemodynamic instability, and is predictable with a complete cardiovascular evaluation. In these patients intraoperative ventilation is still usually possible, but complications generally occur on emergence and the postoperative period. With a tight airway lesion it can be difficult to prevent hyperinflation of the compressed side because of dynamic gas trapping, similar to a ball-valve effect associated with foreign bodies in the airway. Great care should be taken to ensure proper ETT placement and ventilation settings. In severely symptomatic patients, general anesthesia should be considered unsafe.[20] It is also worth noting that lesions may compress greater than 50% of the trachea, but positive pressure ventilation (PPV) may be initiated if an ETT can be passed past the lesion.

Regardless of technique used, if spontaneous respiration is attempted to maintain airway patency, it is often difficult to maintain without added respiratory support, because of the effect of general anesthesia.[21–23] Preoperative tests are usually unhelpful, but flow-volume loops with a mixed pattern of obstruction and restriction have been shown to be predictive of postoperative respiratory complications.[18] Many studies have shown pulmonary function tests to correlate poorly with outcome.[20,24] Even with spontaneous respiration, the loss of muscle tone and functional residual capacity is enough to worsen the obstruction, and one should not be lulled into thinking spontaneous respiration will prevent problems.[7,25] One published option that might limit loss of functional residual capacity and muscle tone involves using ketamine and dexmedetomidine as anesthetics.[6] Whatever anesthetic agents are used, if spontaneous ventilation is attempted and if during the process a patient is forced to generate a strong negative pressure breath because of higher than normal resistance, respiratory problems will ensue and will undoubtedly fail. This problem is amplified, and has been published with regard to diagnostic flexible bronchoscopy procedures[26] during which resistance to spontaneous respiration is high.

In the presented case, the tumor was seen to displace and compress the trachea approximately 50%. Because the obstruction was not fixed, it was anticipated that a reinforced endobronchial tube could easily be passed into the LMB, effectively bypassing the tumor. To prevent hyperinflation of the right lung, isolation of the left lung was considered essential owing to the near 100% obstruction of the right mainstem bronchus. In addition, ventilation of the right lung was anticipated to provide little benefit, owing to the severely compromised state of the right lung and its corresponding compressed pulmonary artery.

Cardiovascular Evaluation

Often neglected in the discussion of mediastinal masses is vascular stability caused by compression of the vena cava, pulmonary arteries, and/or pericardium.[6,10,27] This evaluation is more important in the adult population, and vascular compression is more likely to lead to hemodynamic collapse (compared with the potential for airway collapse) on induction. Of particular concern are patients with pericardial effusions for whom spontaneous respiration may not be adequate to maintain stability.[6,17] This situation introduces the concept of mediastinal mass syndrome,[5,17] which describes immediate right heart failure secondary to vascular compression when PPV is initiated. When PPV is introduced, excess pressure is transmitted through to the already severely compressed vessels (and airways), making the degree of compression even worse. As these patients are preload sensitive, any changes brought on by induction, PPV, or blood loss can be deleterious. Maintenance of preload is critical, and one published approach that can alleviate the effects of poor preload in patients with SVC syndrome is axillofemoral venous bypass.[28,29]

Ventilation-perfusion mismatch caused by compression of a bronchus and the contralateral pulmonary artery has been shown to be fatal.[30] This term refers to asymmetric obstruction of respiratory and vascular structures. For example, LMB compression in the presence of compression of the right pulmonary artery can result in severe shunt, leading to cardiovascular collapse. Treatments need to be tailored on an individual basis by critically evaluating structures that are affected to predict stability after induction. Risk-stratification schemes have been proposed by Blank and de Souza[6] who have published a concise approach, which is presented in **Table 1**. **Fig. 3** is a new proposed algorithm that could be used to guide the decision-making process.

One example of a textbook perioperative plan for a case like this would be to institute CPB[30–32] or, as some case studies have reported, extracorporeal membrane oxygenation[33] before induction. Many physicians would agree that instituting CPB is conceptually simple but quite difficult to execute, especially in an emergency setting,[6,13,20,34] and has little benefit in the management of these patients. Elective CPB can be successfully initiated without difficulty.

CPB was discussed in this case and was deemed unnecessary after careful examination of the airway and vascular structures. The natural progression of leiomyoma tumor growth is very slow, which explains how it was able to become so large before symptom development; this also provided an explanation of why there were only minor signs of SVC syndrome. Fortunately, there was no evidence of pericardial effusion. The lack of SVC symptoms was further reinforced during the elective C-section 1 week before the mediastinal mass resection, when only minor hemodynamic changes were observed with 700 mL blood loss. From an airway perspective, it was anticipated that the LMB could be intubated. Because the left and main pulmonary arteries were patent and the right pulmonary artery was compressed, it was concluded that ventilation-perfusion matching was adequate and CPB would be unnecessary. To further justify this approach, the author's surgical experience has shown that when tumors are resected while on bypass, blood loss can be severe, with high rates of mortality. A rescue plan was predetermined in case the patient became unstable, and included placing the patient in the right lateral decubitus position.[35] This position was chosen based on the known right-sided tumor location; anticipating gravity would

Table 1	
Risk stratification for patients with mediastinal mass	
Low risk	Asymptomatic or mildly symptomatic, without postural symptoms or radiographic evidence of significant compression of structures
Intermediate risk	Mild to moderate postural symptoms, tracheal compression <50%
High risk	Severe postural symptoms, stridor, cyanosis, tracheal compression >50% or tracheal compression with associated bronchial compression, pericardial effusion or SVC syndrome

Data from Blank RS, de Souza DG. Anesthetic management of patients with an anterior mediastinal mass: continuing professional development. Can J Anaesth 2011;58(9):853–67.

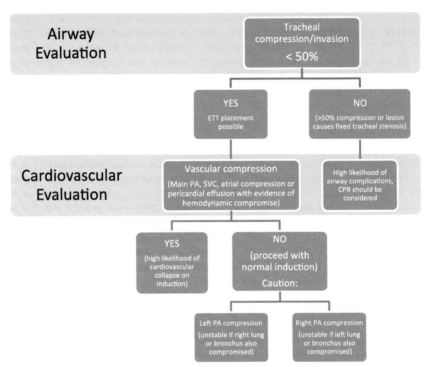

Fig. 3. Proposed algorithm for clinical decision making with mediastinal masses. CPB, cardio-pulmonary bypass; ETT, endotracheal tube; PA, pulmonary artery; SVC, superior vena cava.

relieve any worsening obstruction. It should also be noted that at all times rigid bronchoscopy was immediately available with the surgeon at the bedside.

CASE SUMMARY

The patient successfully made it to 32 weeks' gestation and Scenario #1 was followed. A routine epidural was placed and the newborn was delivered by routine C-section. The patient's blood pressure dropped briefly with delivery of the newborn, but this was stabilized with fluid boluses and small doses of phenylephrine. The procedure was otherwise uneventful and the newborn was healthy.

Two thoracic anesthesiologists were assigned to the mediastinal mass resection surgery 1 week postpartum. An antecubital large bore intravenous and left radial arterial line were inserted for induction. Drugs used were midazolam 2 mg, remifentanil 40 mcg, propofol 80 mg and rocuroniuim 50 mg. One dose of phenylephrine 200 mcg was given prophylactically to help maintain preload. A reinforced endobronchial tube was placed, initially above the carina and then into them LMB. The tube was placed without difficulty and under bronchoscopic guidance was observed easily displacing the tumor compressing the LMB. Central lines (7 French) under ultrasound guidance were then placed above and below the diaphragm, in the left internal jugular and femoral veins respectively. The right internal jugular was intentionally avoided due to the mass' location. A left femoral arterial line was also inserted. The patient's stretcher was left in the operating room in the event she needed to be stabilized with positional changes. Cardiorespiratory stability was maintained easily, and the patient underwent successful tumor resection through a routine sternotomy. The source of the tumor was found to be the posterior wall of the innominate vein, in keeping with leiomyoma. After the innominate vein was sacrificed, 2 subclavian-right atrial conduits were created. SVC syndrome developed, but this subsided as collateral circulation became more dominant in the postoperative period. She was taken to the ICU, and after two days was successfully extubated with mild stridor, likely secondary to right recurrent laryngeal resection. This resolved within 24 hours and she was transferred out of the ICU on postoperative day #4. She has since remained disease free.

REFERENCES

1. Ferrari LR, Bedford RF. Anterior mediastinal mass in a pregnant patient: anesthetic management and considerations. J Clin Anesth 1989;1(6):460–3.
2. Martin WJ. Cesarean section in a pregnant patient with an anterior mediastinal mass and failed supradiaphragmatic irradiation. J Clin Anesth 1995;7(4):312–5.
3. Boyne IC, O'Connor R, Marsh D. Awake fibreoptic intubation, airway compression and lung collapse in a parturient: anaesthetic and intensive care management. Int J Obstet Anesth 1999;8(2):138–41.
4. Gothard JW. Anesthetic considerations for patients with anterior mediastinal masses. Anesthesiology 2008;26(2):305–14, vi.
5. Erdos G, Tzanova I. Perioperative anaesthetic management of mediastinal mass in adults. Eur J Anaesthesiol 2009;26(8):627–32.
6. Blank RS, de Souza DG. Anesthetic management of patients with an anterior mediastinal mass: continuing professional development. Can J Anaesth 2011; 58(9):853–67.
7. Greengrass R. Anaesthesia and mediastinal masses. Can J Anaesth 1990;37(5): 596–7.
8. Anderson DM, Dimitrova GT, Awad H. Patient with posterior mediastinal mass requiring urgent cardiopulmonary bypass. Anesthesiology 2011;114(6):1488–93.
9. Yoneda KY, Louie S, Shelton DK. Mediastinal tumors. Curr Opin Pulm Med 2001; 7(4):226–33.
10. Narang S, Harte BH, Body SC. Anesthesia for patients with a mediastinal mass. Anesthesiol Clin North America 2001;19(3):559–79.
11. Neuman GG, Weingarten AE, Abramowitz RM, et al. The anesthetic management of the patient with an anterior mediastinal mass. Anesthesiology 1984;60(2): 144–7.
12. Hack HA, Wright NB, Wynn RF. The anaesthetic management of children with anterior mediastinal masses. Anaesthesia 2008;63(8):837–46.
13. Hammer GB. Anaesthetic management for the child with a mediastinal mass. Paediatr Anaesth 2004;14(1):95–7.
14. Pullerits J, Holzman R. Anaesthesia for patients with mediastinal masses. Can J Anaesth 1989;36(6):681–8.
15. Halpern S, Chatten J, Meadows AT, et al. Anterior mediastinal masses: anesthesia hazards and other problems. J Pediatr 1983;102(3):407–10.
16. Shamberger RC, Holzman RS, Griscom NT, et al. CT quantitation of tracheal cross-sectional area as a guide to the surgical and anesthetic management of children with anterior mediastinal masses. J Pediatr Surg 1991;26(2):138–42.
17. Luckhaupt-Koch K. Mediastinal mass syndrome. Paediatr Anaesth 2005;15(5): 437–8.
18. Bechard P, Letourneau L, Lacasse Y, et al. Perioperative cardiorespiratory complications in adults with mediastinal mass: incidence and risk factors. Anesthesiology 2004;100(4):826–34 [discussion: 825A].

19. Goh MH, Liu XY, Goh YS. Anterior mediastinal masses: an anaesthetic challenge. Anaesthesia 1999;54(7):670–4.

20. Slinger P, Karsli C. Management of the patient with a large anterior mediastinal mass: recurring myths. Curr Opin Anaesthesiol 2007;20(1):1–3.

21. Westbrook PR, Stubbs SE, Sessler AD, et al. Effects of anesthesia and muscle paralysis on respiratory mechanics in normal man. J Appl Phys 1973;34(1):81–6.

22. Bergman NA. Reduction in resting end-expiratory position of the respiratory system with induction of anesthesia and neuromuscular paralysis. Anesthesiology 1982;57(1):14–7.

23. Wahba RW. Perioperative functional residual capacity. Can J Anaesth 1991;38(3): 384–400.

24. Hnatiuk OW, Corcoran PC, Sierra A. Spirometry in surgery for anterior mediastinal masses. Chest 2001;120(4):1152–6.

25. Asai T. Emergency cardiopulmonary bypass in a patient with a mediastinal mass. Anaesthesia 2007;62(8):859–60.

26. Gardner JC, Royster RL. Airway collapse with an anterior mediastinal mass despite spontaneous ventilation in an adult. Anesth Analg 2011;113(2):239–42.

27. Wynne J, Markis JE, Grossman W. Extrinsic compression of the heart by tumor masquerading as cardiac tamponade. Cathet Cardiovasc Diagn 1978;4(1):81–5.

28. Shimokawa S, Yamashita T, Kinjyo T, et al. Extracorporeal venous bypass: a beneficial device in operation for superior vena caval syndrome. Ann Thorac Surg 1996;62(6):1863–4.

29. Radauceanu DS, Dunn JO, Lagattolla N, et al. Temporary extracorporeal jugulosaphenous bypass for the peri-operative management of patients with superior vena caval obstruction: a report of three cases. Anaesthesia 2009;64(11):1246–9.

30. Takeda S, Miyoshi S, Omori K, et al. Surgical rescue for life-threatening hypoxemia caused by a mediastinal tumor. Ann Thorac Surg 1999;68(6):2324–6.

31. Inoue M, Minami M, Shiono H, et al. Efficient clinical application of percutaneous cardiopulmonary support for perioperative management of a huge anterior mediastinal tumor. J Thorac Cardiovasc Surg 2006;131(3):755–6.

32. Tempe DK, Arya R, Dubey S, et al. Mediastinal mass resection: femorofemoral cardiopulmonary bypass before induction of anesthesia in the management of airway obstruction. J Cardiothorac Vasc Anesth 2001;15(2):233–6.

33. Gourdin M, Dransart C, Delaunois L, et al. Use of venovenous extracorporeal membrane oxygenation under regional anesthesia for a high-risk rigid bronchoscopy. J Cardiothorac Vasc Anesth 2012;26(3):465–7.

34. Turkoz A, Gulcan O, Tercan F, et al. Hemodynamic collapse caused by a large unruptured aneurysm of the ascending aorta in an 18 year old. Anesth Analg 2006;102(4):1040–2.

35. Choi WJ, Kim YH, Mok JM, et al. Patient repositioning and the amelioration of airway obstruction by an anterior mediastinal tumor during general anesthesia -a case report. Korean J Anesthesiol 2010;59(3):206–9.

Pulmonary Pathophysiology and Lung Mechanics in Anesthesiology: A Case-Based Overview

Marcos F. Vidal Melo, MD, PhD[a,b], Guido Musch, MD[a,b],
David W. Kaczka, MD, PhD[a,c],*

KEYWORDS

- Integrative physiology • Pulmonary mechanics • Ventilation • Pulmonary circulation
- Gas exchange

KEY POINTS

- Alterations in patient condition and unpredictable requirements of surgery affect critical respiratory function and mechanics.
- Altered physiology of acute and chronic cardiopulmonary disease results in extreme changes in lung volumes, mechanics, and control of breathing.
- The anesthesiologist must integrate and apply a thorough understanding of basic respiratory physiology and mechanics under a variety of changing constraints to optimize anesthetic delivery to patients.

INTRODUCTION

In the operating room, with the induction and maintenance of anesthesia and the requirements of surgery, respiratory physiology and lung mechanics present a diverse and dynamic set of challenges for the anesthesiologist. For example, changing from spontaneous to controlled ventilation, reduced chest wall recoil with muscle relaxation, increased intra-abdominal pressure from laparoscopic insufflation or retractor placement, as well as the loss of airway tone and hypoxic pulmonary vasoconstriction from inhaled anesthetics, all contribute to changing ventilation distribution and poor ventilation-to-perfusion ($\dot{V}/\dot{Q}$) matching. Blood loss and fluid resuscitation, patient

Conflicts of interest: Nil.

This work was partially supported by NIH HL086827 (MFVM), HL094639 (GM), and HL089227 (DWK).

[a] Department of Anaesthesia, Harvard Medical School, Boston, MA, USA; [b] Department of Anesthesia, Critical Care and Pain Medicine, Massachusetts General Hospital, Gray-Bigelow 444, 55 Fruit Street, Boston, MA 02114, USA; [c] Department of Anesthesia, Critical Care, and Pain Medicine, Beth Israel Deaconess Medical Center, 330 Brookline Avenue, Dana 717A, Boston, MA 02215, USA

* Corresponding author. Department of Anesthesia, Critical Care, and Pain Medicine, Beth Israel Deaconess Medical Center, 330 Brookline Avenue, Dana 717A, Boston, MA 02215.

E-mail address: dkaczka@bidmc.harvard.edu

Anesthesiology Clin 30 (2012) 759–784

http://dx.doi.org/10.1016/j.anclin.2012.08.003

anesthesiology.theclinics.com

positioning requirements, surgical stress and inflammation, infections and sepsis, cardiopulmonary bypass (CPB), regional anesthesia, changing composition of inhaled gases, and many other issues arise during surgery that affect pulmonary function. Moreover, patients present with the full spectrum of cardiopulmonary disorders of varying causes and severities.

This article takes a case-based approach to discuss the complex interactions that affect respiratory physiology and mechanics. First it considers an elderly patient with advanced chronic obstructive pulmonary disease (COPD) requiring a lung resection for cancer. Preoperative risk stratification and prediction of postoperative pulmonary function, physiologic considerations of lung isolation and lateral positioning to facilitate surgery, and the impact of anesthetic technique on gas exchange, lung mechanics, $\dot{V}/\dot{Q}$ matching, and postoperative pain control are addressed. Next, the example of a patient undergoing coronary artery bypass grafting under CPB is used to discuss mechanical ventilation, as well as the complex impact of CPB on lung inflammation, gas exchange, and mechanics, and postoperative pulmonary dysfunction.

CASE I: LUNG RESECTION IN A PATIENT WITH COPD

A 67-year-old woman with a 50-pack-year smoking history is diagnosed with a recurrence of lung cancer. Two years ago, the patient presented with right lower lobe adenocarcinoma for which she underwent a segmentectomy, because results from pulmonary function testing were deemed too poor for a lobectomy. Because her cancer has recurred, the decision is now made to perform a completion right lower lobectomy. Her forced expiratory volume in 1 second (FEV$_1$) is 0.96 L (46% of predicted), and lung diffusion capacity for carbon monoxide (DLCO) is 28% of predicted. Her peripheral oxygen saturation on room air is 96% at rest, and 88% with mild exercise.

Risk Stratification and Prediction of Postoperative Pulmonary Function After Lung Resection

One goal of preoperative risk stratification is to identify patients at risk for perioperative pulmonary complications and long-term pulmonary disability. Smoking is a significant risk factor for both lung cancer and COPD, and patients who present for lung resection often have impaired pulmonary function and increased risk of intraoperative and postoperative respiratory complications. Spirometry in this patient revealed a pattern consistent with severe obstructive disease, because her FEV$_1$ was markedly reduced. This is mainly caused by loss of lung recoil and by the tethering forces that keep intrapulmonary airways open during expiration. This dynamic airway compression occurs during exhalation, resulting in a so-called equal-pressure point along the airway tree in which extramural pressure equals intraluminal pressure. These airways thus behave as Starling resistors.[1] In this situation, expiratory flow becomes independent of pleural pressure, and cannot be increased with greater expiratory muscle effort. This phenomenon is known as expiratory flow limitation. Reduced FEV$_1$ is thus a measure of decreased ventilatory function. Patients with FEV$_1$ less than 1 to 2 L are at increased risk for pulmonary morbidity and mortality following lung resection, with the lower limit applying to minor resections (such as segmentectomies) and the higher limit to pneumonectomies.[2–4] To account for patient age, stature, and gender, these limits are usually compared with predicted normal values. Perioperative risk increases substantially for FEV$_1$ of 40% to 70% of the predicted normal value.[5,6] DLCO less than 50% to 60% of predicted is similarly associated with increased perioperative morbidity and mortality.[7,8]

Patients with impaired pulmonary function tests may also undergo split lung function studies to better estimate postoperative pulmonary function. These studies may predict residual pulmonary function following resection according to the formula:

Predicted postoperative (PPO) FEV_1 = Preoperative FEV_1 × (1 − fraction of lung function lost after resection)

The functional portion of resected lung has been estimated using several methods. Bronchospirometry was used in early studies in which a double-lumen endobronchial tube was inserted in the awake subject to selectively measure right and left pulmonary function.[9,10] Less invasive methods are now available with radionuclide lung scanning. These techniques allow determination of the fraction of ventilation (as measured with inhaled ^{133}Xe[11–15]) or perfusion (as measured with ^{99m}Tc-macroaggregates[16–18]) of the lung portion to be resected. PPO FEV_1 has been shown to predict postoperative complications in one large study.[19] Perioperative morbidity and mortality may be substantial when PPO FEV_1 is less than 1 L or 40% of predicted.[15,20,21] Operability should be regarded with skepticism when PPO FEV_1 is less than 0.7 L or 30% of predicted.[5,20] Long-term disability, as shown by the need for home oxygen, is also increased when PPO FEV_1 is less than 40%.[22] In the same way as FEV_1, PPO DLCO can be calculated from whole lung measurement of DLCO and regional measurements of ventilation or perfusion. Markos and colleagues[20] found that PPO DLCO less than 40% of predicted is associated with increased postoperative complications. Lung volume reduction surgery, in which emphysematous lung tissue is resected to restore parenchymal recoil, improve chest wall mechanics, and increase expiratory flow, has shown that patients with preoperative FEV_1 of 25% to 30% of predicted can undergo successful resection under certain conditions.[23,24] In addition, preoperative hypercapnia with $Paco_2$ greater than 45 mm Hg has been associated with increased risk of postoperative pulmonary complications, thus it is not likely to be an independent risk factor,[19] but rather is a marker of impaired ventilatory function. Preoperative hypoxemia with arterial oxygen saturation lower than 90% has also been associated with increased risk of postoperative complications,[25] as has arterial desaturation greater than 4% during exercise testing.[20,25–28] Based on these criteria, this patient could be classified as being at extremely high risk for pulmonary resection because of her low FEV_1, DLCO lower than 30% of predicted, and arterial oxygen desaturation of 8% during mild exercise.

Before surgery, an epidural catheter is placed between the sixth and seventh thoracic vertebrae for intraoperative and postoperative analgesia. After induction of general anesthesia, the patient is intubated with a left-sided double-lumen endobronchial tube, which allows independent lung ventilation. After intubation, the ventilator circuit is connected and a continuously increasing exhaled CO_2 pattern is observed. Furthermore, an expiratory flow-volume pattern showing a marked upper concavity and significant end-expiratory flow despite a prolonged expiratory time is observed, similar to that reproduced in **Fig. 1**. The patient is ventilated with 100% oxygen, her arterial oxygen saturation is 100%, with plateau airway pressures of 25 cm H_2O. Anesthesia is maintained with isoflurane. The patient is turned into lateral decubitus position with her right side up for thoracotomy. Unilateral ventilation of the left lung is initiated by occluding the right arm of the double-lumen tube, with the operative lung emptied to atmosphere.

Five minutes after the start of unilateral ventilation and thoracotomy, oxygen saturation slowly decreases to 89%, and end-tidal CO_2 concentration increases. Increasing the plateau pressures and respiratory rate are not successful at relieving hypercapnia. During the operation, a branch of the right pulmonary artery is inadvertently severed,

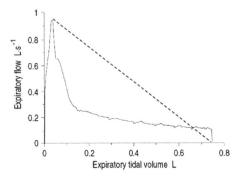

Fig. 1. Expiratory flow-volume curve of an anesthetized mechanically ventilated patient with severe COPD. Note the marked upper concavity and an end-expiratory flow of approximately 0.1 L/s. Both these features indicate heterogeneous emptying of alveolar units. Units with higher resistance and longer time constants are still emptying when the mechanical ventilator initiates the next inspiration. This flow-volume pattern is consistent with the steadily increasing exhaled CO_2 capnogram that was observed in the patient undergoing lung resection. The dashed line represents a hypothetical expiratory flow-volume pattern expected in a subject without pulmonary disease. (*Adapted from* Musch G, Foti G, Cereda M, et al. Lung and chest wall mechanics in normal anesthetized subjects and in patients with COPD at different PEEP levels. Eur Respir J 1997;10(11):2550; with permission.)

resulting in a brisk blood loss of approximately 3 L. Crystalloid is administered and a phenylephrine infusion is initiated to promote vasoconstriction and counteract the hypotension. Oxygen saturation initially increases to 96%, and then to 100% when the surgeon clamps the right pulmonary artery to control bleeding. To repair the vascular tear, the surgeon extends the resection to a bi-lobecotomy, removing both the lower and middle right lobes.

Lung Isolation: Methods, Physiology, and Mechanics

Methods of lung isolation

Lung isolation prevents ventilation to the operative lung to facilitate surgical exposure. Double-lumen endobronchial tubes have two channels: one extends into either the left or right bronchus, and the other terminates in the trachea. Separate inflatable cuffs seal each of these airflow pathways, and using clamps it is possible to ventilate either lung separately or both together. These tubes add substantial resistance in series to the lung's airway resistance, because of the small inner diameter and increased length of each channel, especially for the bronchial lumen. This resistance may enhance the effects of increased airway resistance in patients with COPD, further slowing expiration and leading to dynamic hyperinflation and air trapping. In this patient, the presence of dynamic hyperinflation can be inferred by the nonzero end-expiratory flow. Moreover, in the presence of expiratory flow limitation, dynamic hyperinflation can be present even when end-expiratory flow is negligible. In this case, the severity of hyperinflation is indicated by the persistence of end-expiratory flow despite prolonged expiratory time. The continuously increasing exhaled CO_2 capnograph reflects the sequential emptying of short to long time constant units. Because units with longer time constants have reduced alveolar ventilation and higher local alveolar CO_2 concentrations, phase III of the capnograph steadily increases, achieving a final value that reflects truncation of expiration by the subsequent inspiration.[29]

In the presence of expiratory flow limitation, dynamic hyperinflation occurs even when end-expiratory flow is low (typically less than 50 mL/s and therefore hard to detect on clinical monitors). Thus, prolonging the expiratory time does not result in meaningful reductions in lung volume. Furthermore, because the flow-limited airway behaves as a Starling resistor, expiratory flow cannot be augmented by increased expiratory effort or decreased pressure at the airway opening. Therefore, dynamic hyperinflation resulting from expiratory flow limitation cannot be effectively controlled by changing the mechanical ventilator's settings. Although dynamic hyperinflation during anesthesia may lead to hypotension caused by increased intrathoracic pressure and decreased venous return, it may also have some favorable consequences. For example, increased end-expiratory lung volume allows higher oxygen reserve, which is advantageous during single-lung ventilation by decreasing the propensity to atelectasis.

Physiologic effects of unilateral ventilation and lateral decubitus position

Unilateral ventilation is accompanied by a reduction of the distribution volume for tidal volume. The left lung normally accounts for 45% of functional residual capacity (FRC) and the right lung for 55%. Previous recommendations were to maintain the same minute ventilation for unilateral ventilation as during bilateral ventilation. To minimize the risk of volutrauma, more recent studies recommend maintaining similar airway plateau pressures for unilateral and bilateral ventilation,[30] with modest increases in respiratory rate. In patients with expiratory flow limitation, higher rates may not be tolerated or may not improve effective alveolar ventilation.[31]

In the lateral decubitus position, the weight of the mediastinum and cephalad displacement of the lower diaphragm caused by increased intra-abdominal pressure reduce FRC and the compliance of the dependent ventilated lung. This reduction may be alleviated by judicious application of positive end-expiration pressure (PEEP) to the dependent lung, which returns it to a more compliant portion of its pressure-volume curve and minimizes atelectasis.[32,33] In COPD, higher expiratory flows are supported by the higher lung volumes resulting from PEEP, and alveolar ventilation improves. Once tidal volume and expiratory time are maximized, residual hypercarbia may be unavoidable. For short periods of time, respiratory acidosis under anesthesia and mechanical ventilation is well tolerated, so long as the hypercarbia is relieved when two-lung ventilation is resumed before spontaneous ventilation and emergence.

Unilateral ventilation is also accompanied by shunt in the nonventilated lung, leading to arterial hypoxemia.[34] Hypoxic pulmonary vasoconstriction (HPV) counteracts this hypoxemia by increasing pulmonary vascular resistance and diverting blood flow to the ventilated lung. Animal studies have shown that such flow diversion occurs within 30 seconds of unilateral bronchial occlusion, and blood flow to the occluded lung is approximately half that during double-lung ventilation by 2 minutes.[35] If HPV is intact, shunt fraction during single-lung ventilation may be only 20% to 30% of cardiac output, as opposed to the 50% that might be expected in its absence.

In lateral decubitus position with a nonventilated nondependent lung, gravity favors blood flow to the dependent lung, further adding to the favorable effects of HPV on perfusion redistribution. However, even the dependent lung may be regionally hypoxic because of compression or absorption atelectasis (the latter favored by the use of high forced inspiratory oxygen [Fio_2] during unilateral ventilation). If these hypoxic compartments are substantial (ie, greater than 70% of the lung), the effectiveness of HPV will be reduced because the normoxic portions of lung are not sufficient to receive diverted blood flow.[32]

The gradual decrease in peripheral arterial oxygen saturation for this patient during unilateral ventilation and thoracotomy can be explained by resorption of oxygen from the nonventilated lung, which becomes progressively atelectatic and shunting. This patient's pulmonary disease was such that HPV and baseline lung function were not sufficient to maintain normal saturation during unilateral ventilation. Her arterial saturation improved after blood loss and vasoconstrictor therapy, most likely because of the reduced shunt fraction associated with decreased cardiac output and pulmonary arterial pressure, because pulmonary hypoperfusion functionally enhances the effects of HPV. The HPV may also have been further potentiated by the vasoconstrictor phenylephrine. The beneficial effect of a reduction in shunt fraction deriving from a reduction in pulmonary perfusion on arterial oxygenation can be offset by a concomitant reduction in mixed venous oxygen tension ($P_{\bar{v}}O_2$), which may accompany a decrease in cardiac output. For a given shunt fraction, lower $P_{\bar{v}}O_2$ results in lower arterial oxygen tension.[36] Augmenting cardiac output through fluid management or inotropic agents could potentially increase $P_{\bar{v}}O_2$ and improve arterial oxygenation in the presence of shunt. Surgical clamping of the right pulmonary artery virtually eliminates all shunt through the nonventilated lung, further improving arterial oxygen saturation.

To restore $\dot{V}/\dot{Q}$ matching and improve gas exchange during unilateral ventilation in the lateral decubitus position, selective application of PEEP to the dependent ventilated lung or continuous positive airway pressure (CPAP) to the nondependent lung have been investigated. The rationale for the use of PEEP is to optimize the function of the ventilated lung by bringing it to a more compliant portion of the pressure-volume curve and, mainly, reverse atelectasis.[33] This technique generally improves alveolar ventilation and reduces shunt flow in this lung. However, excessive PEEP can also increase the vascular resistance of the dependent lung, thus diverting blood flow back to the nonventilated lung and increasing shunt, especially if additional recruitment of atelectatic parenchyma does not occur.[37] The global effects of PEEP to the dependent lung thus represent the trade-off between these two opposing effects. Some studies have shown PEEP to improve oxygenation during unilateral ventilation,[34] whereas others have shown no improvement or even worsening of oxygenation.[38,39]

Another remedy for hypoxemia during unilateral ventilation is application of low levels of CPAP with 100% oxygen to the nondependent lung. By applying $\sim$5 cm H_2O of CPAP to the nonventilated lung, it is possible to use this lung for apneic oxygenation and thus reduce hypoxemia. Although selective application of CPAP to the nondependent lung is generally more reliable than application of PEEP to the dependent lung for improving hypoxemia, to be maximally effective it must be applied before the nonventilated lung is allowed to deflate completely.[40] CPAP may also interfere with surgical exposure. Some investigators have combined the application of PEEP to the dependent lung and CPAP to the nondependent lung, although it is controversial whether this strategy offers any advantages compared with PEEP or CPAP alone.[34,39] As a mitigating maneuver, intermittent insufflation of oxygen at low pressure into the conducting airways of the operative lung may provide enough apneic oxygenation to allow surgery to continue without compromising surgical exposure. If these maneuvers fail to improve oxygenation and saturation decreases to a dangerous level, urgent reexpansion of the operative lung should be considered, depending on the stage of surgery. Clamping of the pulmonary artery to the operative lung should also be considered.

Modulation of HPV

Inhalational anesthetics inhibit HPV because of their vasodilatory effect. However, this effect seems to be more pronounced *in vitro* and *ex vivo* than in the intact respiratory system. Domino and colleagues[41] showed a dose-response relation between isoflurane concentration and inhibition of HPV in vivo during canine single-lung ventilation. This effect seems to be small, because one minimum alveolar concentration (MAC) of isoflurane causes an increase in shunt fraction of only 4%, which rarely compromises clinical management. These values agree with clinical measurements performed by Spies and colleagues.[42] Intravenous anesthetics, in particular propofol, seem to have even less (if any) of an inhibitory effect on HPV during unilateral ventilation.[42–45] It is therefore possible that this patient's hypoxemia would have been less with intravenous rather than inhalational anesthesia, although the effect of isoflurane on arterial oxygenation in patients with emphysema undergoing unilateral ventilation in the lateral decubitus position seems to be minimal.[46]

Inflammation, as caused by systemic sepsis or localized pneumonia, is another potent inhibitor of HPV,[47–50] and it exacerbates the hypoxemia caused by shunt. Pharmacologic agents such as almitrine (which augments HPV) and inhaled nitric oxide (a selective pulmonary arterial vasodilator) have been shown both separately and in concert to improve oxygenation during single-lung ventilation,[51] although these are not typically used in clinical practice.

At the end of the operation, the patient is transported to the intensive care unit intubated. Overnight, she is hemodynamically stabilized and an epidural infusion of bupivacaine 0.1% with hydromorphone 20 µg/mL is started for pain control. On the following day, she is successfully extubated and remains pain free with epidural analgesia.

Regional Thoracic Anesthesia and Lung Mechanics

Thoracic epidural analgesia (TEA) is an effective method to relieve pain after thoracotomy. Effective pain relief is critical in facilitating deep breathing and coughing to minimize atelectasis and clear secretions. However, two potential concerns arise in the application of TEA to patients with severe COPD. First, local anesthesia may cause partial respiratory motor blockade, thus further impairing ventilatory function. Second, it may also result in pulmonary sympathetic blockade, which could theoretically lead to increased bronchial tone and airway resistance, as well as decreased pulmonary vasoconstrictor response. Groeben and colleagues[52] showed that TEA leads to a ~11% decrease of FEV_1 and ~15% decrease of vital capacity (VC) in women with severe COPD or asthma. Because the ratio of FEV_1 to VC increased by 4%, they concluded that the decrease of FEV_1 and VC was caused by mild motor blockade of respiratory muscles rather than increased airway resistance resulting from increased bronchial tone caused by pulmonary sympathetic blockade. They hypothesized that systemic absorption of local anesthetic from the epidural space was responsible for a direct bronchodilatory effect of TEA that overrode the indirect bronchoconstrictor effect.

Garutti and colleagues[53] showed that, when TEA was added to general anesthesia during unilateral ventilation for thoracic surgery, Pao_2 and shunt fraction were slightly worse (by ~60 mm Hg and 5%, respectively) compared with general anesthesia alone. They hypothesized that this was caused by the inhibition of HPV resulting from sympathetic blockade of the noradrenergic innervation to the pulmonary vasculature. Despite these possible limitations, the advantages of improved pulmonary function from effective pain control, without the sedation and respiratory depression that occurs with systemic opioids, has made the use of TEA a virtual standard of care in patients with severe emphysema undergoing lung volume reduction surgery.[54,55]

CASE II: CARDIAC SURGERY

A 69-year-old woman with history of severe three-vessel coronary artery disease and COPD is scheduled to undergo coronary artery bypass graft (CABG) surgery using 4 distal anastomosis, including a left internal mammary artery (LIMA) graft to the left anterior descending coronary artery. The patient is preoxygenated by breathing 100% oxygen through a mask before induction of anesthesia.

Preoxygenation and Induction of Anesthesia

Preoxygenation at the beginning of general anesthesia is intended to avoid hypoxemia during the period of apnea required to obtain endotracheal intubation. The increased time constant inequalities present in COPD lungs[56] require longer preoxygenation times to achieve similar end-expiratory oxygen fractions in COPD than in normal lungs.[57] General anesthesia and muscle paralysis result in decreased FRC, cross-sectional chest area, and thoracic volume, with a concomitant cranial shift of the diaphragm.[58,59] These changes are associated with atelectasis and airway closure[60] in dependent lung regions caused by tissue compression,[61] as well as loss of respiratory muscle tone and gas resorption[62,63] resulting in increased intrapulmonary shunt and regions of low $\dot{V}/\dot{Q}$.[64,65]

The risk of hypoxemia in a patient with critical coronary artery stenosis takes precedence over the minor risks from breathing 100% oxygen, such as the increased likelihood of absorption atelectasis[66] or short-term risks of oxygen toxicity.[62] Use of moderate PEEP (ie, 6–10 cm H_2O) during induction of anesthesia prevents atelectasis and improves oxygenation.[67,68] A diagnosis of COPD in this patient suggests increased $\dot{V}/\dot{Q}$ heterogeneity with anesthesia and positive pressure ventilation. However, she will be less prone than a healthy patient to develop atelectasis and shunt because of the reduced elastic recoil and air trapping in COPD.[69]

A direct laryngoscopy is performed, the patient is endotracheally intubated, and mechanical ventilation is initiated.

Mechanical Ventilation During Cardiac Surgery

Mechanical ventilation during cardiac surgery requires considerations of factors promoting ventilator-induced lung injury, similar to patients at risk for acute lung injury. Respiratory complications are frequent after cardiac surgery,[70–72] and mechanical ventilation for more than 48 hours is one of the most frequent complications,[73,74] although development of acute respiratory distress is rare.[75]

Mechanical ventilation can produce lung injury,[76] and ventilator settings can influence patient morbidity and mortality in intensive care units (ICUs).[77,78] Furthermore a two-hit condition, in which the mechanical ventilation insult is accompanied by an inflammatory or other cellular-level injurious stimulus, can significantly aggravate the lung injury.[79,80] Surgical trauma, exposure to CPB,[81,82] endotoxemia,[83,84] ischemia-reperfusion of the lung[85] (including reduction of bronchial perfusion),[86–88] and frequent blood transfusion[89] are some of the mechanisms associated with the inflammatory response in cardiac surgery that may amplify lung injury during mechanical ventilation.[90] These processes are particularly important because the physiologic mechanisms that produce ventilator-associated lung injury (ie, tidal recruitment and overinflation) are frequently present in patients with and without previous lung disease undergoing cardiac surgery.[91]

Previous studies suggest that intraoperative use of protective modes of ventilation, with higher PEEP values (10 cm H_2O) and lower tidal volumes (6–8 mL/kg of predicted body weight), reduce the inflammatory response and improve pulmonary mechanics in patients after cardiac surgery (**Fig. 2**).[92,93] In one of these studies, the protective mode explicitly included a recruitment maneuver by increasing peak inspiratory pressure to 40 cm H_2O for 15 seconds. The inflammatory response for the cases of protective ventilation was characterized by lower levels of interleukin IL-6 and IL-8 in plasma and bronchoalveolar lavage (BAL) fluid. Protective ventilation did not prevent adverse

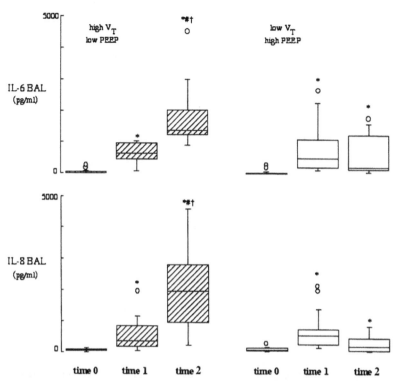

Fig. 2. The effect of high tidal volume (V_T)/low PEEP versus low V_T/high PEEP ventilation strategies on lung inflammation as indicated by bronchioalveolar lavage (BAL) fluid interleukin IL-6 and IL-8 concentrations at 3 time points during cardiac surgery. Time 0, before sternotomy; time 1, during CPB; and time 2, 6 hours after resuming mechanical ventilation. (*Reprinted from* Zupancich E, Paparella D, Turani F, et al. Mechanical ventilation affects inflammatory mediators in patients undergoing cardiopulmonary bypass for cardiac surgery: a randomized clinical trial. J Thorac Cardiovasc Surg 2005;130(2):380; with permission.)

effects of CPB in the lungs in one study,[94] but these investigators used a PEEP of 5 cm H_2O in their protective mode in contrast with 10 cm H_2O used in other studies. This finding suggests that low lung volumes may be an important component of ventilator-induced lung injury during cardiac surgery.

The fraction of inspired oxygen (Fio_2) during cardiac surgery involves a balance between maximizing oxygenation and minimizing oxidative stress, absorption atelectasis, and ventilator-induced lung injury. The use of $Fio_2 = 1.0$ compared with $Fio_2 = 0.5$ throughout surgery is associated with delayed recovery of oxygenation and increased levels of tumor necrosis factor-α in BAL.[95] Despite these considerations, outcome data for specific ventilator settings during cardiac surgery are still lacking.

After intubation, placement of central venous access, and positioning, the patient is prepped, draped, the skin incision is made, and sternotomy is performed.

Opening of the chest results in partial reduction of the contribution of the chest wall to the impedance of the respiratory system.[96] This reduction is partial because the chest wall is not completely separated from the lungs but instead is usually spread at the sternum, with remaining contact of lung and chest wall in dorsal and lateral areas. This technique may result in increased inflation of the lung FRC,[97] with decreased elastance and resistance of the respiratory system and an inadvertently increased delivered tidal volume if pressure-controlled ventilation is used.

The LIMA is dissected in order to be used as a graft to the left anterior descending coronary artery.

The LIMA (also called internal thoracic artery) branches from the subclavian artery near its origin, and travels downward on the inside of the chest wall, approximately a centimeter from the sides of the sternum, and medial to the nipple. Because of its anatomic position, dissection of the LIMA usually involves the opening of the left pleura and packing of the left lung to facilitate exposure. Temporary reduction of tidal volume for better visualization and surgical manipulation may be required. Such interventions can cause significant left lung atelectasis and respiratory dysfunction that persist into the postoperative period.[98–100] Worsening of lung mechanics after CABG surgery is more marked when pleurotomy is performed.[100–102] Imaging studies using computed tomography showed significantly more densities after surgery in the left lung of patients having CABG than patients undergoing mitral valve repair,[103] potentially a result of left internal mammary harvesting.

The aorta and right atrium are cannulated and the patient is placed on extracorporeal circulation with CPB for the performance of the bypass grafting.

For many decades, pulmonary complications were a major cause of death following CPB.[104] Acute respiratory distress following CPB is now unusual, but milder forms of acute lung injury are more frequently observed after cardiac surgery[75,105] and can be critical in the patient at risk.[106,107]

Lung Histology After CPB

Lung parenchyma following CPB usually reveals mild changes. Although data on histopathologic changes after CPB are limited because of the difficulty in obtaining samples, microbiopsies performed 20 minutes following CPB show poorly aerated alveoli, different degrees of alveolar edema, thickening of alveolar septa, alveolar capillaries with perivascular halo, and alveolar flooding.[108] Neutrophils are found in the interstitium and alveolar space, with large alveolar macrophages containing numerous vacuoles indicating activation. Electron microscopy may show additional details on injury to the alveolar-capillary barrier. In some cases, only edema of the endothelial cells is found, whereas both endothelial and type I epithelial cells may be swollen in other cases. In severe cases, there may be necrosis of epithelial cells with denuded basement membranes. Alveolar capillaries are often congested with signs of leakage (ie, airspaces filled with edema fluid). Many polymorphonuclear neutrophils are found in blood vessels. Pulmonary surfactant seems to be normal in well-aerated alveoli, although not in fluid-filled alveoli.[108]

Lung Management During CPB

During CPB, the lungs are either opened to atmosphere, kept at a constant positive airway pressure, or ventilated at a slow rate. That management of the lungs during CPB could have an effect on post-CPB pulmonary function was recognized decades ago with the finding of improved compliance and shunt in calves when lungs were not ventilated during CPB.[109] Using inert gases, Loeckinger and colleagues[110] showed that 10 cm H_2O of CPAP during CPB resulted in more perfusion to areas with normal $\dot{V}/\dot{Q}$, with significantly less shunt and low $\dot{V}/\dot{Q}$ perfusion 4 hours following CPB. This result was accompanied by improved postoperative oxygenation. In contrast, CPAP of 5 cm H_2O during CPB did not improve lung function when used in patients[111] or pigs.[112] More recently, experiments in pigs suggested that a slow ventilatory rate

(5 per min) may lead to even better postoperative outcome because of a reduction in ischemic injury (**Fig. 3**).[113]

Bypass of the pulmonary artery flow produces lung ischemia and respiratory dysfunction.[86] This mechanism has recently been explored with use of pulsatile pulmonary perfusion during experimental CPB, which further reduced the inflammatory response in pigs.[114] Also potentially contributing to this effect is a reduction of bronchial artery blood flow during CPB, which increases the risk of lung ischemia, and a tissue-level constriction in response to hypocapnia that develops when there is ventilation in the absence of pulmonary blood flow.[115]

Inflammatory Response to CPB

Exposure of blood to foreign surfaces, ischemia-reperfusion, and endotoxemia during CPB trigger a strong inflammatory response and the complement system, the cytokine cascade, the coagulation-fibrinolytic system, the cellular-immune system, and the endothelium are all activated.[90] Gene array and multiplex protein analysis suggest that circulating leukocytes overexpress adhesion and signaling factors after CPB, which could facilitate their trapping in the lungs and promote a subsequent tissue-associated inflammatory response.[116] There is evidence of lung-specific inflammatory responses after CPB,[82,117] underscoring the relevance of addressing compromised pulmonary function in patients at risk.

Off-pump CABG Surgery

Because of the marked inflammatory response to CPB, cardiac surgery without CPB ("off-pump" surgery) has been theorized to reduce respiratory impairment after surgery.[118–120] Off-pump CPB yields lower levels of several inflammatory markers, such as cytokines, polymorphonuclear elastase, thrombin-antithrombin III complex, and complement factor (C3a), oxidative stress, and blood endotoxin than on-pump CPB.[121–124]

Although some studies report improvement in shunting and hypoxemia,[125] other studies partitioning lung and chest wall mechanics do not support a significant effect of off-pump CABG on respiratory dysfunction.[126] Studies using the forced oscillation technique (FOT) found that off-pump CABG does not affect airway mechanics, but still

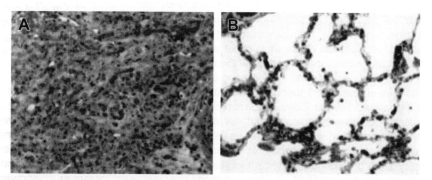

Fig. 3. Lung tissue light micrographs depicting alveolar regions 90 minutes after CPB. (*A*) When the lung was either open to the atmosphere or received 5 cm H_2O CPAP there was significant atelectasis and pulmonary edema. (*B*) Low-frequency ventilation (5 breaths per minute) led to normal-appearing lung tissue. (*Modified from* Imura H, Caputo M, Lim K, et al. Pulmonary injury after cardiopulmonary bypass: beneficial effects of low-frequency mechanical ventilation. J Thorac Cardiovasc Surg 2009;137(6):1535; with permission.)

impairs the parenchymal tissues to degrees similar to those occurring with CPB.[127] Although it is hypothesized that off-pump CABG improves outcomes in patients at risk for respiratory dysfunction, such as patients with COPD,[128] it is questionable whether off-pump CABG results in better outcomes overall.[107,120,129]

Once the grafts are finished, the lungs are reexpanded and mechanical ventilation resumed as part of the sequence of procedures preceding the discontinuation of extracorporeal circulation.

Optimal ways to reexpand the lungs have been studied. Based on animal data for CPB[130] and human data under anesthesia and mechanical ventilation,[131] some investigators suggest recruiting the lungs using Fio_2 less than 1.0. For instance, Fio_2 of 0.4 has been used to prevent alveolar derecruitment through reabsorption atelectasis following experimental CPB.[130] Expansion to pressures of 35 cm H_2O for 15 seconds with $Fio_2 = 0.4$ before separation from CPB, combined with a second VC maneuver within 20 to 30 minutes after arrival in the ICU ($Fio_2 = 0.4$, inflation pressure = 30 cm H_2O for 5 seconds) reduces hypoxemia in the first 24 hours after surgery,[132] and a single VC maneuver after CPB may lead to improved intraoperative oxygenation and shorter times to extubation.[133]

Following discontinuation of CPB, mechanical ventilation is resumed with settings of $Fio_2 = 1.0$, PEEP = 5 cm H_2O, tidal volume = 8 mL/kg predicted body weight, and a respiratory rate of 12 per minute. After a few minutes of mechanical ventilation, peak inspiratory pressure increases to 35 cm H_2O, plateau pressure to 28 cm H_2O, and the expiratory flow curves show nonzero flow at the end of exhalation. Direct inspection of the lungs shows slow deflation.

Effects of Cardiac Surgery and CPB on Respiratory Mechanics

Deterioration of lung mechanics is frequently encountered following cardiac surgery[134] and can exacerbate the already compromised respiratory function commonly found in patients undergoing cardiac surgery caused by preexisting cardiac disease, smoking habits, and other comorbidities.[135] Lung resistance and elastance are usually increased after cardiac surgery.[101,136–140] Immediately after anesthesia induction and endotracheal intubation for CABG surgery, frequency and tidal volume dependence of elastance and resistance are similar to those observed in seated healthy subjects.[141] After CABG surgery, lung elastance and resistance markedly decrease with increasing tidal volume, whereas resistance shows a greater dependence on frequency compared with presurgical conditions.[137] Reductions in FRC,[142] as well as increases in airway and tissue heterogeneity,[143,144] may contribute to such enhanced frequency and tidal volume dependencies. Changes in chest wall mechanics caused by cardiac surgery with CPB are inconsistent in other studies.[126,135,137,145,146] Pleurotomy and positive fluid balance accentuate the deterioration of lung mechanics.[101,138]

Changes in respiratory mechanics following heart surgery seem to depend on the specific cardiac disease. Comparison of mechanically ventilated patients with ischemic versus valvular disease indicated that valvular patients had significantly higher lung elastance (but not chest wall elastance), as well as higher lung resistance that was associated with uneven time constants (stress relaxation and pendelluft).[135,146] After surgery, both groups had significant increases in lung elastance, whereas chest wall elastance was not modified.[135] These changes may represent increases in extravascular lung water, capillary volume, and/or alveolar collapse. Both groups also showed postoperative decrease in lung resistance and increase in chest wall resistance.[135] Decreases in lung resistance are postulated to be related to release of smooth muscle active substances such as prostaglandin E2, pulmonary hypoxia, and lung interdependence with collapse leading to remote bronchial distension. Presence of preoperative pulmonary hypertension in valvular patients, a factor relieved at least partially after surgery, may also contribute to alterations in lung mechanics.[135,147,148]

Human studies addressed the discrimination between airway and parenchymal tissue contributions to the deterioration of perioperative lung mechanics. The forced oscillation method[140] was used to measure lung and respiratory system impedance (Z_{rs}), based on the observation that frequency dependency at low oscillation frequencies is different for the airways and the parenchyma, allowing the separation of their contributions to total lung impedance.[149–152] Babik and colleagues[140] found that cardiac surgery with extracorporeal circulation increased tissue elastance, tissue damping, and airway resistance, and significantly reduced airway inertance (**Fig. 4**). Inhomogeneous narrowing of peripheral airways from mucosal thickening or release of inflammatory mediators seems to be the main mechanism producing CPB-induced increase in airways resistance. Restrictive processes caused by lung derecruitment also contribute to alterations in elastance and tissue damping. Dopamine, an adrenergic inotrope frequently administered during cardiac surgery, counteracted the bronchoconstriction seen in patients who undergo CPB (see **Fig. 4**). These observations seem to be independent from increases in extravascular lung water and in the pulmonary circulation.[140]

Measurements of Z_{rs} and its components after extubation and the first postoperative week showed that airway resistance increased immediately after extubation and gradually decreased to baseline values at postoperative day 5.[127] Worsening of elastance peaked at postoperative day 2 and persisted at higher than baseline levels for the whole first postoperative week. Peak increase in elastance was higher and its increase lasted longer in patients undergoing CPB than those undergoing off-pump CABG.[127] The total volume of fluids administered to patients seems to also play a role in the respiratory mechanics. Positive fluid balance was associated with worsening in respiratory mechanics and indices of oxygenation.[101]

Together with the changes in respiratory mechanics, the patient develops hypoxemia with arterial oxygen saturation (Sao_2) = 90% to 92%.

During the critical period immediately following discontinuation of CPB, even mild hypoxemia is undesirable because it reduces oxygen transport to the newly revascularized heart, as well as to other tissues. To manage this issue, it is important to realize that there are multiple causes for lung dysfunction during and after cardiac surgery including accumulation of extravascular fluid in the alveolar-capillary membrane,[153] alveolar collapse,[154,155] a decrease in FRC,[97] retention of airway secretion, or insufficient cough as a consequence of pain (after surgery).

Effects of Cardiac Surgery and CPB on Gas Exchange

Increases in venous admixture and physiologic dead space, worsening of blood gas tensions, and reduction in FRC after CPB persisting for days after surgery have been reported for decades.[156–158] These changes are usually short lived, with modest effect on the postoperative clinical course.[159] They gain relevance in the management of patients with additional respiratory disease or risk factors.[106,160]

Despite complex and rapid changes in cardiopulmonary function on separation from bypass, atelectasis is still the main mechanism producing gas exchange impairment in the perioperative period of cardiac surgery.[155,161] An estimated average of 24% of lung tissue is collapsed 2.5 hours after the end of uncomplicated cardiac surgery.[162] Atelectasis following cardiac surgery is significantly greater than that observed after abdominal and lower extremity surgery on the first postoperative day.[163,164] This difference is attributed to the aforementioned effects of inflammation, internal mammary harvest, opening of the pleural space, ventilatory management, surfactant dysfunction, and

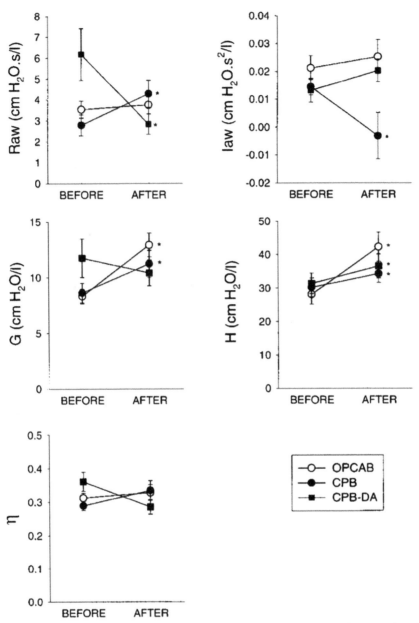

Fig. 4. Changes in airway and lung tissue mechanical properties in patients undergoing off-pump CABG (OPCAB) surgery, or with CPB. Group CPB-DA also had intravenous dopamine administered. G, tissue damping coefficient; H, tissue elastance coefficient; I_{aw}, airways inertance; R_{aw}, airways resistance; η, tissue hysteresivity. (*Reprinted from* Babik B, Asztalos T, Petak F, et al. Changes in respiratory mechanics during cardiac surgery. Anesth Analg 2003;96(5):1284; with permission.)

changes in lung recoil from pulmonary edema. The lungs after CPB exhibit poor $\dot{V}/\dot{Q}$ matching, in addition to the true shunt caused by atelectasis. Increases in $\dot{V}/\dot{Q}$ heterogeneity are associated with the inflammatory response to CPB, likely because of both the local redistribution of perfusion and of ventilation (although little is known about the regional characteristics of this $\dot{V}/\dot{Q}$ distribution following CPB). Gas exchange impairment improves along the first 24 hours after surgery, with low $\dot{V}/\dot{Q}$ regions comprising 11% and shunt 7.5% of total gas exchange regions, as measured with inert gases reported at 21 hours after cardiac surgery.[165–167]

Sequential intraoperative measurements showed that airway dead space increases with sternotomy by 32%.[168] Airway dead space is reduced following extracorporeal circulation and sternal closure. However, by the end of surgery, alveolar dead space increases significantly. Airway dead space at this stage can be smaller compared with the preoperative state, and so there is no net change in the physiologic dead space fraction at the end of surgery.[168] Despite such findings, some groups failed to find an increase in the arterial end-tidal gradient of P_{CO_2} after CPB.[169,170]

Although the magnitude of atelectasis has not been found to be different between CABG and mitral valve surgery, it seems that control of regional blood flow may differ in those conditions.[103,171] Atelectasis measured with computed tomography was better correlated with global shunt measured with oxygen in the first postoperative day after mitral valve replacement or repair than after CABG surgery. Effective HPV would be expected to reduce blood flow in regions of alveolar collapse, resulting in a limited relationship between lung collapse and shunt. These results suggest reduction in the effect of HPV to optimize gas exchange in mitral cases, perhaps related to the associated increased pulmonary vascular pressures.

A recruitment maneuver is performed by inflating the lungs to 30 cm H_2O for 30 seconds. During this procedure, systemic blood pressure is carefully monitored, because such increased intrathoracic pressure reduces venous return and cardiac output. Endotracheal suctioning is performed. The inspiratory/expiratory ratio in the mechanical ventilator is increased to 1:3.5 and PEEP of 5 cm H_2O is added. Incomplete deflation persists, and a β-agonist (albuterol) is delivered through inhalation. Following these interventions, the Sao_2 increases to 100%.

Perioperative Respiratory Dysfunction and Mechanical Ventilation in Patients with COPD

Patients with COPD have early changes in the topographic distribution of regional perfusion that contribute to increased $\dot{V}/\dot{Q}$ mismatch.[172–174] This perfusion redistribution can compound the aforementioned perioperative factors to accentuate gas exchange dysfunction. Such patients present with loss of elastic recoil and longer regional time constants. They also have lower vertical gradients in aeration and ventilation during spontaneous breathing compared with normal subjects.[174] Such characteristics seem to make them less prone to the development of reabsorption atelectasis during spontaneous breathing and mechanical ventilation,[69,174,175] and worsening of lung mechanics and gas exchange during cardiac surgery.[176]

Although use of PEEP during mechanical ventilation of patients with COPD is not standard, in selected cases it can help with reduction of airway closure and work of breathing, relief of lung overinflation, and improving respiratory system time constants.[177] The presence of sticky airway closure, alterations in intraparenchymal tethering forces, and increases in airway wall rigidity caused by PEEP are possible mechanisms. A priori information regarding disease, respiratory mechanics, or ventilatory settings does not predict the response. As a consequence, an empirical PEEP trial investigating plateau pressure response was suggested as a strategy to guide use of PEEP in patients with COPD during mechanical ventilation.[178]

Significant bronchoconstriction is sometimes observed at the end of the CPB period.[179,180] Because patients with COPD have a chronic lung inflammation and higher airway resistances, bronchoconstriction in these patients can be particularly critical. Bronchodilators, such as β-agonists, are administered either by inhalation or intravenously in these cases. In some cases of bronchospasm, inhaled nitric oxide may be considered with the aim of reducing pulmonary artery pressures, unloading the right ventricle, and relieving bronchospasm while improving $\dot{V}/\dot{Q}$ matching.[181–183] However, use of inhaled nitric oxide in patients with COPD can lead to deterioration of gas exchange. This deterioration is caused by $\dot{V}/\dot{Q}$ imbalances rather than by shunt, likely because of impaired hypoxic regulation of the matching between ventilation and perfusion.[184]

In addition, it has been recognized that patients with COPD have distinct elements of the inflammatory response in the perioperative period of cardiac surgery. For example, release of cysteinyl leukotrienes increases during cardiac surgery with CPB and is larger in patients with than without COPD.[185] This may be related to higher lung and airway production of cysteinyl leukotrienes and neutrophil activation, which could contribute to the postoperative deterioration in lung function.

The sternotomy is closed with stainless-steel wires, and the remaining tissue planes and skin are also closed. The peak inspiratory pressure is noticed to increase from 24 to 37 cm H_2O. Arterial blood gas at the end of the case shows that $Pao_2/Fio_2 = 287$ mm Hg. The patient is transferred to the ICU while still intubated. Respiratory mechanics and gas exchange are still marginal at ICU arrival but improved 16 hours after surgery, allowing patient extubation.

Closure of the chest results in the restoration of the contribution of the chest wall to the impedance of the respiratory system. As a consequence, increases in the inspiratory pressures are expected. Deleterious effects to gas exchange and respiratory mechanics can occur because of increased derecruitment of dependent and subdiaphragmatic lung regions. Resistance is increased because of the chest wall contribution and likely, at least partially, because of interdependence, in which the collapse of alveolar units reduces traction on the small airways allowing a reduction in their diameter. FRC after chest closure can be lower than that at the beginning of surgery.[97] The observed Pao_2/Fio_2 ratio, within the range defined for mild acute lung injury, is frequently found and tends to improve in the hours and days following admission to the ICU.[106,145]

SUMMARY

Nowhere more than in the operating room or delivery suite do rapid changes in a patient's condition and the dynamic and unpredictable requirements of surgery affect critical respiratory function and mechanics. Instrumentation of the airway, inhalation of halogenated hydrocarbon anesthetics, motor block resulting from neuraxial anesthesia, CPB, and single-lung ventilation have significant effects on respiratory function. The altered physiology of acute and chronic cardiopulmonary disease may result in extreme changes in lung volumes, mechanics, and control of breathing. Anesthetic challenges range from common problems of reducing atelectasis and maintaining ventilated lung volume, to mitigating changes in ventilation-to-perfusion matching, to reducing the risk of ventilator-associated lung injury in response to inflammation and iatrogenic ischemia-reperfusion injury. The anesthesiologist must integrate and apply a sound understanding of basic physiologic principles under a wide variety of changing constraints to balance life support and optimize the delivery of safe and effective anesthesia with minimal risk to each patient.

ACKNOWLEDGMENTS

The authors thank Dr Brett Simon for his helpful criticism during the preparation of this article.

REFERENCES

1. Bates JH. Physics of expiratory flow limitation. Physiologic basis of respiratory disease. Hamilton (Ontario): BC Decker; 2005. p. 55–60.
2. Bolliger CT, Perruchoud AP. Functional evaluation of the lung resection candidate. Eur Respir J 1998;11(1):198–212.
3. Gilbreth EM, Weisman IM. Role of exercise stress testing in preoperative evaluation of patients for lung resection. Clin Chest Med 1994;15(2):389–403.
4. Beckles MA, Spiro SG, Colice GL, et al. The physiologic evaluation of patients with lung cancer being considered for resectional surgery. Chest 2003; 123(Suppl 1):105S–14S.
5. Pate P, Tenholder MF, Griffin JP, et al. Preoperative assessment of the high-risk patient for lung resection. Ann Thorac Surg 1996;61(5):1494–500.
6. Mittman C. Assessment of operative risk in thoracic surgery. Am Rev Respir Dis 1961;84:197–207.
7. Ferguson MK, Little L, Rizzo L, et al. Diffusing capacity predicts morbidity and mortality after pulmonary resection. J Thorac Cardiovasc Surg 1988;96(6): 894–900.
8. Nagasaki F, Flehinger BJ, Martini N. Complications of surgery in the treatment of carcinoma of the lung. Chest 1982;82(1):25–9.
9. Carlens E. A new flexible double-lumen catheter for bronchospirometry. J Thorac Surg 1949;18(5):742–6.
10. Jacobaeus HC, Frenckner P, Björkman S. Some attempts at determining the volume and function of each lung separately. Acta Med Scand 1932;79: 174–215.
11. Neuhaus H, Cherniack NS. A bronchospirometric method of estimating the effect of pneumonectomy on the maximum breathing capacity. J Thorac Cardiovasc Surg 1968;55:144–8.
12. Ali MK, Mountain CF, Ewer MS, et al. Predicting loss of pulmonary function after pulmonary resection for bronchogenic carcinoma. Chest 1980;77(3):337–42.
13. Tonnesen KH, Dige-Petersen H, Lund JO, et al. Lung split function test and pneumonectomy. A lower limit for operability. Scand J Thorac Cardiovasc Surg 1978;12(2):133–6.
14. Kristersson S, Arborelius M Jr, Jungquist G, et al. Prediction of ventilatory capacity after lobectomy. Scand J Respir Dis 1973;54(6):315–25.
15. Kristersson S, Lindell SE, Svanberg L. Prediction of pulmonary function loss due to pneumonectomy using 133 Xe-radiospirometry. Chest 1972;62(6):694–8.
16. Ellis DA, Hawkins T, Gibson GJ, et al. Role of lung scanning in assessing the resectability of bronchial carcinoma. Thorax 1983;38(4):261–6.
17. Boysen PG, Harris JO, Block AJ, et al. Prospective evaluation for pneumonectomy using perfusion scanning: follow-up beyond one year. Chest 1981;80(2):163–6.
18. Olsen GN, Block AJ, Tobias JA. Prediction of postpneumonectomy pulmonary function using quantitative macroaggregate lung scanning. Chest 1974;66(1): 13–6.
19. Kearney DJ, Lee TH, Reilly JJ, et al. Assessment of operative risk in patients undergoing lung resection. Importance of predicted pulmonary function. Chest 1994;105(3):753–9.

20. Markos J, Mullan BP, Hillman DR, et al. Preoperative assessment as a predictor of mortality and morbidity after lung resection. Am Rev Respir Dis 1989;139(4): 902–10.
21. Olsen GN, Block AJ, Swenson EW, et al. Pulmonary function evaluation of the lung resection candidate: a prospective study. Am Rev Respir Dis 1975; 111(4):379–87.
22. Cerfolio RJ, Allen MS, Trastek VF, et al. Lung resection in patients with compromised pulmonary function. Ann Thorac Surg 1996;62(2):348–51.
23. Edwards MA, Hazelrigg S, Naunheim KS. The national emphysema treatment trial: summary and update. Thorac Surg Clin 2009;19(2):169–85.
24. Ingenito EP, Evans RB, Loring SH, et al. Relation between preoperative inspiratory lung resistance and the outcome of lung-volume-reduction surgery for emphysema. N Engl J Med 1998;338(17):1181–5.
25. Ninan M, Sommers KE, Landreneau RJ, et al. Standardized exercise oximetry predicts postpneumonectomy outcome. Ann Thorac Surg 1997;64(2):328–33.
26. Ribas J, Diaz O, Barbera JA, et al. Invasive exercise testing in the evaluation of patients at high-risk for lung resection. Eur Respir J 1998;12(6):1429–35.
27. Pierce RJ, Copland JM, Sharpe K, et al. Preoperative risk evaluation for lung cancer resection: predicted postoperative product as a predictor of surgical mortality. Am J Respir Crit Care Med 1994;150(4):947–55.
28. BTS guidelines: guidelines on the selection of patients with lung cancer for surgery. Thorax 2001;56(2):89–108.
29. Gravenstein JS, Paulus DA, Hayes TJ. Capnography in clinical practice. Boston: Butterworth Publishers; 1989.
30. Fernandez-Perez ER, Keegan MT, Brown DR, et al. Intraoperative tidal volume as a risk factor for respiratory failure after pneumonectomy. Anesthesiology 2006;105(1):14–8.
31. Musch G, Foti G, Cereda M, et al. Lung and chest wall mechanics in normal anaesthetized subjects and in patients with COPD at different PEEP levels. Eur Respir J 1997;10(11):2545–52.
32. Benumof JL. One-lung ventilation and hypoxic pulmonary vasoconstriction: implications for anesthetic management. Anesth Analg 1985;64(8):821–33.
33. Valenza F, Ronzoni G, Perrone L, et al. Positive end-expiratory pressure applied to the dependent lung during one-lung ventilation improves oxygenation and respiratory mechanics in patients with high FEV1. Eur J Anaesthesiol 2004; 21(12):938–43.
34. Fujiwara M, Abe K, Mashimo T. The effect of positive end-expiratory pressure and continuous positive airway pressure on the oxygenation and shunt fraction during one-lung ventilation with propofol anesthesia. J Clin Anesth 2001;13(7): 473–7.
35. Johansen B, Melsom MN, Flatebo T, et al. Time course and pattern of pulmonary flow distribution following unilateral airway occlusion in sheep. Clin Sci (Lond) 1998;94(4):453–60.
36. Vidal Melo MF. Effect of cardiac output on pulmonary gas exchange: role of diffusion limitation with VA/Q mismatch. Respir Physiol 1998;113(1):23–32.
37. Musch G, Harris RS, Vidal Melo MF, et al. Mechanism by which a sustained inflation can worsen oxygenation in acute lung injury. Anesthesiology 2004;100(2): 323–30.
38. Katz JA, Laverne RG, Fairley HB, et al. Pulmonary oxygen exchange during endobronchial anesthesia: effect of tidal volume and PEEP. Anesthesiology 1982; 56(3):164–71.

39. Cohen E, Eisenkraft JB, Thys DM, et al. Oxygenation and hemodynamic changes during one-lung ventilation: effects of CPAP10, PEEP10, and CPAP10/PEEP10. J Cardiothorac Anesth 1988;2(1):34–40.
40. Slinger P, Triolet W, Wilson J. Improving arterial oxygenation during one-lung ventilation. Anesthesiology 1988;68(2):291–5.
41. Domino KB, Borowec L, Alexander CM, et al. Influence of isoflurane on hypoxic pulmonary vasoconstriction in dogs. Anesthesiology 1986;64(4):423–9.
42. Spies C, Zaune U, Pauli MH, et al. [A comparison of enflurane and propofol in thoracic surgery]. Anaesthesist 1991;40(1):14–8.
43. Benumof JL, Wahrenbrock EA. Local effects of anesthetics on regional hypoxic pulmonary vasoconstriction. Anesthesiology 1975;43(5):525–32.
44. Kellow NH, Scott AD, White SA, et al. Comparison of the effects of propofol and isoflurane anaesthesia on right ventricular function and shunt fraction during thoracic surgery. Br J Anaesth 1995;75(5):578–82.
45. Abe K, Shimizu T, Takashina M, et al. The effects of propofol, isoflurane, and sevoflurane on oxygenation and shunt fraction during one-lung ventilation. Anesth Analg 1998;87(5):1164–9.
46. Satoh D, Sato M, Kaise A, et al. Effects of isoflurane on oxygenation during one-lung ventilation in pulmonary emphysema patients. Acta Anaesthesiol Scand 1998;42(10):1145–8.
47. Easley R, Mulreany D, Lancaster C, et al. Redistribution of pulmonary blood flow impacts thermodilution-based extravascular lung water measurements in a model of acute lung injury. Anesthesiology 2009;111(5):1065–74.
48. Easley RB, Fuld MK, Fernandez-Bustamante A, et al. Mechanism of hypoxemia in acute lung injury evaluated by multidetector-row CT. Acad Radiol 2006;13(7): 916–21.
49. Gust R, Kozlowski J, Stephenson AH, et al. Synergistic hemodynamic effects of low-dose endotoxin and acute lung injury. Am J Respir Crit Care Med 1998; 157(6 Pt 1):1919–26.
50. Ichinose F, Zapol W, Sapirstein A, et al. Attenuation of hypoxic pulmonary vaso-constriction by endotoxemia requires 5-lipoxygenase in mice. Circ Res 2001; 88(8):832–8.
51. Silva-Costa-Gomes T, Gallart L, Vallès J, et al. Low- vs high-dose almitrine combined with nitric oxide to prevent hypoxia during open-chest one-lung venti-lation. Br J Anaesth 2005;95(3):410–6.
52. Groeben H, Schafer B, Pavlakovic G, et al. Lung function under high thoracic segmental epidural anesthesia with ropivacaine or bupivacaine in patients with severe obstructive pulmonary disease undergoing breast surgery. Anesthe-siology 2002;96(3):536–41.
53. Garutti I, Quintana B, Olmedilla L, et al. Arterial oxygenation during one-lung ventilation: combined versus general anesthesia. Anesth Analg 1999;88(3): 494–9.
54. Brister N, Barnette R, Kim V, et al. Anesthetic considerations in candidates for lung volume reduction surgery. Proc Am Thorac Soc 2008;5(4):432–7.
55. Hillier J, Gillbe C. Anaesthesia for lung volume reduction surgery. Anaesthesia 2003;58(12):1210–9.
56. Guerin C, Coussa ML, Eissa NT, et al. Lung and chest wall mechanics in me-chanically ventilated COPD patients. J Appl Physiol 1993;74(4):1570–80.
57. Samain E, Biard M, Farah E, et al. Monitoring expired oxygen fraction in preox-ygenation of patients with chronic obstructive pulmonary disease. Ann Fr Anesth Reanim 2002;21(1):14–9.

58. Hedenstierna G, Strandberg A, Brismar B, et al. Functional residual capacity, thoracoabdominal dimensions, and central blood volume during general anesthesia with muscle paralysis and mechanical ventilation. Anesthesiology 1985; 62(3):247–54.

59. Hedenstierna G, Strandberg A, Brismar B, et al. What causes the lowered FRC during anaesthesia? Clin Physiol 1985;5(Suppl 3):133–41.

60. Rothen HU, Sporre B, Engberg G, et al. Airway closure, atelectasis and gas exchange during general anaesthesia. Br J Anaesth 1998;81(5):681–6.

61. Brismar B, Hedenstierna G, Lundquist H, et al. Pulmonary densities during anesthesia with muscular relaxation–a proposal of atelectasis. Anesthesiology 1985;62(4):422–8.

62. Davis WB, Rennard SI, Bitterman PB, et al. Pulmonary oxygen toxicity. Early reversible changes in human alveolar structures induced by hyperoxia. N Engl J Med 1983;309(15):878–83.

63. Edmark L, Kostova-Aherdan K, Enlund M, et al. Optimal oxygen concentration during induction of general anesthesia. Anesthesiology 2003;98(1):28–33.

64. Tokics L, Hedenstierna G, Strandberg A, et al. Lung collapse and gas exchange during general anesthesia: effects of spontaneous breathing, muscle paralysis, and positive end-expiratory pressure. Anesthesiology 1987;66(2):157–67.

65. Tokics L, Hedenstierna G, Svensson L, et al. V/Q distribution and correlation to atelectasis in anesthetized paralyzed humans. J Appl Physiol 1996;81(4): 1822–33.

66. Dantzker DR, Wagner PD, West JB. Proceedings: instability of poorly ventilated lung units during oxygen breathing. J Physiol (Lond) 1974;242(2):72P.

67. Coussa M, Proietti S, Schnyder P, et al. Prevention of atelectasis formation during the induction of general anesthesia in morbidly obese patients. Anesth Analg 2004;98(5):1491–5.

68. Rusca M, Proietti S, Schnyder P, et al. Prevention of atelectasis formation during induction of general anesthesia. Anesth Analg 2003;97(6):1835–9.

69. Gunnarsson L, Tokics L, Lundquist H, et al. Chronic obstructive pulmonary disease and anaesthesia: formation of atelectasis and gas exchange impairment. Eur Respir J 1991;4(9):1106–16.

70. Athanasiou T, Al-Ruzzeh S, Del Stanbridge R, et al. Is the female gender an independent predictor of adverse outcome after off-pump coronary artery bypass grafting? Ann Thorac Surg 2003;75(4):1153–60.

71. Daganou M, Dimopoulou I, Michalopoulos N, et al. Respiratory complications after coronary artery bypass surgery with unilateral or bilateral internal mammary artery grafting. Chest 1998;113(5):1285–9.

72. Taggart DP, el-Fiky M, Carter R, et al. Respiratory dysfunction after uncomplicated cardiopulmonary bypass. Ann Thorac Surg 1993;56(5):1123–8.

73. Hammermeister KE, Burchfiel C, Johnson R, et al. Identification of patients at greatest risk for developing major complications at cardiac surgery. Circulation 1990;82(Suppl 5):IV380–9.

74. Sundar S, Novack V, Jervis K, et al. Influence of low tidal volume ventilation on time to extubation in cardiac surgical patients. Anesthesiology 2011;114(5): 1102–10.

75. Milot J, Perron J, Lacasse Y, et al. Incidence and predictors of ARDS after cardiac surgery. Chest 2001;119(3):884–8.

76. Webb HH, Tierney DF. Experimental pulmonary edema due to intermittent positive pressure ventilation with high inflation pressures. Protection by positive end-expiratory pressure. Am Rev Respir Dis 1974;110(5):556–65.

77. Amato MB, Barbas CS, Medeiros DM, et al. Effect of a protective-ventilation strategy on mortality in the acute respiratory distress syndrome. N Engl J Med 1998;338(6):347–54.
78. The Acute Respiratory Distress Syndrome Network. Ventilation with lower tidal volumes as compared with traditional tidal volumes for acute lung injury and the acute respiratory distress syndrome. N Engl J Med 2000; 342(18):1301–8.
79. Altemeier WA, Matute-Bello G, Frevert CW, et al. Mechanical ventilation with moderate tidal volumes synergistically increases lung cytokine response to systemic endotoxin. Am J Physiol Lung Cell Mol Physiol 2004;287(3):L533–42.
80. Costa EL, Musch G, Winkler T, et al. Mild endotoxemia during mechanical ventilation produces spatially heterogeneous pulmonary neutrophilic inflammation in sheep. Anesthesiology 2010;112(3):658–69.
81. Bruins P, te Velthuis H, Yazdanbakhsh AP, et al. Activation of the complement system during and after cardiopulmonary bypass surgery: postsurgery activation involves C-reactive protein and is associated with postoperative arrhythmia. Circulation 1997;96(10):3542–8.
82. Massoudy P, Zahler S, Becker BF, et al. Evidence for inflammatory responses of the lungs during coronary artery bypass grafting with cardiopulmonary bypass. Chest 2001;119(1):31–6.
83. Andersen LW, Baek L, Degn H, et al. Presence of circulating endotoxins during cardiac operations. J Thorac Cardiovasc Surg 1987;93(1):115–9.
84. Riddington DW, Venkatesh B, Boivin CM, et al. Intestinal permeability, gastric intramucosal pH, and systemic endotoxemia in patients undergoing cardiopulmonary bypass. JAMA 1996;275(13):1007–12.
85. Kuratani T, Matsuda H, Sawa Y, et al. Experimental study in a rabbit model of ischemia-reperfusion lung injury during cardiopulmonary bypass. J Thorac Cardiovasc Surg 1992;103(3):564–8.
86. Chai PJ, Williamson JA, Lodge AJ, et al. Effects of ischemia on pulmonary dysfunction after cardiopulmonary bypass. Ann Thorac Surg 1999;67(3):731–5.
87. Dodd-O JM, Welsh LE, Salazar JD, et al. Effect of bronchial artery blood flow on cardiopulmonary bypass-induced lung injury. Am J Physiol Heart Circ Physiol 2004;286(2):H693–700.
88. Schlensak C, Doenst T, Preusser S, et al. Cardiopulmonary bypass reduction of bronchial blood flow: a potential mechanism for lung injury in a neonatal pig model. J Thorac Cardiovasc Surg 2002;123(6):1199–205.
89. Koch CG, Li L, Sessler DI, et al. Duration of red-cell storage and complications after cardiac surgery. N Engl J Med 2008;358(12):1229–39.
90. Laffey JG, Boylan JF, Cheng DC. The systemic inflammatory response to cardiac surgery: implications for the anesthesiologist. Anesthesiology 2002; 97(1):215–52.
91. Carvalho AR, Ichinose F, Schettino IA, et al. Tidal lung recruitment and exhaled nitric oxide during coronary artery bypass grafting in patients with and without chronic obstructive pulmonary disease. Lung 2011;189(6):499–509.
92. Chaney MA, Nikolov MP, Blakeman BP, et al. Protective ventilation attenuates postoperative pulmonary dysfunction in patients undergoing cardiopulmonary bypass. J Cardiothorac Vasc Anesth 2000;14(5):514–8.
93. Zupancich E, Paparella D, Turani F, et al. Mechanical ventilation affects inflammatory mediators in patients undergoing cardiopulmonary bypass for cardiac surgery: a randomized clinical trial. J Thorac Cardiovasc Surg 2005;130(2): 378–83.

94. Koner O, Celebi S, Balci H, et al. Effects of protective and conventional mechanical ventilation on pulmonary function and systemic cytokine release after cardiopulmonary bypass. Intensive Care Med 2004;30(4):620–6.

95. Pizov R, Weiss YG, Oppenheim-Eden A, et al. High oxygen concentration exacerbates cardiopulmonary bypass-induced lung injury. J Cardiothorac Vasc Anesth 2000;14(5):519–23.

96. Barnas GM, Gilbert TB, Watson RJ, et al. Respiratory mechanics in the open chest: effects of parietal pleurae. Respir Physiol 1996;104(1):63–70.

97. Jonmarker C, Nordstrom L, Werner O. Changes in functional residual capacity during cardiac surgery. Br J Anaesth 1986;58(4):428–32.

98. Guizilini S, Gomes WJ, Faresin SM, et al. Influence of pleurotomy on pulmonary function after off-pump coronary artery bypass grafting. Ann Thorac Surg 2007; 84(3):817–22.

99. Peng MJ, Vargas FS, Cukier A, et al. Postoperative pleural changes after coronary revascularization. Comparison between saphenous vein and internal mammary artery grafting. Chest 1992;101(2):327–30.

100. Singh NP, Vargas FS, Cukier A, et al. Arterial blood gases after coronary artery bypass surgery. Chest 1992;102(5):1337–41.

101. Gilbert TB, Barnas GM, Sequeira AJ. Impact of pleurotomy, continuous positive airway pressure, and fluid balance during cardiopulmonary bypass on lung mechanics and oxygenation. J Cardiothorac Vasc Anesth 1996;10(7): 844–9.

102. Gullu AU, Ekinci A, Sensoz Y, et al. Preserved pleural integrity provides better respiratory function and pain score after coronary surgery. J Cardiovasc Surg 2009;24(4):374–8.

103. Hachenberg T, Tenling A, Hansson HE, et al. The ventilation-perfusion relation and gas exchange in mitral valve disease and coronary artery disease. Implications for anesthesia, extracorporeal circulation, and cardiac surgery. Anesthesiology 1997;86(4):809–17.

104. Pennock JL, Pierce WS, Waldhausen JA. The management of the lungs during cardiopulmonary bypass. Surg Gynecol Obstet 1977;145(6):917–27.

105. Messent M, Sullivan K, Keogh BF, et al. Adult respiratory distress syndrome following cardiopulmonary bypass: incidence and prediction. Anaesthesia 1992;47(3):267–8.

106. Apostolakis E, Filos KS, Koletsis E, et al. Lung dysfunction following cardiopulmonary bypass. J Cardiovasc Surg 2010;25(1):47–55.

107. Ng CS, Wan S, Yim AP, et al. Pulmonary dysfunction after cardiac surgery. Chest 2002;121(4):1269–77.

108. Wasowicz M, Sobczynski P, Drwila R, et al. Air-blood barrier injury during cardiac operations with the use of cardiopulmonary bypass (CPB). An old story? A morphological study. Scand Cardiovasc J 2003;37(4):216–21.

109. Stanley TH, Liu WS, Gentry S. Effects of ventilatory techniques during cardiopulmonary bypass on post-bypass and postoperative pulmonary compliance and shunt. Anesthesiology 1977;46(6):391–5.

110. Loeckinger A, Kleinsasser A, Lindner KH, et al. Continuous positive airway pressure at 10 cm H_2O during cardiopulmonary bypass improves postoperative gas exchange. Anesth Analg 2000;91(3):522–7.

111. Berry CB, Butler PJ, Myles PS. Lung management during cardiopulmonary bypass: is continuous positive airways pressure beneficial? Br J Anaesth 1993; 71(6):864–8.

112. Magnusson L, Zemgulis V, Wicky S, et al. Effect of CPAP during cardiopulmonary bypass on postoperative lung function. An experimental study. Acta Anaesthesiol Scand 1998;42(10):1133–8.
113. Imura H, Caputo M, Lim K, et al. Pulmonary injury after cardiopulmonary bypass: beneficial effects of low-frequency mechanical ventilation. J Thorac Cardiovasc Surg 2009;137(6):1530–7.
114. Siepe M, Goebel U, Mecklenburg A, et al. Pulsatile pulmonary perfusion during cardiopulmonary bypass reduces the pulmonary inflammatory response. Ann Thorac Surg 2008;86(1):115–22.
115. Simon BA, Tsuzaki K, Venegas JG. Changes in regional lung mechanics and ventilation distribution after unilateral pulmonary artery occlusion. J Appl Physiol 1997;82(3):882–91.
116. Tomic V, Russwurm S, Moller E, et al. Transcriptomic and proteomic patterns of systemic inflammation in on-pump and off-pump coronary artery bypass grafting. Circulation 2005;112(19):2912–20.
117. Friedman M, Sellke FW, Wang SY, et al. Parameters of pulmonary injury after total or partial cardiopulmonary bypass. Circulation 1994;90(5 Pt 2):II262–8.
118. Al-Ruzzeh S, Hoare G, Marczin N, et al. Off-pump coronary artery bypass surgery is associated with reduced neutrophil activation as measured by the expression of CD11b: a prospective randomized study. Heart Surg Forum 2003;6(2):89–93.
119. Al-Ruzzeh S, Nakamura K, Athanasiou T, et al. Does off-pump coronary artery bypass (OPCAB) surgery improve the outcome in high-risk patients?: a comparative study of 1398 high-risk patients. Eur J Cardiothorac Surg 2003;23(1):50–5.
120. Staton GW, Williams WH, Mahoney EM, et al. Pulmonary outcomes of off-pump vs on-pump coronary artery bypass surgery in a randomized trial. Chest 2005;127(3):892–901.
121. Aydin NB, Gercekoglu H, Aksu B, et al. Endotoxemia in coronary artery bypass surgery: a comparison of the off-pump technique and conventional cardiopulmonary bypass. J Thorac Cardiovasc Surg 2003;125(4):843–8.
122. Cavalca V, Sisillo E, Veglia F, et al. Isoprostanes and oxidative stress in off-pump and on-pump coronary bypass surgery. Ann Thorac Surg 2006;81(2):562–7.
123. Hazama S, Eishi K, Yamachika S, et al. Inflammatory response after coronary revascularization: off-pump versus on-pump (heparin-coated circuits and poly2methoxyethylacrylate-coated circuits). Ann Thorac Cardiovasc Surg 2004;10(2):90–6.
124. Wan S, Izzat MB, Lee TW, et al. Avoiding cardiopulmonary bypass in multivessel CABG reduces cytokine response and myocardial injury. Ann Thorac Surg 1999;68(1):52–6 [discussion: 56–7].
125. Tschernko EM, Bambazek A, Wisser W, et al. Intrapulmonary shunt after cardiopulmonary bypass: the use of vital capacity maneuvers versus off-pump coronary artery bypass grafting. J Thorac Cardiovasc Surg 2002;124(4):732–8.
126. Roosens C, Heerman J, De Somer F, et al. Effects of off-pump coronary surgery on the mechanics of the respiratory system, lung, and chest wall: comparison with extracorporeal circulation. Crit Care Med 2002;30(11):2430–7.
127. Albu G, Babik B, Kesmarky K, et al. Changes in airway and respiratory tissue mechanics after cardiac surgery. Ann Thorac Surg 2010;89(4):1218–26.
128. Guler M, Kirali K, Toker ME, et al. Different CABG methods in patients with chronic obstructive pulmonary disease. Ann Thorac Surg 2001;71(1):152–7.

129. Moller CH, Perko MJ, Lund JT, et al. No major differences in 30-day outcomes in high-risk patients randomized to off-pump versus on-pump coronary bypass surgery: the best bypass surgery trial. Circulation 2010;121(4):498–504.
130. Magnusson L, Zemgulis V, Tenling A, et al. Use of a vital capacity maneuver to prevent atelectasis after cardiopulmonary bypass: an experimental study. Anesthesiology 1998;88(1):134–42.
131. Rothen HU, Sporre B, Engberg G, et al. Influence of gas composition on recurrence of atelectasis after a reexpansion maneuver during general anesthesia. Anesthesiology 1995;82(4):832–42.
132. Minkovich L, Djaiani G, Katznelson R, et al. Effects of alveolar recruitment on arterial oxygenation in patients after cardiac surgery: a prospective, randomized, controlled clinical trial. J Cardiothorac Vasc Anesth 2007;21(3):375–8.
133. Murphy GS, Szokol JW, Curran RD, et al. Influence of a vital capacity maneuver on pulmonary gas exchange after cardiopulmonary bypass. J Cardiothorac Vasc Anesth 2001;15(3):336–40.
134. Prakash O, Meij S, Bos E, et al. Lung mechanics in patients undergoing mitral valve replacement. The value of monitoring of compliance and resistance. Crit Care Med 1978;6(6):370–2.
135. Auler JO Jr, Zin WA, Caldeira MP, et al. Pre- and postoperative inspiratory mechanics in ischemic and valvular heart disease. Chest 1987;92(6):984–90.
136. Andersen NB, Ghia J. Pulmonary function, cardiac status, and postoperative course in relation to cardiopulmonary bypass. J Thorac Cardiovasc Surg 1970;59(4):474–83.
137. Barnas GM, Watson RJ, Green MD, et al. Lung and chest wall mechanical properties before and after cardiac surgery with cardiopulmonary bypass. J Appl Physiol 1994;76(1):166–75.
138. Ghia J, Andersen NB. Pulmonary function and cardiopulmonary bypass. JAMA 1970;212(4):593–7.
139. Prakash O, Meij S, v d Borden B, et al. Cardiorespiratory monitoring during open heart surgery. Crit Care Med 1981;9(7):530–5.
140. Babik B, Asztalos T, Petak F, et al. Changes in respiratory mechanics during cardiac surgery. Anesth Analg 2003;96(5):1280–7.
141. Barnas GM, Mills PJ, Mackenzie CF, et al. Dependencies of respiratory system resistance and elastance on amplitude and frequency in the normal range of breathing. Am Rev Respir Dis 1991;143(2):240–4.
142. Heldt GP, Peters RM. A simplified method to determine functional residual capacity during mechanical ventilation. Chest 1978;74(5):492–6.
143. Kaczka DW, Hager DN, Hawley ML, et al. Quantifying mechanical heterogeneity in canine acute lung injury: impact of mean airway pressure. Anesthesiology 2005;103(2):306–17.
144. Kaczka DW, Brown RH, Mitzner W. Assessment of heterogeneous airway constriction in dogs: a structure-function analysis. J Appl Physiol 2009;106(2):520–30.
145. Ranieri VM, Vitale N, Grasso S, et al. Time-course of impairment of respiratory mechanics after cardiac surgery and cardiopulmonary bypass. Crit Care Med 1999;27(8):1454–60.
146. Zin WA, Caldeira MP, Cardoso WV, et al. Expiratory mechanics before and after uncomplicated heart surgery. Chest 1989;95(1):21–8.
147. Garzon AA, Seltzer B, Lichtenstein S, et al. Influence of open-heart surgery on respiratory work. Dis Chest 1967;52(3):392–6.

148. Habre W, Schutz N, Pellegrini M, et al. Preoperative pulmonary hemodynamics determines changes in airway and tissue mechanics following surgical repair of congenital heart diseases. Pediatr Pulmonol 2004;38(6):470–6.

149. Hantos Z, Daroczy B, Suki B, et al. Input impedance and peripheral inhomogeneity of dog lungs. J Appl Physiol 1992;72(1):168–78.

150. Hantos Z, Petak F, Adamicza A, et al. Differential responses of global airway, terminal airway, and tissue impedances to histamine. J Appl Physiol 1995; 79(5):1440–8.

151. Lutchen KR, Hantos Z, Petak F, et al. Airway inhomogeneities contribute to apparent lung tissue mechanics during constriction. J Appl Physiol 1996; 80(5):1841–9.

152. Suki B, Petak F, Adamicza A, et al. Airway and tissue constrictions are greater in closed than in open-chest conditions. Respir Physiol 1997;108(2):129–41.

153. Royston D, Minty BD, Higenbottam TW, et al. The effect of surgery with cardiopulmonary bypass on alveolar-capillary barrier function in human beings. Ann Thorac Surg 1985;40(2):139–43.

154. Hachenberg T, Lundquist H, Tokics L, et al. Analysis of lung density by computed tomography before and during general anaesthesia. Acta Anaesthesiol Scand 1993;37(6):549–55.

155. Magnusson L, Zemgulis V, Wicky S, et al. Atelectasis is a major cause of hypoxemia and shunt after cardiopulmonary bypass: an experimental study. Anesthesiology 1997;87(5):1153–63.

156. Nahas RA, Melrose DG, Sykes MK, et al. Post-perfusion lung syndrome: effect of homologous blood. Lancet 1965;2(7406):254–6.

157. Nahas RA, Melrose DG, Sykes MK, et al. Post-perfusion lung syndrome: role of circulatory exclusion. Lancet 1965;2(7406):251–4.

158. Rea HH, Harris EA, Seelye ER, et al. The effects of cardiopulmonary bypass upon pulmonary gas exchange. J Thorac Cardiovasc Surg 1978;75(1):104–20.

159. Weiss YG, Merin G, Koganov E, et al. Postcardiopulmonary bypass hypoxemia: a prospective study on incidence, risk factors, and clinical significance. J Cardiothorac Vasc Anesth 2000;14(5):506–13.

160. Apostolakis EE, Koletsis EN, Baikoussis NG, et al. Strategies to prevent intraoperative lung injury during cardiopulmonary bypass. J Cardiothorac Surg 2010; 5(1):1.

161. Groeneveld AB, Jansen EK, Verheij J. Mechanisms of pulmonary dysfunction after on-pump and off-pump cardiac surgery: a prospective cohort study. J Cardiothorac Surg 2007;2:11.

162. Hachenberg T, Tenling A, Nystrom SO, et al. Ventilation-perfusion inequality in patients undergoing cardiac surgery. Anesthesiology 1994;80(3):509–19.

163. Lindberg P, Gunnarsson L, Tokics L, et al. Atelectasis and lung function in the postoperative period. Acta Anaesthesiol Scand 1992;36(6):546–53.

164. Strandberg A, Tokics L, Brismar B, et al. Atelectasis during anaesthesia and in the postoperative period. Acta Anaesthesiol Scand 1986;30(2):154–8.

165. Anjou-Lindskog E, Broman L, Broman M, et al. Effects of oxygen on central haemodynamics and VA/Q distribution after coronary bypass surgery. Acta Anaesthesiol Scand 1983;27(5):378–84.

166. Anjou-Lindskog E, Broman L, Broman M, et al. Effects of nitroglycerin on central haemodynamics and VA/Q distribution during ventilation with FIO2 = 1.0 in patients after coronary bypass surgery. Acta Anaesthesiol Scand 1984;28(1): 27–33.

167. Anjou-Lindskog E, Broman L, Holmgren A. Effects of nitroglycerin on central haemodynamics and VA/Q distribution early after coronary bypass surgery. Acta Anaesthesiol Scand 1982;26(5):489–97.

168. Fletcher R, Malmkvist G, Niklason L, et al. On-line measurement of gas-exchange during cardiac surgery. Acta Anaesthesiol Scand 1986;30(4):295–9.

169. Fletcher R, Veintemilla F. Changes in the arterial to end-tidal PCO_2 differences during coronary artery bypass grafting. Acta Anaesthesiol Scand 1989;33(8): 656–9.

170. Myles PS, Story DA, Higgs MA, et al. Continuous measurement of arterial and end-tidal carbon dioxide during cardiac surgery: Pa-ETCO2 gradient. Anaesth Intensive Care 1997;25(5):459–63.

171. Tenling A, Hachenberg T, Tyden H, et al. Atelectasis and gas exchange after cardiac surgery. Anesthesiology 1998;89(2):371–8.

172. Barbera JA, Ramirez J, Roca J, et al. Lung structure and gas exchange in mild chronic obstructive pulmonary disease. Am Rev Respir Dis 1990;141(4 Pt 1): 895–901.

173. Peinado VI, Barbera JA, Ramirez J, et al. Endothelial dysfunction in pulmonary arteries of patients with mild COPD. Am J Physiol 1998;274(6 Pt 1):L908–13.

174. Vidal Melo MF, Winkler T, Harris RS, et al. Spatial heterogeneity of lung perfusion assessed with (13)N PET as a vascular biomarker in chronic obstructive pulmonary disease. J Nucl Med 2010;51(1):57–65.

175. Wagner PD, Dantzker DR, Dueck R, et al. Ventilation-perfusion inequality in chronic obstructive pulmonary disease. J Clin Invest 1977;59(2):203–16.

176. Vidal Melo MF, Ichinose F, Walker J, et al. Intraoperative changes in respiratory function during on-pump CABG in COPD patients. Anesthesiology 2006;105: A1221.

177. Kaczka DW, Ingenito EP, Body SC, et al. Inspiratory lung impedance in COPD: effects of PEEP and immediate impact of lung volume reduction surgery. J Appl Physiol 2001;90(5):1833–41.

178. Caramez MP, Borges JB, Tucci MR, et al. Paradoxical responses to positive end-expiratory pressure in patients with airway obstruction during controlled ventilation. Crit Care Med 2005;33(7):1519–28.

179. Kawahito S, Kitahata H, Tanaka K, et al. Bronchospasm induced by cardiopulmonary bypass. Ann Thorac Cardiovasc Surg 2001;7(1):49–51.

180. Morel DR, Zapol WM, Thomas SJ, et al. C5a and thromboxane generation associated with pulmonary vaso- and broncho-constriction during protamine reversal of heparin. Anesthesiology 1987;66(5):597–604.

181. Gwyn DR, Lindeman KS, Hirshman CA. Inhaled nitric oxide attenuates bronchoconstriction in canine peripheral airways. Am J Respir Crit Care Med 1996; 153(2):604–9.

182. Lindeman KS, Aryana A, Hirshman CA. Direct effects of inhaled nitric oxide on canine peripheral airways. J Appl Physiol 1995;78(5):1898–903.

183. Matera MG. Nitric oxide and airways. Pulm Pharmacol Ther 1998;11(5–6): 341–8.

184. Barbera JA, Roger N, Roca J, et al. Worsening of pulmonary gas exchange with nitric oxide inhalation in chronic obstructive pulmonary disease. Lancet 1996; 347(8999):436–40.

185. de Prost N, El-Karak C, Avila M, et al. Changes in cysteinyl leukotrienes during and after cardiac surgery with cardiopulmonary bypass in patients with and without chronic obstructive pulmonary disease. J Thorac Cardiovasc Surg 2011;141(6): 1496–502.

Index

Note: Page numbers of article titles are in **boldface** type

Anesthesiology Clin 30 (2012) 785–794
http://dx.doi.org/10.1016/S1932-2275(12)00119-X
1932-2275/12/$ – see front matter © 2012 Elsevier Inc. All rights reserved.
anesthesiology.theclinics.com

United States Postal Service

Statement of Ownership, Management, and Circulation
(All Periodicals Publications Except Requestor Publications)

1. Publication Title	2. Publication Number	3. Filing Date
Anesthesiology Clinics	0 0 0 - 2 7 7 7	9/14/12

4. Issue Frequency	5. Number of Issues Published Annually	6. Annual Subscription Price
Mar, Jun, Sep, Dec	4	$313.00

7. Complete Mailing Address of Known Office of Publication (Not printer) (Street, city, county, state, and ZIP+4®)

Elsevier Inc.
360 Park Avenue South
New York, NY 10010-1710

Contact Person
Stephen R. Bushing
Telephone (Include area code)
215-239-3688

8. Complete Mailing Address of Headquarters or General Business Office of Publisher (Not printer)

Elsevier Inc., 360 Park Avenue South, New York, NY 10010-1710

9. Full Names and Complete Mailing Addresses of Publisher, Editor, and Managing Editor (Do not leave blank)

Publisher (Name and complete mailing address)

Kim Murphy, Elsevier, Inc., 1600 John F. Kennedy Blvd. Suite 1800, Philadelphia, PA 19103-2899

Editor (Name and complete mailing address)

Pamela Hetherington, Elsevier, Inc., 1600 John F. Kennedy Blvd. Suite 1800, Philadelphia, PA 19103-2899

Managing Editor (Name and complete mailing address)

Sarah Barth, Elsevier, Inc., 1600 John F. Kennedy Blvd, Suite 1800, Philadelphia, PA 19103-2899

10. Owner (Do not leave blank. If the publication is owned by a corporation, give the name and address of the corporation immediately followed by the names and addresses of all stockholders owning or holding 1 percent or more of the total amount of stock. If not owned by a corporation, give the names and addresses of the individual owners. If owned by a partnership or other unincorporated firm, give its name and address as well as those of each individual owner. If the publication is published by a nonprofit organization, give its name and address.)

Full Name	Complete Mailing Address
Wholly owned subsidiary of	1600 John F. Kennedy Blvd, Ste. 1800
Reed/Elsevier, US holdings	Philadelphia, PA 19103-2899

11. Known Bondholders, Mortgagees, and Other Security Holders Owning or Holding 1 Percent or More of Total Amount of Bonds, Mortgages, or Other Securities. If none, check box ☐ None

Full Name	Complete Mailing Address
N/A	

12. Tax Status (For completion by nonprofit organizations authorized to mail at nonprofit rates) (Check one)
The purpose, function, and nonprofit status of this organization and the exempt status for federal income tax purposes:
☐ Has Not Changed During Preceding 12 Months
☐ Has Changed During Preceding 12 Months (Publisher must submit explanation of change with this statement)

PS Form 3526, September 2007 (Page 1 of 3 (Instructions Page 3)) PSN 7530-01-000-9931 PRIVACY NOTICE: See our Privacy policy in www.usps.com

---

13. Publication Title	14. Issue Date for Circulation Data Below
Anesthesiology Clinics	September 2012

15. Extent and Nature of Circulation			Average No. Copies Each Issue During Preceding 12 Months	No. Copies of Single Issue Published Nearest to Filing Date
a. Total Number of Copies (Net press run)			918	850
b. Paid Circulation (By Mail and Outside the Mail)	(1)	Mailed Outside-County Paid Subscriptions Stated on PS Form 3541. (Include paid distribution above nominal rate, advertiser's proof copies, and exchange copies)	349	314
	(2)	Mailed In-County Paid Subscriptions Stated on PS Form 3541 (Include paid distribution above nominal rate, advertiser's proof copies, and exchange copies)		
	(3)	Paid Distribution Outside the Mails Including Sales Through Dealers and Carriers, Street Vendors, Counter Sales, and Other Paid Distribution Outside USPS®	288	294
	(4)	Paid Distribution by Other Classes Mailed Through the USPS (e.g. First-Class Mail®)		
c. Total Paid Distribution (Sum of 15b (1), (2), (3), and (4))			637	608
d. Free or Nominal Rate Distribution (By Mail and Outside the Mail)	(1)	Free or Nominal Rate Outside-County Copies Included on PS Form 3541	73	62
	(2)	Free or Nominal Rate In-County Copies Included on PS Form 3541		
	(3)	Free or Nominal Rate Copies Mailed at Other Classes Through the USPS (e.g. First-Class Mail)		
	(4)	Free or Nominal Rate Distribution Outside the Mail (Carriers or other means)		
e. Total Free or Nominal Rate Distribution (Sum of 15d (1), (2), (3) and (4))			73	62
f. Total Distribution (Sum of 15c and 15e)			710	670
g. Copies not Distributed (See instructions to publishers #4 (page #3))			208	180
h. Total (Sum of 15f and g)			918	850
i. Percent Paid (15c divided by 15f times 100)			89.72%	90.75%

16. Publication of Statement of Ownership

☐ If the publication is a general publication, publication of this statement is required. Will be printed in the December 2012 issue of this publication. ☐ Publication not required

17. Signature and Title of Editor, Publisher, Business Manager, or Owner	Date
Stephen R. Bushing Stephen R. Bushing – Inventory Distribution Coordinator	September 14, 2012

I certify that all information furnished on this form is true and complete. I understand that anyone who furnishes false or misleading information on this form or who omits material or information requested on the form may be subject to criminal sanctions (including fines and imprisonment) and/or civil sanctions (including civil penalties).

PS Form 3526, September 2007 (Page 2 of 3)

Moving?

Make sure your subscription moves with you!

To notify us of your new address, find your **Clinics Account Number** (located on your mailing label above your name), and contact customer service at:

Email: journalscustomerservice-usa@elsevier.com

800-654-2452 (subscribers in the U.S. & Canada)
314-447-8871 (subscribers outside of the U.S. & Canada)

Fax number: 314-447-8029

Elsevier Health Sciences Division
Subscription Customer Service
3251 Riverport Lane
Maryland Heights, MO 63043

ELSEVIER

Printed and bound by CPI Group (UK) Ltd, Croydon, CR0 4YY

14/10/2024

01773668-0002